Beyond Evidence-Based Medicine

Ralph Junckerstorff • Sharmayne Brady
Ar Kar Aung
Editors

Beyond Evidence-Based Medicine

Clinical Pearls from Experienced Physicians

Springer

Editors
Ralph Junckerstorff
Infectious Diseases and General Medicine
Monash Health
Melbourne, VIC, Australia

Sharmayne Brady
Rheumatology
Alfred Health
Melbourne, VIC, Australia

Ar Kar Aung
General Medicine and Infectious Diseases
Alfred Health
Melbourne, VIC, Australia

ISBN 978-981-99-4439-2 ISBN 978-981-99-4440-8 (eBook)
https://doi.org/10.1007/978-981-99-4440-8

This Springer imprint is published by the registered company Springer Nature Singapore Pte Ltd.
The registered company address is: 152 Beach Road, #21-01/04 Gateway East, Singapore 189721, Singapore

Paper in this product is recyclable.

Prologue

Evidence-based medicine (EBM) and clinical guidelines help us choose the best management and treatment options for our patients. They are based on robust clinical studies, often in the form of well-designed randomised controlled trials or systematic reviews and meta-analyses.

However, the art and mastery of practicing medicine is complex and there is more to clinical medicine than EBM. In fact, there are many aspects of medicine that have not been tested in a clinical trial, nor are easily amenable to research. It is the years of clinical experience, constant self-reflection, striving for empathetic patient-centred care, and the acquisition of cumulative wisdom that have been passed down through generations of physicians, through which a clinician's gestalt and acumen is honed.

With the belief that the best clinical practice is indeed a combination of evidence-based medicine and collective anecdotal wisdom gathered from seasoned clinicians, *Beyond Evidence-Based Medicine: Clinical Pearls from Experienced Physicians* offers a unique perspective to the practice of medicine.

In this book, we have invited authors, many of whom are renowned clinicians, medical educators, researchers, and subject experts in their respective fields, across Australia, New Zealand, and the USA, to carefully curate pearls of wisdom from their clinical experience, which they think are important and useful to daily clinical practice. These pearls are illustrated in a case-based format, followed by a brief discussion/explanation with relevant evidence-based references. At the end of each case, the authors have included closely related teaching points as 'Other Gems' or didactic summary points as 'Take-Home Messages'. This book presents a wide range of diseases, clinical syndromes, and diagnostic/management conundrums from various medical specialties, organised into specific chapters. Some of the cases also discuss broader perspectives in clinical medicine such as a patient-centred approach, ethical decision making, end-of-life discussions, choosing cost-effective investigations and treatment, patient safety, and clinical reasoning.

As the editors, it has been our utmost pleasure to assemble this book of clinical pearls and through the process, we have gained a lot more knowledge and insights than we could have hoped for. We believe that this book will also benefit many readers, from medical students to physician trainees to practicing physicians, who are aspiring to become reflective, thoughtful, and artful clinicians.

Ralph Junckerstorff
Sharmayne Brady
Ar Kar Aung

Contents

About the Editors

Ralph Junckerstorff is an Internal Medicine and Infectious Diseases physician at Monash Health in Melbourne, Victoria. He graduated from undergraduate medicine from the University of Western Australia in 2000 and became a fellow of the Royal Australasian College of Physicians in 2010. He also holds a Diploma of Tropical Medicine from the University of Liverpool (UK).Dr. Junckerstorff has been involved in undergraduate and postgraduate teaching throughout his entire career. He strongly believes in evidence-based medicine but also feels that the knowledge gained from clinical experience is invaluable. He believes that excellence in teaching and mentorship has the power to shape and inspire.

Sharmayne Brady is a senior staff specialist in Rheumatology at Alfred Health in Melbourne, Victoria. She studied undergraduate medicine at Monash University and finished her degree with first class honours. She completed an additional, elective, research degree in the subject of cardiovascular risk factors in patients with rheumatoid arthritis, working with leaders in the fields of rheumatology and general medicine at the Alfred Hospital in Melbourne. She trained in adult general medicine at Alfred Health and completed her rheumatology specialist training at both the Alfred and Western Hospitals in Melbourne. Dr. Brady completed her PhD in 2021 with Monash University, working with internationally renowned osteoarthritis experts. She was supported by a prestigious National Health and Medical Research Council (NHMRC) Clinical Postgraduate Research Scholarship. She has published 15 papers in leading peer-reviewed journals in the fields of rheumatoid arthritis, osteoarthritis, back pain, and vasculitis. Dr. Brady has presented her research in several leading international and national conferences over the past 10 years. She is also involved in teaching, mentoring, and supervising medical students, physicians, and rheumatology trainees. She has also recently co-edited a medical textbook for junior doctors called *Clinical Integration: Medicine*, which was published in 2021.

Ar Kar Aung is a General and Infectious Diseases physician at Alfred Health in Melbourne, Victoria. He graduated from the University of Melbourne in 2004 and attained his Fellowship of the Royal Australasian College of Physicians (FRACP) in 2012 and Fellowship of the Royal College of Physicians (Edinburgh) (FRCP Edin) in 2022. He completed Master of Public Health and Tropical Medicine at James Cook University in 2015. He currently holds an adjunct clinical associate professor position at Monash University. Dr. Aung has strong interests in medical education, clinical medicine, quality improvement research, health service and clinical research, medication safety, and adverse drug reactions. He was the former Chair of the Australian General and Acute Care Medicine Advance Training Committee at the Royal Australasian College of Physicians (RACP), and former Director of Physician Education at Alfred Health. He also supervised and coordinated General and Acute Care Medicine advance training program at Alfred Health from

2015 to 2019. He has also served in various local and national leadership roles, including as a Board Director on the Internal Medicine Society of Australia and New Zealand (IMSANZ) from 2018 to 2020, as the head of General Medicine research, and as the Chair of Adverse Drug Reaction Review Committee at Alfred Health. He is currently the Chair of IMSANZ Research Network and Victorian metropolitan representative at the IMSANZ Council. He has published more than 50 peer-reviewed articles, numerous clinical guidelines, and book chapters and co-edited a medical textbook *Clinical Integration: Medicine*.

Part I
Internal Medicine

Consider Adverse Drug Reactions in Undifferentiated Presentations

Chris Cameron

1 Clinical Pearl

When admitting patients with undifferentiated illness, always consider whether this is a typical or atypical presentation of a known adverse effect of one of their medications.

2 Clinical Case

Mr. S, a newly retired man in his late 70s, was referred acutely by his General Practitioner (GP) for a 6-week history of diarrhoea, an 11 kg weight loss and agitation/anxiety. He denied fevers or night sweats and had a normal appetite without nausea or vomiting. He had experienced diarrhoea 5 to 6 times a day for the last 5 weeks, without any blood, mucous or melaena.

Mr. S reported that he had been finding it difficult to initiate sleep and would then sleep for only 2 hours at a time.

The patient's past medical history included stable chronic lymphocytic leukaemia (CLL), hypertension and "obsessive tendencies". He drank 2 to 4 standard alcoholic drinks per week and was a lifelong non-smoker.

His medications included cilazapril 1.25 mg daily, zopiclone 7.5 mg daily (recently started for insomnia), atorvastatin 40 mg daily and fluoxetine 20 mg daily. Fluoxetine, a selective serotonin reuptake inhibitor (SSRI), had been prescribed 8 weeks ago by his GP for "worsening functioning" exposed by the COVID-19 lockdown. The patient was struggling with managing Zoom lecturing, and ruminating about his 10 vintage cars, stored all over the city in rented garages, which he was unable to attend to.

C. Cameron (✉)
Wellington Hospital, Wellington, New Zealand

R. Junckerstorff et al. (eds.), *Beyond Evidence-Based Medicine*,
https://doi.org/10.1007/978-981-99-4440-8_1

He had been reviewed by a neurologist in private practice 2 weeks prior, after an urgent GP referral for a "rapid decline in cognition" and dangerous driving. An urgent CT scan of the brain was reported as within normal limits for his age. The working diagnosis from the neurologist was an early dementing process, but anxiety was felt to be an important component of this. It was recommended that he resign from his professional post and retire, which he had done.

Examination findings were notable for signs suggestive of sympathetic nervous system activation and weight loss. He was tachycardic (heart rate 120 bpm) and hypertensive (188/98 mmHg), tremulous and appeared very thin. His clothing was loose. He was somewhat irritable and difficult to direct.

Investigations revealed abnormal liver enzyme tests in a mixed pattern with ALT 400 U/L (Normal range: 5–40), AST 359 U/L (10–35), GGT 246 U/L (10–50) and ALP 270 U/L (30–150). His Thyroid Stimulating Hormone (TSH) was slightly elevated at 3.9 mIU/L (0.4–3.8), but T4 was within the normal range. Pancreatic amylase was slightly elevated at 57 U/L (8–53). Faecal calprotectin was not requested, nor was faecal elastase.

When reviewed on the ward round, the history from the patient and his wife was of a man who had been a highly functioning 77-year-old, still lecturing and maintaining several hobbies and his own finances. During COVID lockdown, he struggled with the new technology that he was expected to manage, and the concern over the state of his vintage cars. He was distressed by these problems. In response to this, his GP had started fluoxetine some 8 weeks prior. Since then, he had experienced multiple partially formed bowel motions daily, lost weight and did not feel that the fluoxetine had helped with his functioning. Examination findings were similar to those of the previous day, and the patient appeared anxious, difficult to direct and irritable over the re-telling of his history. Repeat liver enzyme tests were similar to those of the previous day, hepatitis viral serology (A, B and C) was negative and other tests to elicit the cause of the abnormal enzymes were pending.

3 Discussion

When taking a history to elicit a diagnosis, the surgical sieve is an important tool, especially for general physicians. When working through the sieve, iatrogenic or drug related adverse effects should be considered. Mr. S had recent contact with his GP and a neurologist for new symptoms and was diagnosed with an organic illness and prescribed medication for this.

The New Zealand formulary states that fluoxetine is a rare cause of liver enzyme abnormalities. More commonly, fluoxetine can cause diarrhoea and worsening of anxiety, insomnia and even mania.

The team caring for Mr. S believed that the timeline was concordant for a Type A adverse drug event (ADE) for fluoxetine, causing extreme anxiety (manifesting as tremor, tachycardia, weight loss and irritability). The drug was slowly withdrawn, to avoid SSRI withdrawal syndrome.

Mr. S was followed up in clinic on three subsequent occasions over the following 2 months. His liver enzymes returned to the normal range, he had spoken with his employer and was now working again (albeit at reduced hours) and had gained 4 kg in weight. His diarrhoea had settled, and his wife described him as "more like his usual hairbrained self". He had been able to reduce the dose of zopiclone down to half a tablet (3.75 mg) at night.

About 5% of patients admitted to General Medicine are there due to an ADE and about 85% of those are Type A, meaning that the ADE is predictable based on the pharmacology of the drug. These ADEs are usually easier to diagnose than the rarer Type B ADE, which may present in such a way that they are not easily identified by the action of the drug.

Rawlins' classification of Adverse Drug Reactions denotes Type A adverse reactions as dose-dependent and related to the pharmacological effect of the drug. Type B adverse reactions are not dose-dependent and classified by Rawlins' as idiosyncratic or an allergic reaction.

SSRIs have many different ADEs, and as they may be prescribed for depression or anxiety, it can be surprising that they may worsen anxiety and cause insomnia in a minority of patients.

Jitteriness is a syndrome of early worsening of anxiety, agitation, and irritability. It is estimated to occur in up to 65% of patients immediately after starting therapy with an SSRI [1].

The lessons to be learned from this case are predominantly around history taking—any recent contact with another health professional must be explored in some depth, especially if there has been a new drug prescribed, even if the course has been completed.

ADEs can be considered as another "great mimicker", along with SLE and HIV. Multiple body systems can be affected, and diagnosis can be elusive, unless the physician is alert to new prescriptions and to potential drug interactions.

4 Other Gems

- Always consider an iatrogenic cause from medications when forming differential diagnoses for patients with an undifferentiated illness.
- SSRIs can have many and varied ADEs affecting many different body systems.
- ADEs can be Type A or Type B—Type A is the most common and can usually be recognised as a known potential exaggerated pharmacological effect of the drug.
- In cases of undifferentiated illness, check with the patient when their most recent contact with a health professional was, and if there was any prescription (including Over-The-Counter medications).
- ADEs are great mimickers, and especially if there are multiple body systems involved, should always be considered in cases of undifferentiated illness.

Reference

1. Sinclair LI, Christmas DM, Hood SD, et al. Antidepressant-induced jitteriness/anxiety syndrome: systematic review. Br J Psychiatry. 2009;194:483–90.

Polypharmacy and Deprescribing

Ian Scott

1 Clinical Pearl

In older multi-morbid patients receiving multiple drugs and who present with ill-defined symptoms, look for potential drug-drug interactions and prescribing cascades.

2 Clinical Case

An 83-year-old was admitted to hospital after presenting with light-headedness and palpitations secondary to recurrent atrial fibrillation (AF) with rapid ventricular response. Her past history comprised hyperlipidaemia, osteoporosis, hypertension, gastro-oesophageal reflux disease (GORD), type 2 diabetes and stage 3A chronic kidney disease. She was commenced on metoprolol succinate at 50 mg daily and verapamil 60 mg daily with prompt normalisation of heart rate. Her other regular medications comprised digoxin, frusemide, atorvastatin, lisinopril, esomeprazole, metformin, gliclazide, apixaban, and vitamin B12 injections.

She was discharged the following day but returned a month later with a presyncopal episode caused by bradycardia and hypotension. Her serum digoxin was noted to be 2.1 ng/ml (reference range 0.8–2.0 ng/ml), serum potassium was elevated at 5.9 mmol/L (reference range 3.5–5.0 mmol/L) and serum magnesium was low at 0.6 mmol/L (reference range 0.8–1.10 mmol/L). Metoprolol, verapamil,

I. Scott (✉)
Internal Medicine and Clinical Epidemiology, Princess Alexandra Hospital, Brisbane, Australia

Centre for Health Services Research, University of Queensland, Brisbane, QLD, Australia

Faculty of Medicine, Queensland University of Technology, Brisbane, QLD, Australia

R. Junckerstorff et al. (eds.), *Beyond Evidence-Based Medicine*,
https://doi.org/10.1007/978-981-99-4440-8_2

digoxin, and potassium were ceased, with metoprolol recommenced some days later at 50 mg daily. A pharmacist reviewed her medications and noted her dose of frusemide had been doubled since her previous admission and potassium supplements added. Her HbA1c was 6.0% and most blood sugar levels in hospital ranged from 4 to 6 mmol/L.

It was thought that verapamil had decreased digoxin clearance which, combined with the β-blocker, led to bradycardia. Verapamil had also caused venous dilation in her lower limbs resulting in leg oedema which had prompted her general practitioner to increase her frusemide which, in turn, caused hypokalaemia leading to the commencement of potassium supplements. Due to the patient's underlying kidney disease, the potassium supplements caused the serum potassium to rise above the normal range. Her blood sugar control was too stringent, aggravated by loss of appetite due to digoxin toxicity. The low serum magnesium and the requirement for B12 injections were thought to be secondary to malabsorption induced by the proton pump inhibitor and metformin respectively, and both were ceased as she was asymptomatic from GORD and her diabetes was well controlled with diet. In light of her renal disease, low LDL-cholesterol (0.6 mmol/L), and absence of cardiovascular disease, her atorvastatin dose was reduced.

3 Discussion

Polypharmacy, defined here as >5 regular prescribed drugs, is common, with nearly 20% of community-dwelling adults older than 65 years prescribed 10 or more medications, with almost half of these patients receiving at least 1 unnecessary medication [1]. Such overprescribing comes with increased risk of adverse drug events (ADEs) in older people due to physiological changes of ageing that alter pharmacokinetic and pharmacodynamic responses to drugs [2]. Observational studies have documented ADEs in at least 15% of older patients [3], contributing to ill health, hospitalisation, and, in some cases, death. The number of drugs that a patient is taking is the single most important predictor of harm [4], and it is estimated that 1 in 5 medications are potentially inappropriate [5].

Deprescribing is a systematic approach for identifying and ceasing, or dose reducing, drugs where actual or potential harm outweighs actual or potential benefit, after accounting for a patients' age, co-morbidities, quality of life and goals of care [6]. The important steps are to match each drug with its putative indication and then for each drug identified, to cease those where the indication no longer exists, or are associated with side effects or high risk of harm, or are proving ineffective or overly burdensome. Deprescribing has been shown to reduce the risk of ADEs [7], and improve patient medication adherence [8]. Deprescribing is safe if selected drugs are ceased or weaned one at a time under close monitoring. They can always be restarted or the dose increased if there is relapse of disease.

4 Other Gems

- Older, frail multi-morbid patients are often excluded from clinical trials of medications and hence the reported benefits seen in the trials may not generalise to this population. Hence caution is required in starting new medications in such patients and 'treat to target' recommendations contained in condition-specific clinical practice guidelines may be inappropriate [9]. For example, aiming for strict blood sugar control (i.e., HbA1c <7%) increases the risk of severe hypoglycaemia in older frail patients.
- Clinicians are often reluctant to cease longstanding medications, despite the potential for harm, because of a fear of: (1) causing an adverse disease-related event ('why rock the boat?'); (2) losing trust of the patient ('are you abandoning me?'); (3) incurring criticism from colleagues who initiated or recommended the medication ('my cardiologist said I should never stop this drug'); and (4) being unable to implement the deprescribing process ('I just don't have the time/skills/resources to do this') [10]. On the other hand, most older patients are willing to stop one or more of their medications if their treating clinician says it is possible, and two thirds report a desire to reduce the number of the medications they are taking. Deprescribing recommendations are deemed acceptable to over 75% of patients and healthcare professionals, with a high level of reported patient and family satisfaction with the deprescribing intervention [6]. Guidelines and resources are available which show how deprescribing can be done safely with patient participation and agreement (available at: Australian Deprescribing Network: www.australiandeprescribingnetwork.com.au)
- Admission to hospital for whatever reason should be taken as an opportunity for physicians to review current medication lists to see if any drug should be considered for deprescribing.

References

1. Hajjar ER, Hanlon JT, Sloane RJ, et al. Unnecessary drug use in frail older people at hospital discharge. J Am Geriatr Soc. 2005;53(9):1518–23.
2. Gnjidic D, Hilmer SN, Blyth FM, et al. Polypharmacy cut-off and outcomes: five or more medicines were used to identify community dwelling older men at risk of different adverse outcomes. J Clin Epidemiol. 2012;65(9):989–95.
3. Opondo D, Eslami S, Visscher S, et al. Inappropriateness of medication prescriptions to elderly patients in the primary care setting: a systematic review. PLoS One. 2012;7(8):e43617.
4. Steinman MA, Miao Y, Boscardin WJ, et al. Prescribing quality in older veterans: a multifocal approach. J Gen Intern Med. 2014;29(10):1379–86.
5. Roughead EE, Anderson B, Gilbert AL. Potentially inappropriate prescribing among Australian veterans and war widows/widowers. Intern Med J. 2007;37(6):402–5.

6. Scott IA, Hilmer SN, Reeve E, et al. Reducing inappropriate polypharmacy – the process of deprescribing. JAMA Intern Med. 2015;175:827–34.
7. Christensen M, Lundh A. Medication review in hospitalised patients to reduce morbidity and mortality. Cochrane Database Syst Rev. 2013;2:CD008986.
8. Reeve E, Wiese MD. Benefits of deprescribing on patients' adherence to medications. Int J Clin Pharm. 2014;36(1):26–9.
9. Boyd CM, Darer J, Boult C, Fried LP, Boult L, Wu AW. Clinical practice guidelines and quality of care for older patients with multiple comorbid diseases: implications for pay for performance. JAMA. 2005;294(6):716–24.
10. Anderson K, Stowasser D, Freeman C, Scott IA. Prescriber barriers and enablers to minimising potentially inappropriate medications in adults: a systematic review and thematic synthesis. BMJ Open. 2014;4:e006544.

Overdiagnosis

Ian Scott

1 Clinical Pearl

> When ordering investigations, be selective and provide a rationale for each one, so as to reduce the risk of overdiagnosis and overtreatment of incidental findings.

2 Clinical Case

A 66-year-old man with diabetes, hypertension, past carotid endarterectomy and peripheral vascular disease presented with fevers, rigors, malaise and headache for 5 days. He was febrile and hypotensive though alert and oriented. Physical examination disclosed findings consistent with cellulitis in his right lower limb. Intravenous penicillin was commenced and blood cultures subsequently grew group G Streptococcus sensitive to β-lactams. However, because a soft systolic murmur was heard for the first time on admission and the patient was considered immunosuppressed, a transthoracic echocardiogram was ordered to exclude bacterial endocarditis. This did not disclose any valvular abnormalities or vegetations, but revealed regional wall abnormalities in the inferior wall of the left ventricle. The patient's exercise tolerance was limited by exercise-induced claudication in his right leg but he described no other limits on activity, reported no chest pain and had no past history of myocardial infarction. A single-photon-emission computed tomographic

---

I. Scott (✉)
Internal Medicine and Clinical Epidemiology, Princess Alexandra Hospital, Brisbane, Australia

Centre for Health Services Research, University of Queensland, Brisbane, QLD, Australia

Faculty of Medicine, Queensland University of Technology, Brisbane, QLD, Australia

R. Junckerstorff et al. (eds.), *Beyond Evidence-Based Medicine*,
https://doi.org/10.1007/978-981-99-4440-8_3

(SPECT) persantin scan revealed normal ejection fraction and no evidence of prior infarction but transient ischemic dilatation was seen in the inferior wall. Given his risk factors, coronary angiography was performed and showed multivessel stenosis: 60% left main, 80% left anterior descending, and 80% posterior descending arteries. He was referred to a cardiothoracic surgeon who recommended coronary artery bypass grafting (CABG). However, given his previous carotid endarterectomy, it was thought prudent prior to the CABG to perform a catheter angiogram of his head and neck to evaluate for any significant stenotic lesions. This revealed stenosis of various segments of the intracerebral arteries but no significant extracranial disease. Unfortunately, three days following the angiogram, the patient presented with acute-onset confusion, word-finding difficulty, and short-term memory deficits. Magnetic resonance imaging of the brain revealed multiple foci of acute ischaemic lesions in different vascular territories consistent with embolic strokes thought to be iatrogenic due to cerebral angiography. He is currently undergoing physical and speech therapy to aid his recovery.

3 Discussion

Overdiagnosis is defined as the diagnosis of a condition or anomaly (often subsequently treated), that would otherwise not cause symptoms or harm to a patient [1]. While it has long been recognised as a consequence of cancer screening, it is increasingly acknowledged as an important consequence of any unjustified diagnostic testing in the absence of symptoms or significant signs of disease [2]. Adverse consequences can arise from such overtesting, either directly from the testing itself, or indirectly from subsequent downstream care cascades, such as invasively investigating incidental but benign findings, or administering treatments that are not indicated or evidence-based. The clinical case above demonstrates all of these effects, from the initial incidental finding of regional wall motion abnormalities in the absence of anginal symptoms, to the questionable undertaking of cerebral angiography in the absence of neurological symptoms and carotid bruits. Harms can be physical, psychological, social, financial and relational (mistrust in clinicians) [3]. Being given unwarranted diagnostic labels can induce anxiety and decrease quality of life and social engagement [4], while providing even potentially beneficial care to patients who do not want it can cause harm, at least psychologically. Reframing overtesting and overdiagnosis as being potentially harmful or wasteful, not just "worth a go" or "better safe than sorry", may incentivise clinicians, patients and organisations to engage more in mitigation efforts [5]. Clinician-directed education programs, clinical guidelines, audit and feedback can reduce overuse of interventions to some degree [6]. However, various sociocognitive biases in clinical reasoning probably drive much of the over-use in current practice for which debiasing strategies may be more effective [7]. Patient-directed strategies which empower care recipients to ask questions of their clinicians as to the need for tests or treatments, their relative benefits and harm, and what alternative options may be possible are also supported by evidence of effectiveness [8].

4 Other Gems

- In recent years, professional societies in various countries have mounted campaigns such as Choosing Wisely (www.choosingwisely.org.au) and EVOLVE (https://evolve.edu.au) to raise awareness among both patients and clinicians of the prevalence and impacts of low value care, and to disseminate recommendations about avoiding overuse of specific tests and treatments in various clinical scenarios.
- Many patients refrain from participating in discussions aimed at avoiding overuse because of a power asymmetry with their clinicians. They sense the need to seek clinician permission to discuss their options, feel they have insufficient knowledge to ask pertinent questions or understand the jargon ("doctor knows best"), and fear repercussions from being seen to challenge clinician credibility (desire to be a 'good patient'). Alternatively, patients may want to avoid responsibility for making a wrong decision they will later regret, or feel unable to participate because of illness symptoms, cognitive impairment, language or cultural barriers, or need for emergency or intensive care [9]. It is the clinician's responsibility to break down these barriers and support patients in shared decision-making.
- Questions which patients should be encouraged to ask are:
  - what is the decision we need to make and why?
  - what are my options?
  - what are potential benefits and harms of each option?
  - what if we do nothing and just watch?
  - are there other things that are important to me and may affect my decision (e.g. costs involved, duration of inability to work or perform social activities, skill and position of those performing a procedure)?

References

1. Brodersen J, Schwartz LM, Heneghan C, et al. Overdiagnosis: what it is and what it isn't. BMJ Evid Based Med. 2018;23(1):1–3.
2. Carter SM, Rogers W, Heath I, et al. The challenge of overdiagnosis begins with its definition. BMJ. 2015;350:h869.
3. Korenstein D, Chimonas S, Barrow B, et al. Development of a conceptual map of negative consequences for patients of overuse of medical tests and treatments. JAMA Intern Med. 2018;178:1401–7.
4. Cotter AR, Vuong K, Mustelin L, et al. Do psychological harms result from being labelled with an unexpected diagnosis of abdominal aortic aneurysm or prostate cancer through screening? A systematic review. BMJ Open. 2017;7:e017565.
5. Liao JM, Schapira MS, Navathe AS, et al. The effect of emphasizing patient, societal, and institutional harms of inappropriate antibiotic prescribing on physician support of financial penalties: a randomized trial. Ann Intern Med. 2017;167:215–6.
6. Colla CH, Mainor AJ, Hargreaves C, et al. Interventions aimed at reducing use of low-value health services: a systematic review. Med Care Res Rev. 2017;74:507–50.

7. Scott IA, Soon J, Elshaug AG, Lindner R. Countering cognitive biases in minimising low value care. Med J Aust. 2017;206:407–11.
8. Sypes EE, de Grood C, Whalen-Browne L, et al. Engaging patients in de-implementation interventions to reduce low-value clinical care: a systematic review and meta-analysis. BMC Med. 2020;18:116.
9. Green AR, Tung M, Segal JB. Older adults' perceptions of the causes and consequences of healthcare overuse: a qualitative study. J Gen Intern Med. 2018;33:892–7.

Chronic Pain Management

Lannie Ho and Benny Katz

1 Clinical Pearl

Chronic pain is not simply acute pain that has persisted. It requires a different therapeutic approach.

2 Clinical Case

JM is a 70-year-old man who presented with a 10-year history of low back pain and bilateral knee pain affecting his mobility. He was only able to walk 150 m before having to stop because of pain, rated at 7/10. He had tried regular paracetamol and non-steroidal inflammatory drugs (NSAIDs) without improvements. An opioid skin patch was not well tolerated as it impacted his cognition and ability to work as an accountant. His past medical history included hypertension and osteoarthritis. He attended a Multidisciplinary Pain Clinic to explore non-surgical options. The program focused on non-pharmacological approaches including pain education, pacing and exercise. After 3 months he was able to walk 500 m before being stopped by pain, rated at 8/10, compared with 150 m and 7/10 respectively prior to the program. Would JM consider this an improvement?

L. Ho
Department of Geriatric Medicine, Austin Hospital, Heidelberg, VIC, Australia

B. Katz (✉)
Department of Geriatric Medicine, St. Vincent's Hospital Melbourne, Fitzroy, VIC, Australia

Faculty of Medicine, Dentistry and Health Sciences, University of Melbourne, Parkville, VIC, Australia

R. Junckerstorff et al. (eds.), *Beyond Evidence-Based Medicine*,
https://doi.org/10.1007/978-981-99-4440-8_4

3 Discussion

Acute and chronic pain are distinct entities and require different management approaches (see Table 1). Acute pain is of recent onset and usually has a close relationship with tissue injury or disease. It is most commonly nociceptive in origin and draws attention to actual or potential tissue damage. Acute pain typically resolves as healing takes place. Typically, it responds to conventional analgesics such as paracetamol, NSAIDs and opioids.

In contrast, chronic pain is defined as pain that has lasted more than 3 months. This is longer than the expected period of recovery from disease or injury. The term persistent pain and chronic pain may be used interchangeably, as the term 'chronic' may have negative connotations [1].

Chronic pain should not be treated as acute pain that has persisted. Acute pain is managed by treatment of the underlying pathology together with provision of pain relief. The underlying cause of chronic pain may not be amenable to treatment, and it does not respond to conventional analgesics such as NSAIDs and opioids in the same manner as acute pain. In this setting the persistence of pain is not always indicative of ongoing tissue damage. Serious pathology such as tumours and infection can usually be eliminated on history and examination, possibly with a few investigations. The focus of treatment shifts from the pain sensation to addressing its functional impact, associated suffering and impact on quality of life. There is an

Table 1 Characteristics and management of acute and chronic pain

	Acute pain	Chronic pain
Characteristics	• Recent onset • Relationship to tissue injury • Pain typically resolves with healing • Most commonly of nociceptive origin	• Defined as pain lasting longer than 3 months • Longer than expected period of recovery of disease • Not always indicative of ongoing tissue injury
Examples	• Finger laceration • Sporting injury • Post operative pain	• Chronic back pain • Osteoarthritis • Diabetic peripheral neuropathy
Risk factors		• Nature of underlying problem (e.g. Osteoarthritis) • Neuropathic pain • Inadequate initial treatment of acute pain • Refusal of treatment • Comorbidities and psychosocial factors (mood disorders)
Management	• Usually improves with time. Typically responds to conventional analgesics	• Less responsive to conventional analgesics • Biopsychosocial approach with goal setting focusing on optimising function and quality of life, not just reduction in pain intensity

expectation that some pain will persist. In this regard chronic pain is best viewed as a multidimensional health problem rather than a symptom of underlying disease [2]. Care should be taken to avoid "over medicalisation" of chronic pain with investigations that will not alter management and/or ongoing trials of analgesics. This may result in false expectations that a cure is possible.

The precise mechanisms that underlie the transition from acute to chronic pain are not always apparent or predictable. Risk factors include the nature of the underlying pathology (e.g., osteoarthritis), neuropathic pain, inadequate initial treatment of acute pain (e.g., post-operative pain), refusal of treatment, comorbidities and psychological factors (e.g., mood disorders).

When chronic pain cannot be managed by treatment of the underlying cause, e.g., joint arthroplasty, a biopsychosocial approach is recommended. This may be delivered by a single health practitioner, but more commonly by a multidisciplinary team. A medication review should take place, discontinuing medications that have not been effective. Just because a medication has not been effective in easing pain does not mean that it does not have side effects. Overemphasis on opioid analgesia in managing chronic pain has contributed to the opioid epidemic of misuse [2].

JM would not consider the pain management program successful if he was expecting complete eradication of pain and full restoration of function. These goals would be reasonable for acute pain, but not for pain that has been present for 10 years. Pain management programs often achieve greater improvements in function and mood than in pain reduction. Realistic treatment goals should be negotiated at the outset. If JM's goal was to be able to walk 500 m to enable him to pick up his grandchild from childcare, then he would consider the program had been successful.

4 Take Home Messages

- Chronic pain is best managed with a biopsychosocial approach. This may be delivered by a single practitioner, but usually requires a multidisciplinary approach.
- The goals of chronic pain management are not simply focused on reduction in pain intensity, but also on optimising function and quality of life.

References

1. Raja SN, Carr DB, Cohen M, et al. The revised International Association for the Study of Pain definition of pain: concepts, challenges, and compromises. Pain. 2020;161:1976–82.
2. Cohen SP, Vase L, Hooten WM. Chronic pain: an update on burden, best practices, and new advances. Lancet. 2021;397(10289):2082–97.

Neuropathic Pain Is a Symptom Not a Diagnosis

Lannie Ho and Benny Katz

1 Clinical Pearl

Neuropathic pain is a clinical description not a diagnosis which requires demonstration of a disease or lesion that satisfies established neurological diagnostic criteria.

2 Clinical Case

MA is an 80-year-old lady who presents with worsening pain that followed a bout of shingles about 18 months ago. Her pain is located in her neck and shoulders, spreading to her trunk and limbs. She has both evoked pain and spontaneous pain described as burning, shooting, and tingling. It affects her sleep and ability to do housework. Her past medical history is significant for shingles in the right T7 dermatome, initially treated with famciclovir, Type 2 diabetes mellitus, insomnia and irritable bladder. Her pain has not been responsive to treatment with oxycodone and pregabalin. Massage makes it worse. She is referred for specialist consultation for management of neuropathic pain.

L. Ho
Department of Geriatric Medicine, Austin Hospital, Heidelberg, VIC, Australia

B. Katz (✉)
Department of Geriatric Medicine, St. Vincent's Hospital Melbourne, Fitzroy, VIC, Australia

Faculty of Medicine, Dentistry and Health Sciences, University of Melbourne, Parkville, VIC, Australia

R. Junckerstorff et al. (eds.), *Beyond Evidence-Based Medicine*,
https://doi.org/10.1007/978-981-99-4440-8_5

3 Discussion

MA was considered to have neuropathic pain based on the description of her pain. Neuropathic pain is a clinical description not a diagnosis. The diagnosis of neuropathic pain requires the diagnosis of a disease or lesion that that satisfies established neurological diagnostic criteria that can account for the pain. Her medical history includes shingles and diabetic mellitus, both conditions that may be associated with neuropathic pain. A careful history reveals that MA's pain is not in the distribution consistent with either diagnosis. She describes widespread pain in her trunk and limbs, with exaggerated response to pressure. A diagnosis of neuropathic pain cannot be confirmed as her symptoms are not explained by a disease or lesion affecting the nervous system.

Fibromyalgia is a better diagnosis. Fibromyalgia is an example of a nociplastic pain. It is characterised by its diffuse nature that is not explained by activation of nociceptors or a lesion or disease of the nervous system. Other examples of nociplastic pain include irritable bowel syndrome, painful bladder syndrome, tension headaches and non-specific low back pain. Fibromyalgia is often associated with other symptoms such as fatigue, irritable bowel and cognitive changes. Nociplastic pain was previously known by various other names such as central sensitisation, hypersensitivity, and pain of unknown origin. A diagnosis of nociplastic pain requires the exclusion of nociceptive and neuropathic causes of pain, however they can co-exist [1].

MA's symptoms are non-specific, and not enough to establish a diagnosis of neuropathic pain. The diagnosis may be established on history and examination possibly supported by diagnostic investigations such as imaging, neurophysiology, biopsies, or laboratory tests. Examples of neuropathic pain include painful diabetic peripheral neuropathy, postherpetic neuralgia, carpal tunnel syndrome, multiple sclerosis, trigeminal neuralgia, and post stroke central pain syndromes.

A different treatment approach is required for neuropathic pain. When appropriately identified, neuropathic pain my give the opportunity for targeted treatments such as carpal tunnel release, nerve root injections for radicular pain, acute antiviral therapy for herpes zoster and optimising diabetic control. For post herpetic neuralgia, topical approaches such as lignocaine or capsaicin may be beneficial with opioids considered third line therapy [2].

Both neuropathic and nociplastic pain are often refractory to conventional analgesics such as paracetamol, NSAIDs and opioids that are used to treat nociceptive pains. They may respond to adjuvant agents such as amitriptyline, gabapentin, pregabalin and duloxetine [3]. Side effects of these medications often limit their use. Patients hope for 100% reduction in pain. In drug trials, a positive response to these agents is defined as a 30% or 50% reduction in pain intensity. Only about 15% of patients achieve this result [4].

There are no specific treatments for nociplastic pains. The emphasis is on symptom management aiming to reduce pain, and to optimise mood, function, and quality of life. It is best managed with a multidisciplinary biopsychosocial approach involving physical therapies, cognitive therapies, and medications. Specialist input

Table 1 Summary of neuropathic and nociplastic pain

	Neuropathic pain	Nociplastic pain
Aetiology	• Lesion or disease affecting the central or peripheral nervous system	• No clear evidence of threatened or actual tissue damage or evidence of disease or lesion of the somatosensory system • Alteration of nociceptive processing or descending inhibition, or both
Characteristics	• Can be non-specific • Typically burning, electric, shooting, tingling	• Diffuse, aching, intense • Often associated with other symptoms including fatigue, irritable bladder, memory and mood disturbance
Diagnosis	• The symptoms should be in a neurologic distribution • Sensory abnormalities are usually present in the affected area • May require investigations to demonstrate the neurologic disease or lesion	• Requires exclusion of nociceptive and neuropathic causes of pain
Examples	• Diabetic neuropathy • Trigeminal neuralgia • Carpel tunnel • Stroke • Multiple sclerosis	• Fibromyalgia (clinical case) • Tension headaches • Irritable bowel syndrome • Irritable bladder syndrome • Non-specific low back pain
Treatment modalities	• Targeted treatments at aetiology (e.g. antiviral therapy for shingles) plus adjuvant analgesics Refractory to standard analgesics such as NSAIDs and opioids, but may respond to adjuvant agents Symptom management to manage pain intensity, mood and functional disturbances Specialist opinion is recommended if complex	• Symptom management Multidisciplinary approach aiming to optimise mood and restore physical function. Less role for medications Avoid opioid analgesia Specialist opinion is recommended for complex cases

such as referral to a geriatrician, rheumatologist, pain specialist or multidisciplinary pain clinic should be considered [5].

A summary of neuropathic and nociplastic pain is provided in Table 1.

4 Take Home Messages

- Neuropathic pain is a symptom not a diagnosis. To make a diagnosis of neuropathic pain requires the confirmation of a neurological disease or lesion that accounts for the pain.

- Nociplastic pain may have similar pain qualities, but the symptoms tend to be more diffuse and not explained by nociceptive or neuropathic mechanisms.
- Appreciating the different mechanisms of pain does assist with choice of therapy and prognostication.

References

1. Fitzcharles M-A, Cohen SP, Clauw DJ, Littlejohn G, Usui C, Häuser W. Nociplastic pain: towards an understanding of prevalent pain conditions. Lancet. 2021;397(10289):2098–110.
2. Derry S, Derry S, Rice ASC, Cole P, Tan T, Moore RA. Topical capsaicin (high concentration) for chronic neuropathic pain in adults. Cochrane Database Syst Rev. 2017;2021(7):CD007393.
3. Moore RA, Chi CC, Wiffen PJ, Derry S, Rice ASC, Moore RA. Oral nonsteroidal anti-inflammatory drugs for neuropathic pain. Cochrane Database Syst Rev. 2015;2019(5):CD010902-CD.
4. Bates D, Schultheis BC, Hanes MC, Jolly SM, Chakravarthy KV, Deer TR, et al. A comprehensive algorithm for management of neuropathic pain. Pain Med. 2019;20(Suppl_1):S2–S12.
5. Cohen SP, Mao J. Neuropathic pain: mechanisms and their clinical implications. BMJ. 2014;348:f7656.

Collaborations in Complexity

Catherine Gibb

1 Clinical Pearl

Phone a friend.

2 Clinical Case

Marie was a 56-year-old lady in good health who presented to her primary care doctor with a left swollen leg. A deep vein thrombosis (DVT) was diagnosed, and she was started on an appropriate dose of anticoagulation. She was due to embark on a much-anticipated holiday for 3 weeks and did not follow up immediately with the suggested investigations to find a cause for her unprovoked DVT.

Unfortunately, when she returned from holidays she had noticed increasing abdominal swelling and a large ovarian mass with inferior vena cava (IVC) compression was diagnosed. Subsequent investigations confirmed ovarian malignancy and a major oophorectomy with hysterectomy and lymph node clearance was planned. She was referred to the perioperative medicine clinic to help plan her perioperative course.

When she presented 2 weeks prior to surgery, her abdomen had increased in girth. She had been on rivaroxaban for about 6 weeks and was felt to have had excellent compliance with the treatment regime. A DVT scan was performed to review any resolution of her clot. Unfortunately she was found to have a rapidly enlarging ovarian lesion with complete occlusion of the IVC, complete occlusion of the left external iliac vein with clot and complete compression of the left external iliac vein.

C. Gibb (✉)
Royal Adelaide Hospital, Adelaide, SA, Australia

R. Junckerstorff et al. (eds.), *Beyond Evidence-Based Medicine*,
https://doi.org/10.1007/978-981-99-4440-8_6

Her right common iliac vein was not visible due to probable compression although the right external iliac vein was patent.

There was only a small portion of the IVC felt to be patent below the liver.

The clinical challenge was to provide the best thromboembolic treatment for this lady to allow her to have the safest possible operation.

Discussions were commenced.

The interventional radiologist contacted the perioperative physician as soon as the ultrasound was performed and advised that there was no possibility of inserting an IVC filter unless it was from the jugular vein and situated above the renal veins.

The haematologist opinion was focussed very much on the medical management of the anticoagulation at the time of surgery, with clear advice as to the transition from rivaroxaban to enoxaparin.

The vascular surgical unit discussed Marie's case at their multidisciplinary meeting. The options of medical management, IVC ligation at the time of surgery or suprarenal IVC filter were discussed. It was agreed that the major risk was at the time of manipulation of the tumour during the surgery. A literature review was conducted during the meeting, and it was agreed that a supra renal IVC filter inserted immediately prior to surgery and removed at 48–72 h after surgery with full reintroduction of anticoagulation was the preferred path.

The intensive care team were contacted and asked to support Marie in the intensive care unit (ICU) after surgery to ensure optimal monitoring of her urine output and renal function with possible need for urgent removal of the suprarenal IVC filter if there were concerns about renal vein thrombosis.

The gynaecological oncology team co-ordinated all the interventions and ensured the timing of the IVC filter, ICU bed flow and subsequent filter removal were arranged to coincide with the surgical date.

Marie was involved in this complex decision making to help her understand the plan that was implemented, allow her to question the decisions and finally to ensure she provided informed consent.

Marie's surgery was complex and involved the formation of a stoma due to sigmoid involvement by the tumour. She however did not have any complications of bleeding and did not develop pulmonary emboli in the immediate postoperative period. She continued to have subsequent treatment for her ovarian malignancy.

3 Discussion

Complexity is an increasing hallmark of modern medicine [1].

When people present with disease that encroaches on multiple domains it is important to ensure that all stakeholders who may support complex decision making are involved [2]. The patient themselves are clearly stakeholders and are integral to making such complex decision.

4 Other Gems

- Decision making can be complex. As a doctor you are never alone and have colleagues who want to support you in finding the best outcome for your patients. As you establish your career, taking time to develop networks of trusted colleagues across multiple specialties will provide support for both you and your patients at difficult times.

References

1. Simpkin AL, Schwartzstein RM. Tolerating uncertainty- the next medical revolution? N Engl J Med. 2016;375(18):1713–5.
2. Glance LG, Osler TM, Neuman MD. Redesigning surgical decision making for high risk patients. N Engl J Med. 2014;370:1379–81.

The Skeleton in the Closet: Preventing Hospital-Associated Malnutrition

Alison M. Mudge, Nicole I. Chan, and Joseph Tan

1 Clinical Pearl

Nutritional status has an important impact on clinical outcomes and should be assessed at admission to identify existing malnutrition. Even those with normal nutrition screening at admission can be at risk of poor intake due to a host of patient and system factors, so rescreening is indicated for those with longer stays.

2 Clinical Case

A 79-year-old ex-plumber is admitted to hospital with increasing breathlessness and fatigue due to exacerbation of heart failure. His medical history includes hypertension and a myocardial infarction 20 years earlier. His heart failure is usually well controlled on perindopril, bisoprolol and frusemide which he titrates based on his weight. He is widowed and lives alone in an independent living unit with fortnightly cleaning assistance. He has a negative Malnutrition Screening Tool at admission. His heart failure improves after 5 days of intensive diuresis with intravenous

A. M. Mudge (✉)
Department of Internal Medicine and Aged Care, Royal Brisbane and Women's Hospital, Herston, QLD, Australia

Medical School, The University of Queensland, Brisbane, QLD, Australia

N. I. Chan
Medical School, The University of Queensland, Brisbane, QLD, Australia

Royal Brisbane and Women's Hospital, Metro North Health, Brisbane, QLD, Australia

J. Tan
Surgical Treatment and Rehabilitation Services, Metro North Health, Brisbane, QLD, Australia

R. Junckerstorff et al. (eds.), *Beyond Evidence-Based Medicine*,
https://doi.org/10.1007/978-981-99-4440-8_7

frusemide infusion and oral spironolactone. He is weaned off oxygen but needs assistance to transfer from bed to chair and requires a four-wheeled walker with assistance for mobility due to fatigue and weakness. He is referred to a rehabilitation unit for convalescence.

Admission assessment by the dietitian on the rehabilitation ward shows moderate malnutrition (Subjective Global Assessment B). On further history, he describes reduced mealtime intake for several weeks before presentation due to fatigue and post-prandial fullness, and reduced appetite in hospital due to dyspnoea and dry mouth from the supplementary oxygen. His albumin has dropped from 29 to 20g/L (normal 35–45g/L) during his admission. He is commenced on Sustagen® supplements and high protein-high energy meals in addition to his physiotherapy program and returns to independent living after 3 weeks.

3 Discussion

Malnutrition is associated with adverse outcomes in hospitalised patients, including sarcopenia and functional decline, prolonged hospital stay and increased mortality. Malnutrition is present in 30–50% of older hospital in-patients and is likely to be under-recognised if routine nutritional screening is not consistently performed at admission [1]. Validated tools such as the Malnutrition Screening Tool [2] use brief screening questions to identify poor eating and recent unplanned weight loss. Positive screening scores can identify patients who require more detailed assessment to confirm malnutrition, using diagnostic tools such as the Subjective Global Assessment [3], which is a multidimensional assessment including body mass index, weight loss, intake, nutrition impact symptoms, physiological stressors, function and fat and muscle distribution. A range of screening and assessment tools have been validated in different clinical populations [4]. However, malnutrition screening and assessment at admission is an unreliable predictor of poor intake in hospital and subsequent hospital-acquired malnutrition [5]. Poor nutritional intake occurs due to a complex interplay of patient factors (e.g., poor appetite, nausea, functional or cognitive impairment), staff factors (e.g. competing priorities at mealtimes, unclear responsibility), mealtime factors (e.g. patient and meal tray positioning, challenging food packaging) and systems factors (e.g. inflexible mealtimes) [6–8].

Meal charts play an important role in providing reliable information about a patient's intake and may aid in preventing muscle loss during hospitalisation. Poor intake requires a team approach to addressing individual barriers (e.g., prescription of pre-meal antiemetics may help nausea; finger foods may help fatigue or incoordination; small, frequent high-density foods or supplements may help fatigue or early satiety). Doctors can help to advocate for a systems approach to organisational and system-level barriers and can set an important example by being more aware of patient mealtimes, encouraging and assisting intake by opening packets or helping position the patient and/or meal tray if they are on the ward at mealtimes, and avoiding interrupting patient meals with non-urgent assessments or activities.

4 Other Gems

- Weight can be an unreliable indicator of nutritional status particularly in patients with large fluid shifts like heart failure, cirrhosis, and renal disease. A full clinical assessment considers nutritional impact symptoms, dietary intake, and assessment of fat stores, muscle mass, oedema and ascites. Lean weight tends to decrease with age, and weight-based diuretic regimens may need to be revised over time.
- Albumin is also an unreliable single measure of nutritional status due to the impact of other diseases, inflammation, and fluid shifts, but may be a useful measure of change in nutritional status over time.

References

1. Cass AR, Charlton KE. Prevalence of hospital-acquired malnutrition and modifiable determinants of nutritional deterioration during inpatient admissions: a systematic review of the evidence. J Hum Nutr Diet. 2022;35:1043–58. https://doi.org/10.1111/jhn.13009.
2. Ferguson M, Capra S, Bauer J, Banks M. Development of a valid and reliable screening tool for adult acute hospital patients. Nutrition. 1999;15:458–64.
3. Detsky AS, McLaughlin JR, Baker JP, et al. What is subjective global assessment of nutritional status? JPEN J Parenter Enteral Nutr. 1986;10:441–5.
4. Mueller C, Compher C, Druyen ME, et al. A.S.P.E.N. clinical guidelines. Nutrition screening, assessment, and intervention in adults. JPEN J Parenter Enteral Nutr. 2011;35:16–24.
5. Young AM, Kidston S, Banks MD, Mudge AM, Isenring EA. Malnutrition screening tools: comparison against two validated nutrition assessment methods in older medical patients. Nutrition. 2013;29(1):101–6.
6. Mudge AM, Ross LJ, Young AM, Isenring EA, Banks MD. Helping understanding nutritional gaps in the elderly (HUNGER): a prospective study of patient factors associated with inadequate nutritional intake in older medical inpatients. Clin Nutr. 2011;30(3):320–5.
7. Ross LJ, Mudge AM, Young AM, Banks MD. Everyone's problem but nobody's job: staff perceptions and explanations for poor nutritional intake in older medical patients. Nutr Diet. 2011;68(1):41–6.
8. Naithani S, Whelan K, Thomas J, Gulliford MC, Morgan M. Hospital inpatients' experiences of access to food: a qualitative interview and observational study. Health Expect. 2008;11(3):294–303.

An Approach to Hyponatraemia

Krita Sridharan and Laila Rotstein

1 Clinical Pearl

Consider low solute intake as a cause for hyponatraemia, especially in elderly patients.

2 Clinical Case

A 92-year-old female from home alone presents with confusion. Blood tests demonstrate a sodium of 121 mmol/L (normal 135–145 mmol/L). On examination she is euvolaemic. There is no other demonstrable cause for her delirium. Her only regular medications are aspirin 100 mg daily and atorvastatin 20 mg daily.

Further results are listed below:

Serum potassium 4.5 mmol/L (normal 3.5–5.2 mmol/L)

Serum bicarbonate 28 mmol/L (normal 22–32 mmol/L)

Serum glucose **8.1** mmol/L (normal 4–7.7 mmol/L)

Serum urea 7.4 mmol/L (normal 3–8 mmol/L)

Serum osmolality **255** mOsmol/kg (normal 280–300 mOsmol/kg)

Urine sodium **<20** mmol/L (normal 40–220 mmol/day)

Urine osmolality 90 mOsmol/kg (normal 50–1200 mOsmol/kg)

Serum creatinine 78 micromol/L (normal 50–110 micromol/L)

eGFR **58** mL/min (normal ≥90 mL/min/1.73 m^2)

The differential diagnosis based on history, examination, and the investigations, in particular the low urine osmolality, is psychogenic polydipsia or low-solute hyponatraemia. Given her age and living circumstances a provisional diagnosis of low

K. Sridharan (✉) · L. Rotstein
Alfred Health and Monash University, Melbourne, VIC, Australia

R. Junckerstorff et al. (eds.), *Beyond Evidence-Based Medicine*,
https://doi.org/10.1007/978-981-99-4440-8_8

solute hyponatraemia is made and she receives 1 litre (L) of 0.9% sodium chloride over 12 hours. Following this and commencement of a normal diet she has a large volume diuresis of approximately 3 L. Repeat serum sodium level 12 hours later is 128 mmol/L. Over the next few days, she is managed with judicious fluid and solute replacement aiming for a slow increment in sodium to avoid osmotic demyelination syndrome. The patient's delirium resolves. On further history it is revealed that she had been experiencing very poor appetite over the previous weeks but had been careful to maintain her water intake. Her diet consisted of one to two pieces of dry toast, one cup of tea, and 3 L of water per day. There was no history of alcohol intake. This confirmed the provisional diagnosis of low solute hyponatraemia.

3 Discussion

The cause for hyponatraemia can be difficult to delineate and requires a careful history, a thorough assessment of fluid status and measurement of serum urea, electrolytes and osmolality in addition to urine sodium and urine osmolality. The following steps are useful in working through the possible diagnoses. Some cases of hyponatraemia are, however, complex and multifactorial.

Step 1: Exclusion of pseudo-hyponatraemia as per Fig. 1.

Step 2: A thorough history is important, considering their age and social circumstances. Current symptoms and approximate duration of symptoms are useful, to determine if the hyponatremia is acute or chronic (≥48 hour duration) [1]. Hyponatraemia associated with long-distance running should be evident from the history. Other symptoms that are important to identify include diarrhoea, vomiting, neurological symptoms (delirium, seizures) and neurological events. A medication

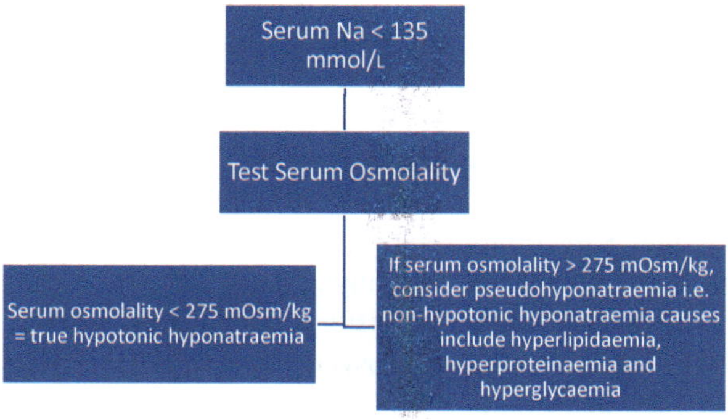

Fig. 1 Pseudohyponatremia can be excluded biochemically by measurement of serum glucose, lipids (the lab may report lipaemic serum) and proteins. It can also be excluded by measurement of serum osmolality. Only hypo-osmolar hyponatraemia (<275 mOsm/kg) is "true hyponatraemia" [1]. Correction for hyperglycaemia can be done with the following formula: measured sodium +0.024 × (Serum glucose in mg/dL—100) [2]. Serum osmolality can be calculated by the following equation: 2 × serum Na + serum glucose + serum urea

history should be taken, with particular focus on the use of thiazide diuretics and drugs associated with increase in anti-diuretic hormone (ADH) e.g., carbamazepine. The current oral (solute) and fluid intake is essential information, as is a history of cardiac, renal or liver disease.

Step 3: A thorough assessment of fluid status and urine sodium measurements will help guide the differential diagnosis as per Fig. 2.

Step 4: For assessment of the euvolaemic and hyponatraemic patient, measure the urine osmolality and interpret according to Fig. 3.

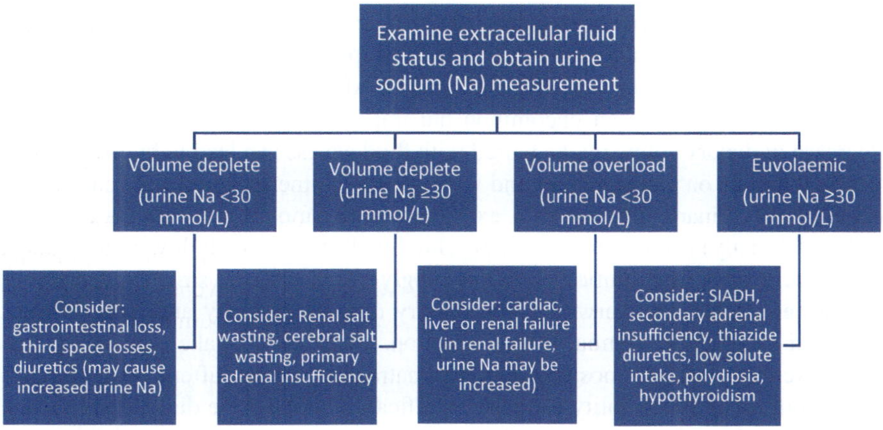

Fig. 2 SIADH: Syndrome of inappropriate antidiuretic hormone ADH release. Note that urine sodium may vary, particularly in patients with multi-factorial hyponatraemia. Diuretic use may be accompanied by euvolaemia, volume depletion or fluid overload and urine sodium may not be interpretable in the setting of diuretic use. Urine sodium is not always interpretable in the presence of severe vomiting due to alkalosis [3]. Low solute intake and polydipsia may be accompanied by low urine sodium [4]. Note that low urine sodium in the presence of low effective circulatory volume occurs in both hypovolaemic and hypervolaemic states (e.g., cardiac failure), due to sodium retention [4]

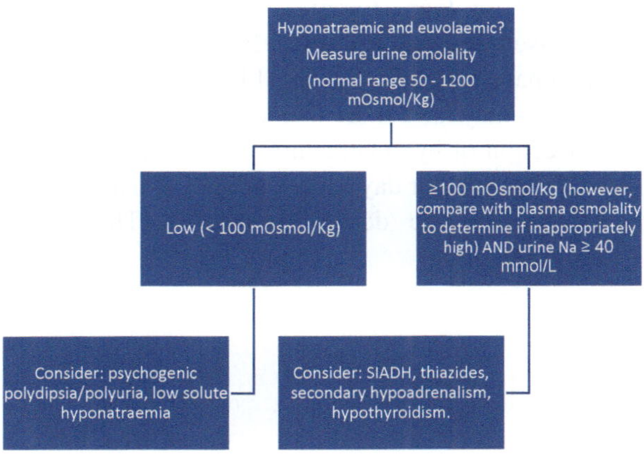

Fig. 3 Urine osmolality <100 mOsmol/Kg suggests suppression of ADH activity [4]. Most cases of hyponatraemia are associated with sustained action of ADH. An exception to this rule is psychogenic polydipsia/polyuria and low solute hyponatraemia where ADH is appropriately suppressed

When considering hyponatraemia, it is important to remember the stimuli for ADH release. The main stimulus for ADH release is high serum osmolality. Hypotension & hypovolaemia also stimulate ADH release through the renin, angiotensin, aldosterone system (RAAS), which overrides osmotic changes. The RAAS responds to true hypovolaemia as well as states of hypervolaemia where tissue perfusion is reduced because of low effective arterial blood volume (despite a state of extracellular fluid accumulation, e.g., heart failure or liver cirrhosis). This explains hyponatraemia during fluid depletion and in heart or liver failure.

Pain, nausea and stress are also stimuli for ADH release, and may contribute to hyponatraemia in the post-operative setting [4]. It is important in this setting to treat the nausea and pain driving the elevation in ADH. Some drugs can also stimulate ADH - examples include carbamazepine, cyclophosphamide and some selective serotonin uptake inhibitors [5]. Alcohol inhibits ADH release [6].

Low-solute intake is an uncommon but important cause of hyponatraemia. A decrease in dietary solute intake paired with fluid excess can lead to hyponatraemia [7]. Individuals on a normal diet and with normal glomerular function have a high capacity for urinary dilution with extremely high amounts of free water intake (~20–25 L daily) [7] required to overwhelm this. With extremely low solute intake, the capacity for urine dilution correspondingly decreases, and smaller amounts of free water intake can overwhelm the urinary dilution capacity and lead to water retention and hyponatraemia. In this situation, once solute intake is restored, free water excretion becomes possible, and hyponatraemia corrects after a brisk diuresis. Urine sodium and osmolality can vary significantly making the diagnosis, in some cases, difficult, which emphasises the importance of a thorough history [8].

4 Other Gems

- While thiazide diuretics commonly cause hyponatraemia, frusemide is an infrequent cause. This is due to their modes of action on different components of the renal tubule.
- Patients on loop diuretics may present with hypernatraemia secondary to increased free water loss [9]. Patients on thiazides who develop hyponatraemia often have a high fluid intake [4].
- Patients may have more than one co-existing cause for hyponatraemia.
- Correction of hyponatraemia, regardless of the cause, must not be greater than 8–10 mmol/L per day and reduced to 4–6 mmol/L per day in patients with a high risk of osmotic demyelination [4]. This is particularly true in chronic hyponatraemia.

References

1. Sahay M, Sahay R. Hyponatremia: a practical approach. Indian J Endocrinol Metab. 2014;18(6):760–71. https://doi.org/10.4103/2230-8210.141320. PMID: 25364669; PMCID: PMC4192979.
2. Hillier TA, Abbott RD, Barrett EJ. Hyponatremia: evaluating the correction factor for hyperglycemia. Am J Med. 1999;106(4):399–403. https://doi.org/10.1016/s0002-9343(99)00055-8. PMID: 10225241.
3. Palmer BF, Clegg DJ. The use of selected urine chemistries in the diagnosis of kidney disorders. Clin J Am Soc Nephrol. 2019;14(2):306–16. https://doi.org/10.2215/CJN.10330818. Epub 2019 Jan 9. Erratum in: Clin J Am Soc Nephrol 2019 Aug 7;14(8):1241. PMID: 30626576; PMCID: PMC6390907.
4. Hoorn EJ, Zietse R. Diagnosis and treatment of hyponatremia: compilation of the guidelines. J Am Soc Nephrol. 2017;28(5):1340–9. https://doi.org/10.1681/ASN.2016101139. Epub 2017 Feb 7. PMID: 28174217; PMCID: PMC5407738.
5. Yasir M, Mechanic OJ. Syndrome of inappropriate antidiuretic hormone secretion. [Updated 2022 May 9]. In: StatPearls [Internet]. Treasure Island, FL: StatPearls Publishing; 2022. Available from: https://www.ncbi.nlm.nih.gov/books/NBK507777/.
6. Epstein M. Alcohol's impact on kidney function. Alcohol Health Res World. 1997;21(1):84–92. PMID: 15706766; PMCID: PMC6826793.
7. Thaler SM, Teitelbaum I, Berl T. "Beer potomania" in non-beer drinkers: effect of low dietary solute intake. Am J Kidney Dis. 1998;31:1028–31.
8. Sanghvi SR, Kellerman PS, Nanovic L. Beer potomania: an unusual cause of hyponatremia at high risk of complications from rapid correction. Am J Kidney Dis. 2007;50:673–80.
9. Liamis G, Milionis HJ, Elisaf M. A review of drug-induced hypernatraemia. NDT Plus. 2009;2(5):339–46. https://doi.org/10.1093/ndtplus/sfp085. Epub 2009 Jul 16. PMID: 25949338; PMCID: PMC4421386.

Part II
Geriatric Medicine

Acopia Is Not a Diagnosis

Emma Hack and Benny Katz

1 Clinical Pearl

Terms such as acopia should not be used. This language implies fault, rather than focusing on the underlying medical and social issues.

2 Clinical Case

A 76-year-old woman was discharged home from the rehabilitation ward following a stroke. Her son was adamant that his mother would not go into a nursing home and quit his job to become her full-time carer. Four weeks later, she arrived in the emergency department with a note from the General Practitioner stating that her son was unable to provide care and requesting admission.

The patient was admitted to hospital with a diagnosis of 'acopia' and referred to the social work department for nursing home admission. The social worker contacted the son who explained that he was coping very well with providing care for his mother but had been called away urgently to provide care for his two infant grandchildren after their mother was injured in a motor vehicle accident. He expected to be able to resume care of his mother after the children's father returned

E. Hack
Department of Geriatric Medicine, St. Vincent's Hospital Melbourne, Fitzroy, VIC, Australia

B. Katz (✉)
Department of Geriatric Medicine, St. Vincent's Hospital Melbourne, Fitzroy, VIC, Australia

Faculty of Medicine, Dentistry and Health Sciences, University of Melbourne, Parkville, VIC, Australia

R. Junckerstorff et al. (eds.), *Beyond Evidence-Based Medicine*,
https://doi.org/10.1007/978-981-99-4440-8_9

home from an overseas business trip in 2 days. The son was apologetic but said that he was unable to arrange urgent respite and following discussion with the General Practitioner, was left with no other option but to send his mother to the Emergency Department.

The patient returned home to her son's care on the third day. Upon seeing the term 'acopia' in the discharge summary, the son lodged a formal complaint to the hospital.

3 Discussion

The term 'acopia' is pejorative and lacks any definition or diagnostic value. The word is ageist and inherently prejudicial, with most of those receiving the label being over the age of 65 years [1]. Other similarly unhelpful labels include 'social admission' and 'bed-blocker' [2]. None of these terms are acceptable as a principal coding diagnosis.

Most people do not want to be in hospital or have their loved ones in hospital. In this case, the admitting doctor had described this as 'acopia' without exploring the facts. The son appeared to be coping very well with his mother's care needs and it was not until he was placed in an impossible situation that he could not continue her care. He should have been offered support and understanding, rather than implying that he was to blame for the admission.

Older people represent the core of hospital admissions, and many are frail and multimorbid. While this case could be described as relating to a social crisis, the clinician should be wary of applying labels that discourage exploration for treatable medical pathology [3]. All patients presenting to hospital should have thorough history, examination and investigation as clinically indicated. Failure to recognise reversible factors may lead to compromised care and poor outcomes [4].

Social issues may co-exist with any hospital admission of any age and background. Caregivers should not be criticised when there are changes in circumstances beyond their control, that result in an inability to provide this care, whether temporary or permanent.

The social worker provided the son with a list of options in the event that urgent respite is required again in the future, however the reality is that the best laid plans do not always work, especially when options are not available when needed.

4 Other Gems

- Avoid unhelpful terminology in the elderly, including ‘acopia’.
  - These terms delegitimise the reason for presenting to hospital, and place blame on the patient and caregiver.
- The clinician should be wary when such terms are seen in documentation, and be vigilant to exclude underlying factors that led to presentation.
  - Ensure all patients undergo a thorough clinical history and examination.
- Don’t be afraid to revisit documentation.
  - Enquire further if a diagnosis seems inaccurate.

References

1. Kee YK, Rippingale C. The prevalence and characteristic of patients with ‘acopia’. Age Ageing. 2009;38(1):103–5.
2. Oliver D. ‘Acopia’ and ‘social admission’ are not diagnoses: why older people deserve better. J R Soc Med. 2008;101(4):168–74.
3. Obeid JL, Ogle SJ. Acopia: a useful term or not? Australas J Ageing. 2000;19(4):195–8.
4. Hodges Z. Diagnosis of “acopia”: prescription for neglect? J Adult Protect. 2021;23(3):191–8.

Observation of Gait in the Older Adult

Nicholas J. Radcliffe and Benny Katz

1 Clinical Pearl

You haven't finished your physical examination until you have observed an older person walk.

2 Clinical Case

A 77-year-old man was reviewed in the hospital Cardiology clinic for aortic stenosis after several recent falls. The cardiologist determined that his valvular pathology was mild, requiring serial surveillance only, and that his falls had been non-syncopal with no injuries to date. The cardiologist requested their accompanying junior doctor to complete the rest of the physical examination.

The junior doctor enthusiastically repeated a bedside cardiac examination with only a soft ejection systolic murmur identified. Having recently completed a Geriatric Medicine term, then proceeded with an assessment of gait by asking the patient to stand from the chair, walk three metres, turn, walk back, and sit down again. The patient was encouraged to use his usual gait aid for the task.

N. J. Radcliffe
Department of Geriatric Medicine, Monash Health, Clayton, VIC, Australia

Monash University, Melbourne, VIC, Australia

Victorian Geriatric Medicine Training Program, Melbourne, VIC, Australia

B. Katz (✉)
Victorian Geriatric Medicine Training Program, Melbourne, VIC, Australia

Department of Geriatric Medicine, St Vincent's Hospital Melbourne, Fitzroy, VIC, Australia

University of Melbourne, Melbourne, VIC, Australia

R. Junckerstorff et al. (eds.), *Beyond Evidence-Based Medicine*,
https://doi.org/10.1007/978-981-99-4440-8_10

The doctor observed multiple abnormalities. The patient was frail and relied on the armrests to rise from a seated position. His movements were slow. He appeared unsteady standing with his single point stick. He walked with short strides and had a reduced arm-swing. This prompted the junior doctor to perform a further neurological examination. There were clear signs of Parkinsonism, with bilateral rigidity but no clear bradykinesia or tremor. The patient was considered to be at risk of further falls.

Reviewing the medical history, the junior doctor noted the patient was on risperidone for schizoaffective disorder and night-time diazepam for insomnia. He consumed approximately one bottle of scotch per week.

The junior doctor dictated a letter to the patient's general practitioner with a copy to his psychiatrist, noting the need to address deconditioning, frailty, choice of gait aid, potential drug-induced Parkinsonism and multiple medications and alcohol contributing to poor balance. Finally, a referral was made to the local Falls and Balance Clinic.

3 Discussion

Gait assessment in the older adult is not overtly onerous nor time consuming and can reveal a wealth of useful information. Whilst further insights may be gained from other specialised tests [1], this should not dissuade from a basic gait observation. All the clinical information identified in this Clinical Case would have helped to prompt meaningful changes to patient management irrespective of the fact that falls were known to be already occurring. Therefore, aim to observe gait in **every** older adult as part of the clinical examination.

Further workup of the older adult with falls is discussed in chapter 12, "Do not use the term mechanical fall".

4 Other Gems

- Frailty is associated with increased risk of falls, hospitalisation, worse outcomes and mortality [2], but may also respond to exercise and/or nutritional-based interventions.
- Observing the patient walk may trigger further evaluation, investigation, or changes in management.
- Look carefully at the whole body including overall pace, use of assistance devices (chair arms, gait aid), stride length, arm swing, turning characteristics, any interruptions, overall balance, and how obstacles are negotiated.

References

1. Barry E, Galvin R, Keogh C, et al. Is the Timed Up and Go test a useful predictor of risk of falls in community dwelling older adults: a systematic review and meta- analysis. BMC Geriatr. 2014;14:14. https://doi.org/10.1186/1471-2318-14-14.
2. Clinical Frailty Scale. https://www.dal.ca/sites/gmr/our-tools/clinical-frailty-scale.html.

Decision-Making Capacity

Nicholas Voon and Benny Katz

1 Clinical Pearl

A strong preference does not always confirm decision-making capacity.

2 Clinical Case

An 82-year-old man with rheumatoid arthritis is admitted to hospital with community acquired pneumonia. On the evening of the third day of admission, he packs his bag and tells his nurse that he is going home. As the doctor covering the evening shift you are asked to see him.

During the first few days following admission he was quiet and drowsy, mainly resting in bed and sleeping during the day. Tonight, he has been restless, pacing the ward and demanding to go home.

He is adamant that he wants to leave the hospital immediately and is not prepared to wait until the morning to speak with his treating doctors.

There is a clinical suspicion that he has a fluctuating delirium. Does he have the capacity to make the decision to leave hospital, or does this indicate impaired decision-making capacity? Should we respect his preference? What is our duty of care?

N. Voon
Department of Geriatric Medicine, Western Health, St Albans, VIC, Australia

B. Katz (✉)
Department of Geriatric Medicine, St. Vincent's Hospital Melbourne, Fitzroy, VIC, Australia

Faculty of Medicine, Dentistry and Health Sciences, University of Melbourne, Melbourne, VIC, Australia

R. Junckerstorff et al. (eds.), *Beyond Evidence-Based Medicine*,
https://doi.org/10.1007/978-981-99-4440-8_11

You assess him. He cannot tell you how he will get home, he does not have a key to the house, and does not acknowledge any risks associated with early hospital discharge. You consider that he does not have decision-making capacity, and as returning home at night would place him at risk, you escort him back into his room with a security guard.

Two hours later, you are informed that he has absconded from hospital. Following hospital procedures, the police are notified to undertake a welfare check. When they arrive at his home the following morning he appears to be managing well and there is no reason to coerce him back to hospital. His family doctor agrees to keep an eye on him. One week later, he appears back to his normal self.

3 Discussion

The patient has demonstrated an ability to express his preference. Does this mean that he has the capacity to make a decision, even if it is a bad one? According to Australian law, anyone aged 18 and over is presumed to have decision-making capacity unless there is evidence to the contrary. If we suspect that he has impaired decision-making capacity and that letting him go home would place him at risk, we have a duty of care to him. He does not have to prove that he retains capacity but rather it is up to the person questioning his capacity to demonstrate the loss of capacity.

Each of us make many decisions every single day. We constantly consciously or subconsciously weigh up options to make decisions. What to eat for lunch. What to wear. Whether to have another drink before driving home. The ability to select an option or express a preference does not prove the person has decision-making capacity. It simply means the person has made a decision – good, bad or otherwise. Making a "good decision" does not prove capacity and making a "bad decision" does not prove loss of capacity. Likewise, if our gentleman has agreed to remain in hospital, this would not equate with proof of capacity.

Capacity assessment includes four key components: understanding of the relevant issues, ability to retain information to make a decision, ability to weigh up the risks and benefits of the options as part of making the decision and the ability to communicate opinions and decisions made whether by speech or other ways. To be deemed to have capacity, an individual needs to meet all four criteria [1]. The fact that he could not recognise any potential risk, nor accept what he was being told about the risk, indicated loss of decision-making capacity.

Although his return home went smoothly, this does not mean that he has decision-making capacity. There are many people managing at home who have impaired decision-making capacity. Often no action needs to be taken unless a significant decision needs to be made, in which case a surrogate decision maker, such as a guardian or administrator, may need to be appointed. Had the police welfare check found that he was not managing and at immediate risk of harm, but still insisting to remain at home, then application for an urgent guardianship order would be considered. The need for intervention is not based on whether a person has decision-making capacity or not, but whether a decision needs to be made. Additionally, capacity is specific to a particular decision and a lack of capacity may be temporary such as due to illness.

4 Other Gems

- Capacity assessment is not always easy. If in doubt seek support of a neuropsychologist, geriatrician or psychiatrist.
- Capacity is actually a legal status, rather than a medical one. Hospitals have legal counsel to assist with complex cases.

References

1. "Can your adult patient consent? (Flowchart)"—Office of the Public Advocate. https://www.publicadvocate.vic.gov.au/resource/file?id=80.

Do Not Use the Term "Mechanical" Fall

Nicholas J. Radcliffe and Benny Katz

1 Clinical Pearl

> The term "mechanical" fall is not a diagnosis and should be avoided. It fails to identify the factors that contributed to the older person falling, and in particular the treatable factors.

2 Clinical Case

An 83-year-old lady presented to the Emergency Department (ED) with her concerned daughter for assessment after a fall. She explained that she was not using her walking stick and slipped on some wet tiles in her bathroom. As she was unable to get off the floor, an ambulance was called. In the ED, serious injury and syncope were excluded and a diagnosis of mechanical fall was made. The Geriatric Medical Registrar was asked to assess whether she was safe to go home or needed admission to hospital.

Multiple factors that had contributed to the fall were identified. The precipitating event was a combination of risk-taking behaviours and environmental factors. These included not using her walking stick, entering the bathroom with the lights off, wet

N. J. Radcliffe
Department of Geriatric Medicine, Monash Health, Clayton, VIC, Australia

Monash University, Melbourne, VIC, Australia

Victorian Geriatric Medicine Training Program, Melbourne, VIC, Australia

B. Katz (✉)
Victorian Geriatric Medicine Training Program, Melbourne, VIC, Australia

Department of Geriatric Medicine, St Vincent's Hospital Melbourne, Fitzroy, VIC, Australia

University of Melbourne, Melbourne, VIC, Australia

R. Junckerstorff et al. (eds.), *Beyond Evidence-Based Medicine*,
https://doi.org/10.1007/978-981-99-4440-8_12

floor tiles and inappropriate footwear. Intrinsic (patient related) factors included postural hypotension and benzodiazepine use for insomnia. The issues could be addressed without the need for hospital admission.

The Geriatric Medical Registrar recommended several environmental and behavioural changes including more suitable footwear, consistent use of her stick and installation of a night-light in the bathroom. Changes were made to her antihypertensive medication and a weaning plan was negotiated for her benzodiazepine. An exercise program and follow-up were arranged in the hospital Falls and Balance Clinic.

3 Discussion

Falls are amongst the most common presentations to hospital and EDs by older adults in Australia and are the leading cause of unintentional injury in older people [1]. They are associated with increased rates of frailty, loss of independence, admission to residential aged care facility, and mortality.

Using the term "mechanical" fall may lead to a less detailed assessment of patient history [2], and hence missed targets for intervention. It may also imply the main driver of a fall is an external factor. In reality, whilst extrinsic (environmental and high-risk activity) factors and precipitating events may contribute, the main drivers in most older people who have fallen are intrinsic factors. Falls are often the interplay of multiple factors. These include cognition, sensory function, balance, strength, and general health status. This usually becomes obvious when you consider why the patient is falling in scenarios where others have not.

4 Other Gems

- Falls are the leading cause of unintentional injuries in older Australians.
- The strongest predictive factor for a future fall is a past fall.
- The first step in falls workup is to exclude syncope and injuries that require immediate attention; however the work up does not stop here.
- The second step should then be to identify treatable risk factors by using the intrinsic, extrinsic and precipitating event structure (see Table 1).
- Consider harm prevention measures, including screening for osteoporosis and vitamin D deficiency in an older person who falls.
- Medication review is an important component of a falls assessment. Medications commonly associated with falls include benzodiazepines, antipsychotics, antidepressants (including SSRIs, tricyclics), antiepileptics, opioids, diuretics and antihypertensives.
- Ensure that footwear is appropriate.

Table 1 Risk factors for falls

Intrinsic risk factors	Extrinsic risk factors	Precipitating factors
Advanced age	Slippery surfaces	Trips and slips
Gender (female > male)	Unsuitable footwear	Dizziness
Previous falls	Stairs	Medication changes
Muscle weakness/sarcopenia	Environmental hazards or clutter (including rugs, electricity cords, pets)	Acute medical illness
Frailty	Poor lighting	
Orthostatic hypotension	Bifocal lenses	
Psychological factors	Restraints	
Neurological conditions (e.g. strokes, parkinsonism, Meniere's disease, peripheral neuropathy)	High risk activities (e.g. ladders, not using gait aid)	
Cognitive impairment (e.g. Alzheimer's disease)		
Living alone		
Urinary incontinence		
Medications and other toxins (including alcohol)		

- Be vigilant for *fear of falling*. This may lead to decreased physical activity and therefore deconditioning, which ironically increases falls risk. Patients with fear of falling should always be referred for follow-up.
- Options for follow-up include Geriatric Outpatients, Falls and Balance Clinics (where available) and specialist rehabilitation services.

References

1. Falls in older Australians 2019–20: hospitalisations and deaths among people aged 65 and over, About [Internet]. Australian Institute of Health and Welfare. https://www.aihw.gov.au/reports/injury/falls-in-older-australians-2019-20-hospitalisation/contents/about. Accessed 7 Apr 2022.
2. Sri-on J, Tirrell GP, Lipsitz LA, Liu SW. Is there such a thing as a mechanical fall? Am J Emerg Med. 2016;34(3):582–5.

Keep an Open Mind: Assessing Unsteadiness in Older People

Nicole I. Chan, Joseph Tan, and Alison M. Mudge

1 Clinical Pearl

Unsteadiness and falls are common presentations in older people. The clinician needs to have a broad range of differential diagnoses and undertake a comprehensive examination, including gait assessment, as the cause is often multifactorial.

2 Clinical Case

A 74-year-old general practitioner presents to the Emergency Department with 'dizziness' 10 days after percutaneous coronary intervention for a myocardial infarction. His symptoms include light-headedness and a feeling of unsteadiness on his feet. He is admitted under the cardiology team, with his symptoms attributed to likely postural hypotension due to his new beta blocker and ACE-inhibitor therapies. Several days into his admission, after the physiotherapist notes concerns about his safety mobilising, the resident performs a full neurological examination which reveals an ataxic gait and dysmetria. Magnetic resonance imaging demonstrates a cerebellar stroke, likely a peri-procedural complication.

N. I. Chan
Royal Brisbane and Women's Hospital, Metro North Health, Brisbane, QLD, Australia

J. Tan
Surgical Treatment and Rehabilitation Services, Metro North Health, Brisbane, QLD, Australia

A. M. Mudge (✉)
Department of Internal Medicine and Aged Care, Royal Brisbane and Women's Hospital, Metro North Health, Brisbane, QLD, Australia

Medical School, The University of Queensland, Brisbane, QLD, Australia

R. Junckerstorff et al. (eds.), *Beyond Evidence-Based Medicine*,
https://doi.org/10.1007/978-981-99-4440-8_13

3 Discussion

Dizziness or unsteadiness are vague terms often reported by patients which carry a wide differential diagnosis. These terms can encompass a broad range of syndromes including vertigo, pre-syncope, autonomic instability, sarcopenia or myopathies, neuropathies and movement disorders as well as medication side effects [1]. It is important to not fixate too early on a potential diagnosis as other serious pathologies can be missed. While the presenting complaint of dizziness is common in patients of all ages, older adults often have more complex considerations due to the accumulation of comorbidities and associated medications.

The clinician should explore the differential diagnoses with a comprehensive history and a thorough examination, including a full cardiovascular examination with postural blood pressures and a full neurological examination with gait assessment. A thorough history establishing a timeline for the unsteadiness and associated symptoms through detailed systems review is key to determining whether the unsteadiness is likely to be a primary neurological complaint or due to another system (e.g. pre-syncope due to volume depletion, cardiac outlet obstruction such as aortic stenosis or vasodilatation due to sepsis). A complete neurological examination should include higher functions (including dyspraxia or executive dysfunction, important for planning movements), cranial nerves (including evidence of nystagmus, central ataxia or weakness) and careful lower limb examination including gait assessment (looking for evidence of incoordination, rigidity, tremor, weakness or sensory impairment). Assessing a patient's mobility not only allows the clinician to evaluate gait and functional status but also helps them to provide the patient with permission and encouragement to maintain mobility on the ward. Physiotherapy involvement can assist the clinician in describing the presenting syndrome and in advising approaches to support safe mobilisation.

4 Other Gems

- It is important to assess patients with their usual mobility aids as this allows a more reliable assessment of their physical ability.
- Having the correct mobility aid available at the patient's bedside helps patients to keep mobile. Extended bedrest detrimentally affects muscle mass and leads to hospital-associated disability. In healthy older adults, it has been shown that 7 days of bedrest results in 1.6 kg loss in lean muscle mass [2]. When this is combined with the catabolic effects of a patient's illness and extended hospital stay, this muscle mass loss can be profound, and 30–40% of older people leave hospital with poorer functional independence than baseline [3].

References

1. Kroenke K, Lucas CA, Rosenberg ML, Scherokman B, Herbers JE Jr, Wehrle PA, et al. Causes of persistent dizziness. A prospective study of 100 patients in ambulatory care. Ann Intern Med. 1992;117(11):898–904.
2. Giogio Di Girolamo F, Fiotti N, Milanovic Z, Situlin R, Mearelli F, Vinci P, et al. The aging muscle in experimental bed rest: a systematic review and meta-analysis. Front Nutr. 2021;8:633987.
3. Loyd C, Markland AD, Zhang Y, Fowler M, Harper S, Wright NC, et al. Prevalence of hospital-associated disability in older adults: a meta-analysis. J Am Dir Assoc. 2020;21(4):455–61.

Right Time and Place: Cognitive Testing in Hospital

Nicole I. Chan, Joseph Tan, and Alison M. Mudge

1 Clinical Pearl

Recognising cognitive impairment in hospital is important for communication, preventive care and discharge planning. The setting, timing and appropriate test selection are important for accurate assessment, as a diagnosis of dementia will have lasting implications for the patient.

2 Clinical Case

A 68-year-old retired truck driver is transferred to the geriatric rehabilitation ward after a prolonged hospital admission for pneumonia. His background includes hearing impairment and chronic obstructive pulmonary disease. He lives alone and independently in the community, with no family nearby. His daughter, attending from interstate, notes that he seems distracted and sometimes their conversations do not make sense, while nursing staff note that he seems withdrawn. The clinical team perform cognitive testing using the Mini Mental State Examination and this reveals

N. I. Chan
Royal Brisbane and Women's Hospital, Metro North Health, Brisbane, QLD, Australia

J. Tan
Surgical Treatment and Rehabilitation Services, Metro North Health, Brisbane, QLD, Australia

A. M. Mudge (✉)
Department of Internal Medicine and Aged Care, Royal Brisbane and Women's Hospital, Metro North Health, Brisbane, QLD, Australia

Medical School, The University of Queensland, Brisbane, QLD, Australia

R. Junckerstorff et al. (eds.), *Beyond Evidence-Based Medicine*,
https://doi.org/10.1007/978-981-99-4440-8_14

multiple errors. His daughter starts to investigate possibilities for residential aged care closer to her home.

The speech pathologist notes that the patient seems to be hearing poorly despite wearing hearing aids and it is discovered that his hearing aids are not working. Cognitive testing is repeated using a simple assisted listening device. The test score is much better, and the patient interacts and participates more actively in his rehabilitation using the listening device. He is discharged home with domestic services, obtains new hearing aids, and continues to actively participate in an outpatient pulmonary rehabilitation group.

3 Discussion

It is common for the older patient to receive a cognitive screen whilst admitted in hospital, as cognition is a vital part of independent functioning. However, the diagnosis of cognitive impairment can have serious and lasting consequences for the older patient and the setting and timing of the cognitive screen should be considered carefully. The clinician should take time to optimise the patient's circumstances prior to performing any cognitive assessment or the patient's baseline function can be misjudged, which could lead to inappropriate discharge planning and perpetuate stereotyping in the older population. Assessments should be undertaken in a well-lit area with background noise minimised. Sensory aids, such as hearing aids and spectacles, should always be in place for testing, but as this case shows, it is important to be confident that they are functioning.

Timing and selection of testing is also important, and consideration of the patient's current clinical status is crucial. Delirium is very common in acute medical and surgical conditions and is under-recognised by clinical staff if formal screening and testing procedures are not in place [1]. Brief screening can be undertaken by any health professional using the 4AT which does not require specific training [2], while slightly longer tools such as the 3D-CAM are more suitable for confirming the diagnosis and rely on brief cognitive questions focussed on attention and orientation accompanied by structured behavioural observations to identify the key diagnostic features [3]. Delirium will result in temporary under-performance on cognitive assessment so it is often appropriate to delay formal cognitive assessment until a patient is stable, often in the outpatient setting. Assessing a patient for dementia during an acute medical illness can lead to inaccurate findings and result in inappropriate referrals or diagnoses [4, 5].

4 Other Gems

- Tests such as the Mini-Mental State Examination (MMSE), Montreal Cognitive Assessment (MoCA) and Addenbrooke's Cognitive Examination–Revised (ACE-R) are cognitive *screens*. To make a diagnosis of dementia, these results must be interpreted in the context of the patient's education, cultural background, clinical condition and a careful collateral history.
- Hearing and listening can be difficult for people even with mild hearing impairment in a hospital setting, where there is substantial background noise. This is especially challenging when healthcare staff are all wearing masks, which muffles speech and reduces the visual cues of lip reading. This adds to patient fatigue and may lead to misunderstanding and/or disengagement with care.
- Check whether a hearing aid is working by cupping your hand around the aid and ear-mould: you should hear a squealing or whistling noise from feedback if it is working. If not, you may need to change the batteries and/or remove any build-up of wax or other material using a tissue.

References

1. Ritter SRF, Cardoso AF, Lins MMP, Zoccoli TLV, Freitas MPD, Camargos EF. Underdiagnosis of delirium in the elderly in acute care hospital settings: lessons not learned. Psychogeriatrics. 2018;18(4):268–75.
2. https://www.the4at.com/. Accessed 24 Nov 2022.
3. Marcantonio ER, Ngo LH, O'Connor M, Jones RN, Crane PK, Metzger ED, et al. 3D-CAM: derivation and validation of a 3-minute diagnostic interview for CAM-defined delirium. Ann Intern Med. 2014;161(8):554–61.
4. Shenkin S, Russ T, Ryan TM, MacLullich A. Screening for dementia and other causes of cognitive impairment in general hospital in-patients. Age Ageing. 2013;43(2):166–8.
5. Phelps A, Kingston B, Wharton RM, Pendlebury ST. Routine screening in the general hospital: what happens after discharge to those identified as at risk of dementia? Clin Med. 2017;17(5):395–400.

First Do No Harm: Beware the Prescribing Cascade

Nicole I. Chan, Joseph Tan, and Alison M. Mudge

1 Clinical Pearl

Polypharmacy is common in older adults and contributes to medication errors, adverse drug events and/or non-compliance. Considering whether new symptoms may be adverse drug events can avoid harmful 'prescribing cascades'. Regular medication review with careful consideration of harms and benefits can reduce medication harm.

2 Clinical Case

A 90-year-old retired schoolteacher is admitted to hospital after a fall at home complicated by acute kidney injury. She describes several months of increasing dizziness, most commonly when standing up after breakfast, and mild nausea without vomiting or change in bowel habit. She also describes stiffness and pain in her left knee which makes her gait unsteady. Medical history includes hypertension and osteoarthritis of the knees, with a right knee replacement 4 years ago complicated by pulmonary embolism. She visits her local GP practice 6 monthly for a 'check-up' and renewed prescriptions. Clinical assessment shows mild dehydration and blood pressure of

N. I. Chan
Royal Brisbane and Women's Hospital, Metro North Health, Brisbane, QLD, Australia

J. Tan
Surgical Treatment and Rehabilitation Services, Metro North Health, Brisbane, QLD, Australia

A. M. Mudge (✉)
Department of Internal Medicine and Aged Care, Royal Brisbane and Women's Hospital, Metro North Health, Brisbane, QLD, Australia

Medical School, The University of Queensland, Brisbane, QLD, Australia

R. Junckerstorff et al. (eds.), *Beyond Evidence-Based Medicine*,
https://doi.org/10.1007/978-981-99-4440-8_15

Table 1 The patient's medications and their clinical indications

Medication	Indication
Aspirin 100 mg mane	Primary prevention of cardiovascular disease
Rosuvastatin 40 mg mane	Primary prevention of cardiovascular disease
Rivaroxaban 20 mg nocte	Pulmonary embolism
Ramipril 5 mg mane	Hypertension
Oxycodone 5 mg tds	Osteoarthritis of knee
Amitriptyline 75 mg nocte	Sleep
Pantoprazole 40 mg nocte	Gastroesophageal reflux
Magnesium 2 tablets bd	Hypomagnesemia
Ergocalciferol 25 μg daily	Vitamin D deficiency
Coloxyl and Senna as required	Constipation
Prochlorperazine as required	PRN for dizziness

145/85 mmHg lying and 125/70 mmHg standing with no evidence of active bleeding. She has limitation to flexion and extension in her left knee with crepitus but no synovial swelling or effusion. Investigations show an acute kidney injury and normal haemoglobin and X-ray of the knee is consistent with osteoarthritis.

She has difficulty recalling all her medications and their indications, and admits that she sometimes gets them mixed up. The junior doctor liaises with the hospital and community pharmacists to compile a current list (Table 1). The treating team commences regular paracetamol and ceases her oxycodone, and the physiotherapist teaches her to use a single point stick to reduce the load on her left knee. Ramipril is withheld and her renal function and postural drop improve with intravenous fluids. All other medications are ceased and her nausea and oral intake improve. She is discharged on slow-release paracetamol only, and the medication changes are discussed with her general practitioner.

3 Discussion

Medication optimisation is a skill that is often overlooked. It requires not only clinical judgement but also a good understanding of the patient's medical history and circumstances, and often requires the treating medical team to review records and gain collateral information, often in collaboration with pharmacists. Polypharmacy is very common in older patients and often reflects a 'prescribing cascade' whereby the first drug prescribed causes adverse effects which leads to prescribing a second drug to treat those effects [1, 2]. In this case, the aspirin likely contributed to gastroesophageal reflux and nausea treated with a proton pump inhibitor, in turn leading to hypomagnesaemia requiring magnesium replacement. Similarly, the anti-hypertensive and anti-cholinergic medications resulted in dizziness, treated inappropriately with prochlorperazine, which in turn may have perpetuated her nausea.

Medications commenced in hospital for an acute but temporary indication are often inadvertently continued in the community. Examples of this include oral anticoagulants for provoked venous thromboembolism, opiates for postoperative pain relief, and antipsychotics prescribed for agitated delirium. If a clear post-discharge plan is not provided by the hospital team, the general practitioner may be reluctant to cease medications started by a specialist team and may continue medications ceased in hospital.

In older patients, medications prescribed for primary prevention should be reviewed to consider the risks versus benefits. This includes medications such as aspirin and statins which are prescribed for prevention of cardiovascular disease [3]. Current guidelines now do not recommend the use of aspirin for primary prevention in adults over the age of 70 years old as the risk of bleeding often outweighs cardiovascular benefits [4]. These medications should be carefully reviewed, and the benefits and risks should be discussed with patients.

4 Other Gems

- The dose of stable long-term medications such as antihypertensive medications may need revising in older age, as loss of fat mass and body water and reduced hepatic and renal function can lead to changes in volume of distribution and clearance [5].
- Recommended therapeutic targets for blood pressure and blood glucose are individualised and often more relaxed in older people with multimorbidity, where the risks of hypotension and hypoglycaemia may outweigh the risk of long-term cardiovascular benefits.
- For patients who are on multiple medications or who have difficulty with medication adherence, Webster packing may help to reduce omissions or duplication of therapies. Liaise with the team pharmacist early to facilitate this.

References

1. Kalisch LM, Caughey GE, Roughead EE, Gilbert AL. The prescribing cascade. Aust Prescr. 2011;34(6):162–6.
2. Ponte ML, Wachs L, Wachs A, Serra HA. Prescribing cascade. A proposed new way to evaluate it. Medicina. 2017;77(1):13–6.
3. Montgomery S, Miedema MD, Dodson JA. Aspirin and statin therapy for primary prevention of cardiovascular disease in older adults. Heart. 2022;108(14):1090–7.
4. Saad M, Abdelaziz HK, Mehta JL. Aspirin for primary prevention in the elderly. Aging (Albany, NY). 2019;11(17):6618–9.
5. Mangoni AA, Jackson SH. Age-related changes in pharmacokinetics and pharmacodynamics: basic principles and practical applications. Br J Clin Pharmacol. 2004;57(1):6–14.

A Delicate Balance: Weighing Risks and Benefits in Frail Patients

Joseph Tan, Nicole I. Chan, and Alison M. Mudge

1 Clinical Pearl

Balancing the benefits and risks of therapies can be challenging, especially in older people with multimorbidity and frailty. Prediction tools can be valuable to inform discussions but must be integrated with individual preferences.

2 Clinical Case

An 85-year-old retired piano teacher is admitted to the geriatric ward with acute confusion and a fall. Her past medical history includes hypertension, dyslipidaemia, stable angina, chronic kidney disease stage IV, osteoarthritis in her hips which limits her mobility, and mild cognitive impairment. She lives with her daughter and reports several falls over the last 6-months despite using a 4-wheel walker. She manages her own medications using a Webster pack and receives assistance from domiciliary nurses for showering three times a week. Clinical assessment shows a moderately frail lady with hypoactive delirium. Admission ECG documents atrial fibrillation

J. Tan
Surgical Treatment and Rehabilitation Services, Metro North Health, Brisbane, QLD, Australia

N. I. Chan
Royal Brisbane and Women's Hospital, Metro North Health, Brisbane, QLD, Australia

A. M. Mudge (✉)
Department of Internal Medicine and Aged Care, Royal Brisbane and Women's Hospital, Metro North Health, Brisbane, QLD, Australia

Medical School, The University of Queensland, Brisbane, QLD, Australia

R. Junckerstorff et al. (eds.), *Beyond Evidence-Based Medicine*,
https://doi.org/10.1007/978-981-99-4440-8_16

with controlled ventricular response at 85 beats per minute. A non-contrast CT of her brain shows mild to moderate generalised atrophy with some evidence of cerebrovascular disease but no stroke. A urine microscopy and culture shows *Escherichia coli* and her delirium resolves after antibiotic therapy, but her atrial fibrillation persists.

In weighing up her risk of a future cerebrovascular event, the treating team calculate an elevated CHA2DS2VAsc score of 5. Her risk of bleeding using the HAS-BLED score is also elevated at 3. They discuss the risks of anticoagulation with the patient and her daughter, who are anxious both about the risk of stroke and of sustaining injuries when she falls, which could each compromise her mobility further. They also have concerns about increasing the complexity of her medical care with warfarin monitoring. After some discussion with the patient's other daughter, they decide to commence apixaban.

3 Discussion

Atrial fibrillation is a major risk factor for thromboembolic complications including stroke, and consequent morbidity and mortality. The CHA2DS2VAsc score is a widely used risk calculator and can help inform discussions of individual risk but must be balanced by considerations of bleeding risk using calculators such as HAS-BLED. These risk tools share several risk factors (including older age, hypertension and previous stroke) so that many older patients are simultaneously at higher risk of stroke without anticoagulation and higher risk of bleeding with treatment. Anticoagulation with warfarin reduces risk of stroke by 30 to 60% [1]. More recent studies have shown similar or better efficacy and safety with direct oral anticoagulants (DOACs) [2].

The risk of falls often deters clinicians from prescribing anticoagulation therapy, despite evidence that benefits usually far outweigh the risks [3]. Whilst DOACs minimise the burden of drug monitoring, some are contraindicated in renal impairment and there have been some concerns about their safety in frail older people because of bleeding risks, although recent data are reassuring [4, 5]. Ultimately a discussion of information about risks and benefits with patients and caregivers allows informed, individualised joint decision-making based on patient preferences and risk appetite or aversion.

4 Other Gems

- The 'right' therapeutic decision is often not clear-cut, for example continuing anticoagulation for mechanical valves in the face of recurrent bleeding risks, 'risk-feeding' in a patient with significant dysphagia or coordinating discharge home for a patient with major concerns about their cognitive or physical function. Clinicians endeavour to do no harm but must also respect patient autonomy. Person-centred discussions are essential to understand our patients' values and their acceptance of risks.

References

1. Hart RG, Benavente O, McBride R, Pearce LA. Antithrombotic therapy to prevent stroke in patients with atrial fibrillation: a meta-analysis. Ann Intern Med. 1999;131(7):492–501.
2. Halvorsen S, Atar D, Yang H, De Caterina R, Erol C, Garcia D, et al. Efficacy and safety of apixaban compared with warfarin according to age for stroke prevention in atrial fibrillation: observations from the ARISTOTLE trial. Eur Heart J. 2014;35(28):1864–72.
3. Gage BF, Birman-Deych E, Kerzner R, Radford MJ, Nilasena DS, Rich MW. Incidence of intracranial hemorrhage in patients with atrial fibrillation who are prone to fall. Am J Med. 2005;118:612–7.
4. Granziera S, Cohen AT, Nante G, Manzato E, Sergi G. Thromboembolic prevention in frail elderly patients with atrial fibrillation: a practical algorithm. JAMDA. 2015;16:358–64.
5. Kim DH, Pawar A, Gagne JJ, Bessette LG, Lee H, Glynn RJ, et al. Frailty and clinical outcomes of direct oral anticoagulants versus warfarin in older adults with atrial fibrillation: a cohort study. Ann Intern Med. 2021;74(9):1214–23.

A Critical Signal: New Atrial Fibrillation in an Inpatient

Nicole I. Chan, Joseph Tan, and Alison M. Mudge

1 Clinical Pearl

Older patients may be less likely to localise symptoms of infection or other serious illness. Subtle and non-specific symptoms and signs such as new fatigue or new atrial fibrillation may be a prelude to acute deterioration and require careful investigation to identify an underlying cause.

2 Clinical Case

During the daily ward round on the geriatric rehabilitation ward, the resident notes 2 hours of self-limiting tachypnoea recorded on the observations of a 90-year-old retired engineer who has been on the ward for 2 weeks for re-conditioning following an episode of community acquired pneumonia. On careful history, the only symptom the patient describes is feeling "a little dopey". All vital signs are within normal limits, although an electrocardiograph shows new atrial fibrillation at a rate of 96 bpm.

N. I. Chan
Royal Brisbane and Women's Hospital, Metro North Health, Brisbane, QLD, Australia

J. Tan
Surgical Treatment and Rehabilitation Services, Metro North Health, Brisbane, QLD, Australia

A. M. Mudge (✉)
Department of Internal Medicine and Aged Care, Royal Brisbane and Women's Hospital, Metro North Health, Brisbane, QLD, Australia

Medical School, The University of Queensland, Brisbane, QLD, Australia

R. Junckerstorff et al. (eds.), *Beyond Evidence-Based Medicine*,
https://doi.org/10.1007/978-981-99-4440-8_17

The following day the patient develops a fever, tachycardia, and hypotension. His urine culture shows >500 leucocytes and growth of *Klebsiella pneumoniae* which responds to intravenous antibiotics.

3 Discussion

Infection is a major cause of morbidity and mortality in older patients. Changes in the immune system result in increased susceptibility to infections with older age, and older adults are at risk of rapid deterioration with an infection if not appropriately identified and treated in a timely manner [1].

Older patients may have poorly localised symptoms of infection and other acute illnesses such as myocardial infarction or gut ischaemia, which therefore may be missed. Subtle new symptoms of fatigue or drowsiness in someone who was previously improving may be the harbinger of serious illness. This issue can be even more challenging in people with cognitive impairment who may be unable to report their symptoms. Clinical signs of serious illness may only be subtle changes in behaviour reported by family members, nursing or residential aged care staff who are familiar with them. Good collateral history and careful reading of nursing notes can provide valuable clues to serious illness [2].

Changes to a patient's physiological parameters are also important to recognise and respond to early, as the older adult in hospital can decline quickly. For example, tachypnoea or acute confusion are common signs of sepsis and new atrial fibrillation with rapid ventricular response can be precipitated by an infection [3]. It is important to not just manage the manifest abnormality (e.g., treating atrial fibrillation with rate controlling drugs) but to also consider and investigate the underlying cause.

4 Other Gems

- More than half of acute atrial fibrillation occurring in the context of acute illness resolves within 48 h [4]. If a patient is hemodynamically stable, efforts should be focused on finding the underlying cause of the atrial fibrillation rather than initial rate or rhythm control.
- Atypical symptoms and signs and delayed or suppressed inflammatory markers can further confound the diagnosis of infection in older adults [5].

References

1. Scott MM, Liang SY. Infections in older adults. Emerg Med Clin North Am. 2021;39(2):379–94.

2. Rowe TA, Jump RL, Anderson BM, Banach DB, Bryant KA, Doernberg SB, et al. Reliability of non-localizing signs and symptoms as indicators of the presence of infection in nursing-home residents. Infect Control Hosp Epidemiol. 2020;43(4):417–26.
3. Vincent JL. The clinical challenge of sepsis identification and monitoring. PLoS Med. 2016;13(5):e1002022.
4. Lip GY, Watson T. Atrial fibrillation (acute onset). BMJ Clin Evid. 2008;2008:0210.
5. Beckett CL, Harbarth S, Huttner B. Special considerations of antibiotic prescription in the geriatric population. Clin Microbiol Infect. 2015;21(1):3–9.

Taboo Clues: Learning from Bodily Functions

Nicole I. Chan, Joseph Tan, and Alison M. Mudge

1 Clinical Pearl

Urination and defecation are essential bodily functions that receive limited attention in standard medical observations but provide important information about hydration status and response to treatment. Urinary retention, constipation and incontinence are common, distressing and can indicate important pathology.

2 Clinical Case

An 85-year-old retired office worker is admitted to the general medical ward for treatment of a community acquired pneumonia and acute on chronic kidney injury. Her medical history includes longstanding type 2 diabetes mellitus, chronic back pain and chronic kidney disease presumed secondary to diabetes. Her usual medications are metformin and gliclazide for diabetes, and controlled release oxycodone/naloxone and amitriptyline for back pain. Renal ultrasound shows no hydronephrosis but a post-void residual volume of 200 mL, for which the urology team advise regular timed voiding.

N. I. Chan
Royal Brisbane and Women's Hospital, Metro North Health, Brisbane, QLD, Australia

J. Tan
Surgical Treatment and Rehabilitation Services, Metro North Health, Brisbane, QLD, Australia

A. M. Mudge (✉)
Department of Internal Medicine and Aged Care, Royal Brisbane and Women's Hospital, Metro North Health, Brisbane, QLD, Australia

Medical School, The University of Queensland, Brisbane, QLD, Australia

R. Junckerstorff et al. (eds.), *Beyond Evidence-Based Medicine*,
https://doi.org/10.1007/978-981-99-4440-8_18

Her acute kidney injury and pneumonia respond well to intravenous fluids and antibiotics, but on day four she develops acute urinary retention with >700 mL in her bladder on bedside ultrasound, requiring an indwelling catheter. The medical team then note that she has had no recorded bowel movement for 4 days, and that no aperients have been charted. She requires multiple aperients and suppositories to resolve her constipation before the catheter can be removed. During this time, she develops delirium which prolongs her hospital stay by several days.

3 Discussion

During medical ward rounds, observation charts with a patient's vital signs are routinely reviewed for physiological derangements (e.g., temperature, haemodynamics and respiration) to identify response to treatment and predict deterioration. However, other important physiological measures including fluid intake, urine output and bowel motions are often overlooked. Patients are often embarrassed to volunteer information about these bodily functions, and may not clearly recall their intake or output, so establishing fluid and bowel charts help to focus nursing and medical attention on these important functions.

Constipation is very common but poorly documented in hospital, and may result from multiple factors including dehydration (due to highly mineralocorticoid-sensitive fluid resorption in the colon), immobility, reduced dietary fibre and medications (e.g. anticholinergics, opiates) [1]. Opiate therapy very commonly causes constipation, and many patients on long-term therapy have well developed dietary (e.g. pear juice, prunes) and aperient routines which can be interrupted during hospitalisation. Constipation can cause abdominal pain and urinary retention, which along with dehydration are risk factors for delirium. Constipation can also lead to overflow incontinence, which is important to recognise as it paradoxically requires an increase in aperients.

4 Other Gems

- Regular aperients (e.g. pegylated ethylene glycol) must always be charted when commencing opiates, and titrated to ensure daily soft stools. Aperients that are not charted as regular medications may not be given if the patient does not request them, leading to delays in recognising and treating their constipation.
- Indwelling catheters should be used for the shortest possible time as they provide a 'tether' that can minimise mobility, cause discomfort and indignity, and provide an environment for iatrogenic infection [2]. Accurate urine output measurement is often possible without a catheter, although may be challenging in patients with urinary incontinence.

- New hospital-acquired incontinence affects 15–20% of older inpatients [3, 4] and is greatly feared by patients [5], but may be minimised by regular toileting, minimising unnecessary incontinence aids, and thoughtful use and timing of intravenous fluids, diuretics and aperients.

References

1. Jani B, Marsicano E. Constipation: evaluation and management. Mo Med. 2018;115(3):236–40.
2. Safdar N, Codispoti N, Purvis S, Knobloch MJ. Patient perspectives on indwelling urinary catheter use in hospital. Am J Infect Control. 2016;44(3):e23–4.
3. Zisberg A, Sinoff G, Gur-Yaish N, Admi H, Sharmi E. In-hospital use of continence aids and new-onset urinary incontinence in adults aged 70 and older. J Am Geriatr Soc. 2011;59:1099–104.
4. Lakhan P, Jones M, Wilson A, Courtney M, Hirdes J, Gray LC. A prospective cohort study of geriatric syndromes among older medical patients admitted to acute care hospitals. J Am Geriatr Soc. 2011;59(11):2001–8.
5. Rubin EB, Buehler AE, Halpern SD. States worse than death among hospitalized patients with serious illnesses. JAMA Intern Med. 2016;176:1557–9.

Part III
Delirium

Prolonged Delirium in the Intensive Care Unit (ICU)

Edward T. H. Fysh

1 Clinical Pearl

Individualised, non-pharmacological management tools such as natural light therapy can be useful for delirium in the ICU.

2 Clinical Case

A 60-year-old professional landscaper presented with abdominal pain and sepsis and was found to have a perforated, obstructed large bowel, secondary to colorectal cancer. He underwent emergency right hemicolectomy, but then developed mesenteric ischaemia and further peritonitis requiring multiple laparotomies, complicated by prolonged septic shock and multiorgan failure. After 12 days of sedation and invasive ventilation he was weaned to a point where extubation was attempted, but he quickly had to be re-sedated and intubated secondary to severe agitation and near dislodgement of essential central venous catheters. Attention was paid throughout to delirium prevention and treatment (such as benzodiazepine avoidance, pain control, family visitation and inclusion). Nevertheless, his Confusion Assessment Method for the Intensive Care Unit (CAM-ICU) score confirmed significant ongoing delirium at 14 days and ongoing sedative infusions were still required despite resolution of septic shock and improved renal function. His family raised concerns that he had spent most of his life outdoors and could become claustrophobic in enclosed environments. He was moved to a room with a large window allowing natural light exposure and a view of a busy street. Within 48 hours he was able to be re-extubated without the need for ongoing sedatives and antipsychotics. As his

E. T. H. Fysh (✉)
Curtin University and St John of God Midland Hospital, Perth, WA, Australia

R. Junckerstorff et al. (eds.), *Beyond Evidence-Based Medicine*,
https://doi.org/10.1007/978-981-99-4440-8_19

cognition improved, the patient stated that the ability to see natural light and glimpse normal life in the outside world helped reorientate him and was key to maintaining a sense of "what was real" when he became confused or scared. Following transfer to rehabilitation, the patient was routinely taken outside for an hour per day, weather and medical condition permitting, and he and his family credited this to improving the speed of his progression to discharge home after 30 days in hospital.

3 Discussion

Delirium is common in patients that require intensive care, affecting up to 82% of invasively ventilated patients. It is associated with increased mortality, requirement for invasive ventilation and prolonged hospital stay, as well as increased likelihood of long-term cognitive impairment [1].

Despite the frequency and impact of delirium in the critically ill, there are few proven treatments. The use of dexmedetomidine as opposed to benzodiazepine sedative infusions has been shown to be beneficial in prevention of delirium [2], however pharmacological therapies ranging from antipsychotics to melatonin have proven disappointing in randomised trials [3, 4]. Adherence to the ABCDEF care bundle (A- assess, prevent and manage pain; B- both spontaneous awakening and breathing trials; C- choice of analgesia and sedation; D- delirium assess, prevent and manage; E- early mobility and exercise; and F- family engagement/empowerment) has been shown to improve mortality and delirium in large prospective observational studies [5], however the individual components are not all evidence-based and are not intended as a "one size fits all approach". Its purpose is to highlight a need to pay attention to and tailor best practice guidelines to individual patients.

Exposure to natural light has been of interest to health professionals caring for patients with delirium for some time. Some studies have shown that natural light has been associated with improved delirium incidence, but overall the data is mixed, possibly because of the difficulty in defining and standardising what constitutes natural light exposure [6].

In the case presented above, the patient had a clear memory of a beneficial response to natural light exposure and ability to see the outside world. Whilst this specific "treatment" won't work in every case, attention to the individual needs and background of our patients can have significant benefits. Moreover, a willingness to listen to the concerns of patients and family members and, if possible, adapt care to their needs can engender a sense of engagement and collaboration in other aspects of the holistic management of the patient.

References

1. Goldberg TE, Chen C, Wang Y, Jung E, Swanson A, Ing C, Garcia PS, Whittington RA, Moitra V. Association of delirium with long-term cognitive decline: a meta-analysis. JAMA Neurol. 2020;77(11):1373–81.
2. Riker RR, Shehabi Y, Bokesch PM, Ceraso D, Wisemandle W, Koura F, Whitten P, Margolis BD, Byrne DW, Ely EW, Rocha MG, SEDCOM (Safety and Efficacy of Dexmedetomidine Compared With Midazolam) Study Group. Dexmedetomidine vs midazolam for sedation of critically ill patients: a randomized trial. JAMA. 2009;301(5):489–99.
3. Girard TD, Exline MC, Carson SS, Hough CL, Rock P, Gong MN, et al. Haloperidol and ziprasidone for treatment of delirium in critical illness. N Engl J Med. 2018;379(26):2506–16.
4. Wibrow B, Martinez FE, Myers E, Chapman A, Litton E, Ho KM, Regli A, Hawkins D, Ford A, van Haren F, Wyer S, McCaffrey J, Rashid A, Kelty E, Murray K, Anstey M. Prophylactic melatonin for delirium in intensive care (pro-MEDIC): a randomized controlled trial. Intensive Care Med. 2022;48(4):414–25.
5. Pun BT, Balas MC, Barnes-Daly MA, Thompson JL, Aldrich JM, Barr J, Byrum D, Carson SS, Devlin JW, Engel HJ, Esbrook CL, Hargett KD, Harmon L, Hielsberg C, Jackson JC, Kelly TL, Kumar V, Millner L, Morse A, Perme CS, Ely EW, et al. Caring for critically ill patients with the ABCDEF bundle: results of the ICU liberation collaborative in over 15,000 adults. Crit Care Med. 2019;47(1):3–14.
6. Vahedian-Azimi A, Bashar FR, Khan AM, Miller AC. Natural versus artificial light exposure on delirium incidence in ARDS patients. Ann Intensive Care. 2020;10(1):15.

Looking for Causes of Delirium

Ian Scott

1 Clinical Pearl

In patients presenting with acute confusion, consider the possibility of delirium and look for background predisposing factors and potentially reversible acute triggers.

2 Clinical Case

A 79-year-old woman with mild cognitive impairment (MCI), type 2 diabetes and chronic kidney disease presented to hospital with 3 days of right-sided neck pain which had affected her right posterior neck and proximal right shoulder on wakening, and then progressed to include the right side of her head. The pain was associated with blurry vision which had resolved by the time of presentation.

Physical examination revealed tenderness on palpation of the strap muscles of her right neck and the right temporal region, in the presence of normal visual acuity. Laboratory investigations showed an elevated erythrocyte sedimentation rate (ESR) of 50 mm/h, and a computed tomographic (CT) scan of the head and neck showed no acute abnormality.

As the patient's live-in son was away for the week and she was alone, and owing to concern for giant cell arteritis (GCA), the patient was admitted to hospital and immediately started on 60 mg/day of oral prednisone while awaiting a temporal artery biopsy.

I. Scott (✉)
Internal Medicine and Clinical Epidemiology, Princess Alexandra Hospital, Brisbane, QLD, Australia

Centre for Health Services Research, University of Queensland, Brisbane, QLD, Australia

Faculty of Medicine, Queensland University of Technology, Brisbane, QLD, Australia

R. Junckerstorff et al. (eds.), *Beyond Evidence-Based Medicine*,
https://doi.org/10.1007/978-981-99-4440-8_20

Oxycodone at a dose of 5 mg q4hourly as required for pain relief was prescribed. As admission occurred at the beginning of a long weekend, the biopsy could not be performed for several days. By day 4, the patient had become restless and agitated, was refusing medicines, and had reduced appetite. Uncontrolled pain from neck spasms, and opiate-induced nausea were thought to be aggravating factors, so baclofen and metoclopramide were added. Her oral fluid intake was noted to be less than a litre a day, urine output was not able to be measured as she had become incontinent, her bowels had not opened for days, and her blood sugars were increasing up to 18 mmol/L. Intravenous (IV) fluids and insulin were administered, an indwelling catheter (IDC) was inserted, and soft mitten restraints were applied to prevent dislodgement of the IV cannula and IDC. At day 6, she underwent the biopsy under local anaesthetic and neuroleptic sedation which subsequently returned a negative result. The prednisone was then ceased and over the next 10 days, the patient made a gradual recovery and was discharged on day 16 to the care of her son. The patient's right-sided neck and temporal pain were ultimately attributed to musculoskeletal strain based on the location of pain and lack of temporal correlation between initiation of corticosteroids and resolution of the pain. Her elevated ESR was attributed to her age and chronic comorbidities.

3 Discussion

The most common hospital-acquired complication affecting up to 1 in 4 older patients is delirium [1], defined as acute onset of disturbance in attention, awareness, and cognition, which can fluctuate over time and is not attributable to other neurocognitive disorders (such as acute stroke). Delirium leads to longer lengths of stay and higher in-hospital mortality and is associated with an increased rate of death, institutionalisation, and development of dementia over succeeding months [2]. These risks are independent of comorbid illness and baseline cognition, indicating that an episode of delirium itself may have permanent deleterious effects on brain function. Up to 30% to 50% of cases of delirium are considered preventable [3], and evidence shows that multicomponent interventions aimed at optimising mobility, nutrition and hydration, sleep, pain management and cognitive and social activities can reduce the incidence of delirium by up to 50% [4, 5]. In the case described, admission to an unfamiliar acute hospital ward without her son, initiation of high dose steroids for a misdiagnosis of GCA, the addition of centrally acting opiates, baclofen and metoclopramide, insertion of IV lines and IDC requiring restraints, inattention to adequate hydration and onset of constipation all compounded to induce and worsen severe delirium in a patient with underlying predisposing factors of age, MCI and co-morbidities.

4 Other Gems

- Hospital-acquired delirium is often subject to delayed recognition in up to 65% of cases, especially as 3 out of 4 cases can be hypoactive delirium (where patients are quietly confused and inactive, and do not attract immediate attention) compared to hyperactive delirium (with agitated behaviour and loud verbalisations) [3].

- Early recognition is aided by the regular use of delirium screening tools, such as the 3D-CAM [6] and the 4-AT [7] which, if screened positive, should initiate a patient review by medical, nursing and allied health staff using the PITCHED checklist (see Fig. 1). The checklist includes all reversible triggers of delirium that, in up to 50% of cases, are potentially amenable to non-pharmacologic intervention.

Pain
- Ensure regular assessment and management of pain
- Assess pain on the Behaviour Observation chart (Verbal scale + PAINAD)

Infection
- Monitor for potential signs and sources of infection
- Pressure injury prevention

Thirst
- Maintain fluid balance and encourage oral intake (water within reach)

Constipation
- Monitor bowels and consider aperients

Hunger
- Maintain nutrition: ensure meal set up, provide dentures & oral care
- Monitor weight
- Consider dietician referral

Environment
- Promote normal sleep/wake patterns
- Promote social & recreational activity (use Cognition Corner)
- Encourage mobility
- Orientation
- Hearing and visual aids
- Sunlight during the day
- Have family provide familiar possessions from home
- Ensure a calm and soothing atmosphere and decrease sensory input

Drugs
- Maintain normal oxygen saturation
- Consider need for pharmacy medication review
- Avoid or minimise psychotropic, sedative or hypnotic drugs

Fig. 1 PITCHED checklist

- Preventing delirium is also aided by screening patients on admission for background risk factors (such as cognitive impairment, hearing and visual impairment, past episodes of delirium, central nervous system (CNS) diseases and CNS acting drugs, depression, older age) and instituting preventive measures that ensure adequate hydration and nutrition, early mobilisation, and engagement in meaningful social activities, while avoiding treatments and other clinical interventions which may trigger delirium.

References

1. Gibb K, Seeley A, Quinn T, et al. The consistent burden in published estimates of delirium occurrence in medical inpatients over four decades: a systematic review and meta-analysis study. Age Ageing. 2020;49(3):352–60.
2. Witlox J, Eurelings LS, de Jonghe JF, et al. Delirium in elderly patients and the risk of post-discharge mortality, institutionalization, and dementia: a meta-analysis. JAMA. 2010;304(4):443–51.
3. Ludolph P, Stoffers-Winterling J, Kunzler AM, et al. Non-pharmacologic multicomponent interventions preventing delirium in hospitalized people. J Am Geriatr Soc. 2020;68(8):1864–71.
4. Burton JK, Craig LE, Yong SQ, et al. Non-pharmacological interventions for preventing delirium in hospitalised non-ICU patients. Cochrane Database Syst Rev. 2021;7(7):CD013307.
5. Mudge A, McRae P, Banks M, et al. Effect of a ward-based program on hospital-associated complications and length of stay for older inpatients: the cluster randomized CHERISH trial. JAMA Intern Med. 2022;182(3):274–82.
6. Marcantonio ER, Ngo LH, O'Connor M, et al. 3D-CAM: derivation and validation of a 3-minute diagnostic interview for CAM-defined delirium: a cross-sectional diagnostic test study. Ann Intern Med. 2014;161(8):554–61.
7. Hendry K, Quinn TJ, Evans J, et al. Evaluation of delirium screening tools in geriatric medical inpatients: a diagnostic test accuracy study. Age Ageing. 2016;45:832–7.

Agitating for Better Care: Minimise Sedatives in Delirium

Alison M. Mudge, Nicole I. Chan, and Joseph Tan

1 Clinical Pearl

Sedation is often requested for patients with agitated delirium, but seldom indicated. The cause of the delirium must be identified, but so must the trigger for the agitated behaviour, which may be the only way a patient can communicate their needs.

2 Clinical Case

An 88-year-old retired nurse is admitted to hospital from a residential aged care facility with vomiting due to an incarcerated hernia requiring laparoscopic surgery. She has moderate dementia (Alzheimer's type) requiring assistance with instrumental activities of daily living but is usually independent with mobility and transfers. Postoperatively she is managed with a nasogastric tube, slow intravenous fluids, and diapers for toileting. She is considered a high falls risk and placed in the high visibility bay near the nurses' station with two unstable patients who require frequent Medical Emergency Response Team reviews. On the second postoperative evening she becomes agitated, removing her intravenous line and nasogastric tube and

A. M. Mudge (✉)
Department of Internal Medicine and Aged Care, Royal Brisbane and Women's Hospital, Metro North Health, Brisbane, QLD, Australia

Medical School, The University of Queensland, Brisbane, QLD, Australia

N. I. Chan
Royal Brisbane and Women's Hospital, Metro North Health, Brisbane, QLD, Australia

J. Tan
Surgical Treatment and Rehabilitation Services, Metro North Health, Brisbane, QLD, Australia

R. Junckerstorff et al. (eds.), *Beyond Evidence-Based Medicine*,
https://doi.org/10.1007/978-981-99-4440-8_21

wandering the ward, intruding into other patients' bed spaces. She becomes increasingly agitated when she is returned to her bed, calling out and trying to get over the bed rails. The covering junior doctor is requested to prescribe sedation.

3 Discussion

Postoperative delirium is a common complication, especially in patients aged over 65 and/or those with underlying cognitive impairment. Delirium often represents the accumulation of several 'triggers' in addition to the acute illness and operation [1]. These include physiological abnormalities such as electrolyte disturbances, new medications, or infection. They also include iatrogenic factors such as dehydration, pain, immobility, restraints (including intravenous lines, drains and indwelling catheters) and sleep disturbance, all of which may have contributed to development of delirium in this case. Systematic approaches to reduce these iatrogenic triggers can significantly reduce hospital-associated delirium [2].

In patients who develop hyperactive delirium, it is important for the attending doctor to make the diagnosis of delirium (using a validated tool such as the 3D-CAM [3]) and seek triggers both for the delirium and for the agitation. People with cognitive impairment may have difficulty expressing their needs verbally, and judgement must be made about whether this patient has pain, hunger, or thirst, which may only become clear by observing behaviour after pain relief or food and fluids are provided. Knowing the person and their usual routines such as preferred foods, ambulation and toileting, or the presence of a family carer or familiar objects from home can be reassuring and reduce anxiety. Knitted 'decoys' to cover intravenous lines can reduce risks of dislodgement.

4 Other Gems

- Pain assessment can be challenging in people with cognitive impairment, although there are several validated tools that rate pain based on non-verbal cues (e.g. the Abbey pain scale). Regularly prescribed analgesia may be more appropriate for patients with cognitive impairment and likely pain, as it does not rely on pain reporting or patient-controlled activation. Patients with cognitive impairment are less likely to receive adequate pain relief [4], and this can contribute to delirium.
- Calling out and wandering are behaviours that may bother staff but are not an appropriate indication for antipsychotics unless there is clear risk to patient or staff [5]. Shared understanding of the patient's biography (through using tools such as This Is Me) can help explain behaviours. For example, this patient may be seeking the toilet as she usually toilets independently, or she may believe she is still a nurse and think she needs to be 'rounding'. Talking to the patient,

validating their emotions (e.g., frustration, hunger or feeling lost), and meeting a need (e.g. taking her to the toilet, providing finger foods that she can manage if she is allowed to resume oral diet or taking her to look out the window) or gently redirecting to another activity (e.g. helping to fold pillowcases or count saline vials) can be helpful.

- Approaching a wandering patient appropriately is also important. Being calm and articulating clearly can minimise the chances of a patient becoming more stressed. Large groups of people, security staff and speaking loudly or rapidly can create greater stress and exacerbate agitated and aggressive behaviour.
- Managing competing priorities is difficult in practice. Although this patient might get more sleep in a quiet single room away from acutely deteriorating patients, she may get less staff interaction (which can provide meaningful orientation) and delayed attention to her fundamental physical care needs like food, drink, mobility, and toileting. Family members familiar with her routines and needs, or skilled assistant staff, can be very valuable assets in care.

References

1. Inouye SK, Westendorp RGJ, Saczynski JS. Delirium in elderly people. Lancet. 2014;383(9920):911–22.
2. Burton J, Craig L, Yong S, Siddiqi N, Teale E, Woodhouse R, et al. Non-pharmacological interventions for preventing delirium in hospitalised non-ICU patients. Cochrane Database Syst Rev. 2021;7(7):CD013307.
3. Marcantonio ER, Ngo LH, O'Connor M, Jones RN, Crane PK, Metzger ED, et al. 3D-CAM: derivation and validation of a 3-minute diagnostic interview for CAM-defined delirium. Ann Intern Med. 2014;161(8):554–61.
4. Graham F, Beattie E, Filelding E. Hospital nurses' management of agitation in older cognitively impaired patients: do they recognise pain-related agitation? Age Ageing. 2022;51(7):afac140.
5. Australian Commission on Safety and Quality in Health Care. Delirium clinical care standard (updated September 2021). Sydney: ACSQHC; 2021. www.safetyandquality.gov.au/our-work/clinical-care-standards/delirium-clinical-care-standard. Accessed September 4 2022.

Antipsychotics and Acute Behavioural Disturbance

Emma Hack and Benny Katz

1 Clinical Pearl

Antipsychotics may not be the best option for an acutely disturbed older person.

2 Clinical Case

A male aged in his mid-80s is admitted to hospital. On the second day, he becomes agitated in the evening and is prescribed an antipsychotic, risperidone. He sleeps most of the following day. At 10 p.m. that night, the covering doctor is called to review the patient.

The patient is distressed and agitated and wanting to go home. He seems inattentive, and nursing staff have been unable to calm or reassure him. The question of using risperidone again is raised. The doctor considers this but decides to look into things further given concerns that antipsychotics might not be the best option. They note there is a history of cognitive impairment, though it is unclear if the behaviour is longstanding, or if it is new and better described as delirium.

The doctor elects to telephone the wife. She reports he has had difficulty sleeping at night for several months and has been taking temazepam every evening.

E. Hack
Department of Geriatric Medicine, St. Vincent's Hospital Melbourne, Fitzroy, VIC, Australia

B. Katz (✉)
Department of Geriatric Medicine, St. Vincent's Hospital Melbourne, Fitzroy, VIC, Australia

Faculty of Medicine, Dentistry and Health Sciences, University of Melbourne, Melbourne, VIC, Australia

R. Junckerstorff et al. (eds.), *Beyond Evidence-Based Medicine*,
https://doi.org/10.1007/978-981-99-4440-8_22

Temazepam is notably absent from the medication chart. The wife asks to speak to her husband, but he cannot hear her speaking as he does not have his hearing aids with him.

3 Discussion

Acute behavioural disturbance in hospital is common, and often occurs 'after hours' or at night. It is often an expression of unmet need, and one may need to act as 'detective' and investigate further. The request for pharmacological therapy is common, the intent being to curb the behaviour and likely cause sedation. In this case, rather than simply prescribing antipsychotic therapy, the doctor identified significant modifiable factors.

History obtained from the wife identified that benzodiazepine withdrawal may be a cause for the agitation, that would be better managed with his usual temazepam, at least in the short term. Benzodiazepines are associated with cognitive decline and dependence, and should not be abruptly discontinued as occurred in this case, as this risks withdrawal symptoms, agitation and seizures [1].

Non-pharmacological management of behavioural disturbance in the elderly should be the first step though is often overlooked, especially when there are staff shortages or competing demands. Reassurance from a trusted and familiar source such as a family member or friends may be help with de-escalation while the situation is reviewed.

The following non-pharmacological management options must first be addressed: ensure history, medication list and examination are accurate; treat pain and constipation, exclude urinary retention; provide the patient with their hearing aids and spectacles; involve family and interpreters to optimise communication; avoid loud noise and harsh lighting, preferably in a single room, and where appropriate; discuss with the ward manager whether the patient might benefit from 1:1 staffing.

Diversional strategies, that might include music or activities suited to the patient should be considered. These and other types of interventions are examples of individualised patient care that prevent delirium [2], though many of these strategies are best implemented during the day by the usual treating team.

Risperidone was not the best option in this scenario. Antipsychotics are overprescribed in the elderly [3], and are associated with potentially serious adverse effects (Fig. 1) including an increased risk of mortality [4].

Should behaviours fail to de-escalate with less-restrictive non-pharmacological attempts, and there is a risk of harm to themselves or others, judicious use of a single dose or short course of antipsychotic medication may be considered, but this should be tapered and ceased at the earliest possibility.

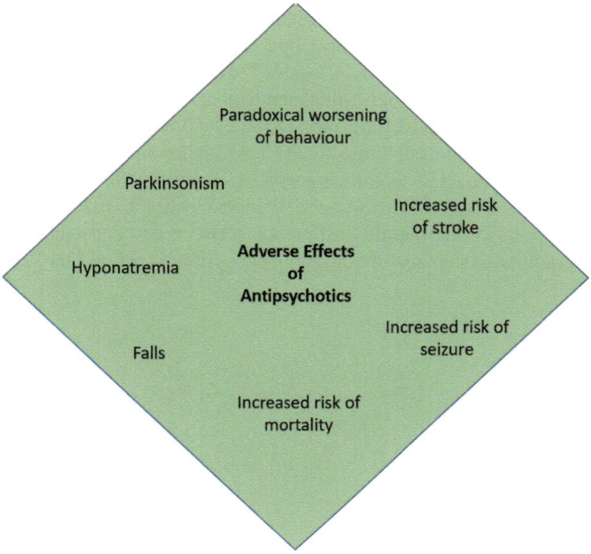

Fig. 1 Adverse effects of antipsychotics

4 Other Gems

- Consider what the patient with behavioural disturbance is trying to tell you
  - Avoid jumping to an assumption that a patient needs antipsychotic medication.
  - Identify the precipitating factors contributing to the behaviour.
- Ask yourself: "Who is the patient?"
  - A person's social, cultural and linguistic background will help you provide a management plan, including behavioural strategies where appropriate.
- Regular visitation from relevant family and caregivers is a key strategy in providing comfort, familiarity and orientation.
- Any use of antipsychotics should be judicious and in consultation with a patient's substitute medical decision maker.
- Delirium is strongly associated with prolonged hospital admission, complications and mortality
  - Early referral to geriatric medicine or aged care psychiatry for assistance with management should be considered.

References

1. Guidance for the use of benzodiazepines in psychiatric practice. Royal Australian & NZ College of Psychiatrists. Professional practice guidelines 5. November 2019. https://www.ranzcp.org/files/resources/college_statements/practice_guidelines/ppg5-use-of-benzodiazepines.

aspx#:~:text=In%20general%2C%20benzodiazepine%20use%20should,based%20pharmacological%20and%20psychological%20treatments.
2. Siddiqi N, Harrison JK, Clegg A, Teale EA, Young J, Taylor J, Simpkins S. Interventions for preventing delirium in hospitalised patients. Cochrane Database Syst Rev. 2016;3(3):CD005563. https://doi.org/10.1002/14651858.CD005563.pub3.
3. Royal Commission into Aged Care Quality and Safety. Final report: care, dignity and respect. Canberra, ACT: Commonwealth of Australia; 2021.
4. Jackson JW, Schneeweiss S, VanderWeele TJ, Blacker D. Quantifying the role of adverse events in the mortality difference between first and second-generation antipsychotics in older adults: systematic review and meta-synthesis. PLoS One. 2014;9(8):e105376.

Urinary Tract Infection May Not Be the Cause of Delirium

Jillian Chau and Benny Katz

1 Clinical Pearl

Both delirium and urinary tract infections (UTIs) are common and may co-exist in older people. However, the UTI may not be the cause of the delirium.

2 Clinical Case

Margaret is in her late 80s and was admitted to hospital with a two-day history of delirium. She has a background of vascular cognitive impairment, Type 2 diabetes mellitus (T2DM), osteoarthritis, heart failure and long-standing urinary incontinence. Her regular medications are paracetamol, metformin, linagliptin, perindopril, bisoprolol, furosemide and spironolactone. She receives intravenous antibiotics for an *E. coli* UTI. Her delirium improves over 48 hours, and she returns home. One week later, Margaret is well, and her general practitioner repeats the urine culture which again grows *E. coli*. Did the UTI cause the delirium?

J. Chau
Department of Geriatric Medicine, Western Health, St Albans, VIC, Australia

B. Katz (✉)
Department of Geriatric Medicine, St. Vincent's Hospital Melbourne, Fitzroy, VIC, Australia

Faculty of Medicine, Dentistry and Health Sciences, University of Melbourne, Melbourne, VIC, Australia

R. Junckerstorff et al. (eds.), *Beyond Evidence-Based Medicine*,
https://doi.org/10.1007/978-981-99-4440-8_23

3 Discussion

Delirium is complex and dynamic; the aetiology is often multifactorial. It is often not possible to identify the factor that precipitated the delirium. In general, any medical condition can precipitate delirium in a susceptible person. The most common causes in older people are fluid and electrolyte disturbances, infections (skin, chest, urinary), medications including medication withdrawal, alcohol and alcohol withdrawal, metabolic disturbances, and postoperative states. Inouye's approach is to consider the interaction between a person's baseline vulnerability (predisposing factors) and the severity of insult (precipitating factors) [1] (Fig. 1).

Asymptomatic bacteriuria is common in elderly people. It is more common in women, in advanced old age and in residential aged care facilities (RACF). In older people, it occurs in up to 50% of women and 40% of men living in RACF [2], which is higher than community-dwelling older people (up to 16% of women and 19% of men) [3].

So, did the UTI cause Margaret's delirium?

Margaret has multiple predisposing factors for developing delirium, including advanced age, pre-existing cognitive impairment, and polypharmacy. In older people like Margaret, who have a high vulnerability to delirium, a minor event such as a UTI may be enough to trigger a delirium. On this occasion, it was appropriate to treat the bacteriuria as a true UTI and monitor her response. The delirium resolved with antibiotics and rehydration. As delirium often resolves over a few days, we cannot be certain whether the improvement was causally related to treatment of the UTI. The delirium can resolve in the same time frame as a course of antibiotics.

The fact that the bacteriuria persisted after antibiotics, and after the delirium had resolved, is suggestive that the bacteriuria was in retrospect asymptomatic, and possibly an incidental finding. Antibiotics to treat asymptomatic bacteriuria do not reduce mortality, morbidity or incontinence [3]. Therefore, if the delirium recurred,

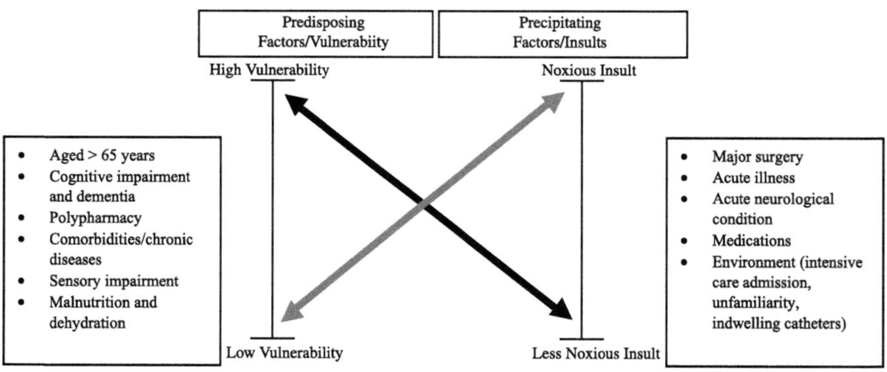

Fig. 1 Predisposing and precipitating factors, vulnerability and insults in delirium. (Adapted from Inouye, 2018 [1])

we would need to consider other reversible causes, such as state of hydration, metabolic disturbances or a new infection, and check for medication changes. A collateral history is helpful to confirm the time course, as fluctuation is a key feature of delirium.

Finally, let's consider Margaret's daughter, who is 65 years old. She does not have diabetes, cognitive impairment, or heart failure and is considered to have low susceptibility for the development of delirium. If a delirium occurred, we would expect it to be in the setting of serious injury or illness, or major surgery. If none of these common causes are apparent, then she should have investigations for less common causes, including brain imaging and possibly cerebral spinal fluid (CSF) studies.

4 Other Gems

- Delirium is common in older people. A screening tool such as the 4AT should be administered on all older people on admission to hospital. https://www.the4at.com/.
- There is insufficient evidence to establish a causative relationship between delirium and asymptomatic bacteriuria, at best the relationship is an association [4].
- As delirium is a risk factor for cognitive impairment and dementia, and people with cognitive impairment or dementia have a higher vulnerability to delirium, it is important to establish the baseline cognitive function and arrange long term cognitive follow up upon delirium resolution.

References

1. Inouye SK. Delirium—a framework to improve acute care for older persons. J Am Geriatr Soc. 2018;66(3):446–51.
2. Nicolle LE, Committee SL-TC. Urinary tract infections in long-term–care facilities. Infect Control Hosp Epidemiol. 2001;22(3):167–75.
3. McKenzie R, Stewart MT, Bellantoni MF, Finucane TE. Bacteriuria in individuals who become delirious. Am J Med. 2014;127(4):255–7.
4. Mayne S, Bowden A, Sundvall P-D, Gunnarsson R. The scientific evidence for a potential link between confusion and urinary tract infection in the elderly is still confusing-a systematic literature review. BMC Geriatr. 2019;19(1):1–15.

Is Delirium Better Managed in Hospital or At Home?

Anna Sigley and Benny Katz

1 Clinical Pearl

Delirium can be managed at home if appropriate care is available in a suitable environment.

2 Clinical Case

A man in his 80s is brought to the Emergency Department with a 3-day history of confusion and a painful right leg. He has a history of memory impairment but is usually independent at home supported by his wife. He is diagnosed with delirium secondary to cellulitis of his right leg. The Emergency Department doctor arranges for him to be admitted to hospital, however the man and his wife insist that he goes home. His daughter asks "is it better for Dad to be cared for by us at home rather than in hospital?"

A. Sigley
Department of Geriatric Medicine, Monash Health, Melbourne, VIC, Australia

B. Katz (✉)
Department of Geriatric Medicine, St. Vincent's Hospital Melbourne, Fitzroy, VIC, Australia

Faculty of Medicine, Dentistry and Health Sciences, University of Melbourne, Melbourne, VIC, Australia

R. Junckerstorff et al. (eds.), *Beyond Evidence-Based Medicine*,
https://doi.org/10.1007/978-981-99-4440-8_24

3 Discussion

There is no correct answer to the daughter's question. Many issues need to be considered and every case is different.

There are many factors favouring managing older people with delirium at home—the familiar environment and people have a positive effect, as does the routine of home life. On the other hand, delirium has the potential to cause behavioural changes such as agitation, aggression and wandering, and adverse medical outcomes such as falls and incontinence. In this case, this man's care needs may be more than his wife can manage.

There are several key issues that need to be explored. The first is explaining delirium and the likely clinical course. Delirium is expected to improve over a short period of time. Once a cause is found (in this case, cellulitis) and treatment started, caregivers should see an improvement in a few days. However, it may take several days, or even weeks, for it to recover completely. It is important to highlight to the caregiver that if the confusion and behaviour get worse or do not improve over this period, further medical assessment is needed.

Exploration of the home environment and the feasibility of delivering care in this environment should be undertaken. This includes the availability of supervision at home and discussing the need for supervision 24 hours per day. It can sometimes be worthwhile to suggest a roster for family members to share this load.

Highlighting the need to pay careful attention to basic care needs is essential. Delirium is associated with an increased risk of falls and injuries. Constipation, dehydration and pressure injuries may lead to prolongation of the delirium after the initial cause has resolved.

After these discussions the doctor, patient and his family come to a shared decision about whether they feel care at home would be the best option.

The doctor then explains the monitoring and follow up needed—including the treatment for cellulitis, hospital at home program, 24/7 emergency contact and the option of returning to hospital if things are not improving. The local General Practitioner is also involved.

4 Other Gems

- There is no specific treatment for delirium - management centres around the reversal of precipitating factors (e.g. drugs, metabolic disturbance, infections) and safe care of the individual until the delirium resolves [1].
- Recent studies have found delirium care at home may be a better option [2], but the benefits of home need to be balanced against the benefits of hospital admission.
- Despite the patient's wish to be cared for at home, this may not be the best option.

- An episode of delirium can be very distressing for both the patient and their carer/family. Not every family/carer will feel comfortable providing care at home during this period.
- Ongoing assessment of delirium is required [3] to ensure it is improving.
- Delirium can persist for many weeks to months in some cases.
- It is important to note that a patient with a delirium should not drive or operate electrical equipment until the delirium has resolved.
- Following an episode of delirium, there is an increased risk of cognitive decline and onset of dementia [4]. A cognitive assessment should be arranged after the delirium has resolved.

References

1. Inouye SK, Westendorp RG, Saczynski JS. Delirium in elderly people. Lancet. 2014;383(9920):911–22.
2. Ford AH. Preventing delirium in dementia: managing risk factors. Maturitas. 2016;92:35–40.
3. Isaia G, Astengo MA, Tibaldi V, et al. Delirium in elderly home-treated patients: a prospective study with 6-month follow-up. Age (Dordr). 2009;31(2):109–17.
4. Fong TG, Davis D, Growdon ME, Albuquerque A, Inouye SK. The interface between delirium and dementia in elderly adults. Lancet Neurol. 2015;14(8):823–32. Erratum in: Lancet Neurol. 2015 Aug;14(8):788.

Part IV
Palliative Care

Advance Care Planning

Ian Scott

1 Clinical Pearl

In older patients with advanced chronic diseases or malignancies, consider the need for advance care planning of end-of-life care.

2 Clinical Case

A 79-year-old man with ischaemic heart disease, chronic obstructive pulmonary disease, heart failure with preserved ejection fraction and chronic kidney disease presents to the emergency department with sudden-onset dyspnoea and is found to be in acute pulmonary oedema. He has had three similar admissions over the last 12 months which respond quickly to intravenous diuretics and result in discharge home. He lives alone in a retirement village and receives twice weekly home help. He has good cognition (Mini Mental State Examination 26/30), is compliant with medications and fluid management plan, and is attended by the heart failure outreach service. On this occasion, despite some improvement in his heart failure, he develops hospital-acquired pneumonia and acute type 1 (hypoxic) respiratory failure and becomes delirious. This patient has no advance care plan or health directive and has not had any end of life care discussions with his son who lives interstate but

I. Scott (✉)
Internal Medicine and Clinical Epidemiology, Princess Alexandra Hospital, Brisbane, QLD, Australia

Centre for Health Services Research, University of Queensland, Brisbane, QLD, Australia

Faculty of Medicine, Queensland University of Technology, Brisbane, QLD, Australia

R. Junckerstorff et al. (eds.), *Beyond Evidence-Based Medicine*,
https://doi.org/10.1007/978-981-99-4440-8_25

who is his enduring power of attorney. When contacted, the son replies, ‘well he has been enjoying life as far as I know and I would be giving him every chance.’ On this basis, the patient is intubated and ventilated as he does not tolerate high flow oxygen by either mask or nasal prongs. His kidney function worsens, and dialysis is initiated, and after several days, total parenteral nutrition is started. Despite these interventions, he continues to require multiorgan system support, and at day 16, his son finally makes the decision to withdraw all life-sustaining treatments, and the patient dies.

3 Discussion

Identifying limits on aggressive and invasive care near the end of life is challenging, especially when patients lose decision-making capacity and are unable to voice their preferences for care. This situation is common, affecting more than 70% of hospitalised patients at times of acute medical crisis when care decisions need to be made [1]. Discussions around goals of care and desirable levels of invasive life support measures need to be undertaken well ahead of such crises, and involve patients, their family or proxy decision-makers, and their treating clinicians. Such discussions may avoid aggressive care at the end of life which often proves non-beneficial [2] and may violate patient preferences. Unfortunately, even in patients with advanced cancer this does not always happen. One study found that more than 1 in 5 patients with advanced malignancy never had any form of end-of-life care discussions which, when they were performed, occurred on average only 4 weeks before death [3].

Advance care planning (ACP) is the iterative process of defining and documenting a person’s values and preferences to guide future healthcare in the event decision-making capacity is lost. Evidence shows that ACP, when performed in a timely fashion, decreases anxiety, grief, decisional conflict and burden for relatives and surrogates [4], enhances clinician adherence to patient preferences, increases use of palliative care, improves patient and family satisfaction with care, and avoids unwanted cardiopulmonary resuscitation (CPR) and life-support treatments [5].

4 Other Gems

- Determining when goals of care should change from a curative focus on prolonging life to one of maximising quality of life can be difficult [6]. Early engagement with ACP-eligible patients can be facilitated by clinicians asking themselves the ‘Surprise’ question: ‘Would I be surprised if this person died over the next 12 months?’ [7]. If the answer is no, then ongoing ACP discussions should be entered into that are relevant to patient needs and cognisant of important inter-

personal relationships. The Surprise question has up to 70% accuracy in predicting patients with life spans shorter than 12 months [7].
- A values-based, standardised Statement of Choices form (available at: https://metrosouth.health.qld.gov.au/acp/queensland-advance-care-planning-forms) serves as a user-friendly, non-legally binding, easy to complete and modify form that details patients' goals of care and preferences for CPR, life-support interventions and other supportive care.
- ACP can be promoted in hospital practice and primary care by whole of community education campaigns, use of skilled ACP facilitators, clinician access to ACP resources and templates, provision of patient information brochures, and embedding of end-of-life care frameworks that clearly define clinician roles and responsibilities for ACP [8, 9]. These strategies help overcome the frequently voiced barriers to ACP which include lack of time, skill, remuneration, organisational support, and patient/family engagement. While as many as 1 in 5 patients may not want to engage in ACP, the remaining 80% need to be given every opportunity to do so [8].

References

1. Silveira MJ, Kim SY, Langa KM. Advance directives and outcomes of surrogate decision making before death. N Engl J Med. 2010;362(13):1211–8.
2. Carter HE, Winch S, Barnett AG, et al. Incidence, duration and cost of futile treatment in end-of-life hospital admissions to three Australian public-sector tertiary hospitals: a retrospective multicentre cohort study. BMJ Open. 2017;7(10):e017661.
3. Mack JW, Cronin A, Taback N, et al. End-of-life care discussions among patients with advanced cancer: a cohort study. Ann Intern Med. 2012;156(3):204–10.
4. Brinkman-Stoppelenburg A, Rietjens JAC, van der Heide A. The effects of advance care planning on end-of-life care: a systematic review. Palliat Med. 2014;28(8):1000–25.
5. MacKenzie MA, Smith-Howell E, Bomba PA, Meghani SH. Respecting choices and related models of advance care planning: a systematic review of published evidence. Am J Hosp Palliat Care. 2018;35(6):897–907.
6. Scott IA, Mitchell GK, Reymond EJ, Daly MP. Difficult but necessary conversations—the case for advance care planning. Med J Aust. 2013;199:662–6.
7. Romo RD, Lynn J. The utility and value of the "surprise question" for patients with serious illness. CMAJ. 2017;189:E1072–3.
8. Scott IA, Rajakaruna N, Shah D, et al. Normalising advance care planning in a general medicine service of a tertiary hospital: an exploratory study. Aust Health Rev. 2016;40(4):391–8.
9. Scott IA, Reymond E, Sansome X, Miller L. A whole of community program of advance care planning for end-of-life care. Aust Health Rev. 2022;46(4):442–9.

Just Because a Treatment Is Available, Does Not Mean That It Must Be Given

Jia Hao Hui and Benny Katz

1 Clinical Pearl

Treat the person who has the disease, not just the disease. The person's values and preference should be given the highest priority.

2 Clinical Case

PL, a frail gentleman in his 80s from a residential aged care facility (RACF), was sent to the emergency department (ED) with productive cough and fever, unable to swallow antibiotics prescribed by his General Practitioner (GP). He was diagnosed with aspiration pneumonia, commenced on 1 g intravenous ceftriaxone, made nil-by-mouth, and referred to the medical team for admission.

His eldest daughter arrived in ED stating that she did not want her father to be treated with antibiotics, as this was his third episode of aspiration pneumonia in the last 6 months. She stated that he had never fully recovered following each episode and had experienced significant physical and functional decline leading to a poor quality of life. PL was too drowsy to engage in the discussion. A copy of his Advance Care Directive (ACD) was obtained from his RACF. It appointed his daughter as his Medical Treatment Decision Maker (MTDM) and stated that he would prefer to

J. H. Hui
Department of Geriatric Medicine, Austin Health, Melbourne, VIC, Australia

B. Katz (✉)
Department of Geriatric Medicine, St. Vincent's Hospital Melbourne, Fitzroy, VIC, Australia

Faculty of Medicine, Dentistry and Health Sciences, University of Melbourne, Melbourne, VIC, Australia

R. Junckerstorff et al. (eds.), *Beyond Evidence-Based Medicine*,
https://doi.org/10.1007/978-981-99-4440-8_26

avoid hospitalisation and did not want any life-prolonging treatments. She also felt that being made nil-by-mouth adversely affected his quality of life and requested that he be permitted to sip water if he asked.

Antibiotics were ceased and he was transferred back to RACF with as-required medications for symptom management and the support of the residential in-reach team. A detailed handover was provided to RACF staff and the patient's GP. He passed away peacefully 2 days later in the presence of his loving family and familiar carers.

3 Discussion

Person-centred care is about treating a person with dignity and respect through active shared decision-making between the patient, their families, and the health-care providers, while taking into consideration their individual values, needs and preferences [1]. It involves clinicians actively seeking out to understand what is important to the person and working in partnership to plan care. Evidence shows that person-centred care improves patients', families' and health professionals' care experience and satisfaction [2].

It is important to remember that the patient is the most crucial person and should always come first. We need to ensure that their voice is heard before others, including that of their substitute decision-makers. A person is presumed to retain decision-making capacity unless there is evidence to the contrary. The presence of cognitive impairment or mental health conditions does not automatically equate to incapacity. A person is deemed to have capacity if they can understand, retain, weigh the information, and communicate their decision. The legal instruments appointing a substitute decision-maker only take effect once the patient has lost decision-making capacity.

If a person is deemed incapable of consenting or refusing treatment, such as the case of our patient, we need to establish whether they have an ACD and determine who their substitute decision-maker is. An ACD is a formal document outlining the individual's preferences for future care along with their beliefs, values and goals. A doctor must not treat a person contrary to the instructions in a valid ACD. It is not sufficient to be told about someone's ACD and its contents without sighting it. It is also recommended to obtain a copy for medical documentation purposes.

A substitute decision-maker may be one legally appointed by the person, an appointed guardian by the tribunal, or someone with a close continuing relationship with the patient (refer to Office of the Public Advocate (OPA) websites for the hierarchy of treatment decision-makers). The legislation and terminologies differ between states and territories in Australia. For instance, an appointed substitute decision-maker is called a MTDM in Victoria but an enduring guardian in News South Wales and Tasmania.

Once the substitute decision-maker is identified, it is the responsibility of health professionals to discuss treatment options, including that of no treatment, and follow their directions. Doctors are not obliged to provide treatment that is unreasonable or thought to be not in line with the patient's wishes. In the presence of conflict, it is recommended to seek further advice from the OPA.

Our patient was not capable of consenting or refusing treatment for pneumonia as he was unable to engage in the discussion. It was apparent from his ACD, and the opinion of his MTDM, that he would have found treatment with antibiotics and being made nil-by-mouth distressing and not consistent with his goals and personal preferences.

4 Other Gems

- Health care professionals are responsible for providing information about the risks, benefits and alternatives of a given treatment so that the person or substitute decision-maker can make an informed decision.
- Primacy of patient's preferences and values stands true even if they do not align with those of the healthcare professionals; it is important to consider and address potential issues related to diversity including their culture (i.e. Aboriginal and Torres Strait Islander people, culturally and linguistically diverse people), sexuality (i.e., LGBTQIA+) and spirituality.
- Written information, diagrams and decision-making tools can be helpful to support the shared decision-making process.
- Goals of care do not simply entail a narrow definition of resuscitation preferences, but should include decisions regarding specific treatments, intensity of treatment, and future care needs.
- There are several communication frameworks that can be helpful in assisting clinicians in having complex and sensitive conversations regarding goals of care, such as the REMAP model [3]:

  - Reframe: Provide the person with a big picture of the current situation including clinical problems, prognosis and available treatment options available with respective risks and benefits.
  - Expect emotion: Acknowledge emotions and express empathy.
  - Map out goals: Encourage the person to think about what is important to them with open-ended questions (i.e., "what matters most to you in life?", "what is an unacceptable outcome for you?").
  - Align with goals: Reflect on the person's goals and offer options aligned with the goals, based on best clinical evidence.
  - Propose plans: With the person's permission, propose a care plan that is in line with their values.

- There are often many options available, including no treatment, and there is no right or wrong decision.

References

1. International Alliance of Patients' Organizations. What is patient-centred health care? A review of definitions and principles. 2nd ed. London: IAPO; 2007. p. 1–34.
2. Australian Commission on Safety and Quality in Health Care. Patient-centred care: improving quality and safety through partnerships with patients and consumers. Sydney: ACSQHC; 2011.
3. Childers JW, Back AL, Tulsky JA, Arnold RM. REMAP: a framework for goals of care conversations. J Oncol Pract. 2017;13(10):e844–50.

Shared Decision Making in the End-of-Life Setting

Catherine Gibb

1 Clinical Pearl

Sometimes the cure is worse than the disease.

2 Clinical Case

Graham was a 68-year-old man. He lived alone and was close to his only daughter who lived a 5-minute drive away.

Graham had a complex medical history. He was a lifelong smoker and had significant chronic obstructive pulmonary disease (COPD) which limited his exercise tolerance to 5 minutes only. He was on treatment for hypertension and used inhaled therapy for his COPD.

He was also a head and neck cancer survivor.

He had undergone a mandibulectomy with bilateral neck dissections and reconstruction with a fibular free flap 10 years ago. He had then experienced a further complication of infection requiring removal of the mandibular plate 5 years later. On both occasions he had spent many weeks in hospital and in recovery. His speech was dysarthric and at times he was difficult to understand. This, along with his concerns about facial disfigurement, significantly limited his social interactions. He was able to maintain his nutrition orally with a soft moist diet, but his body mass index (BMI) had only reached a maximum of 22 since his surgery 10 years ago.

Graham had recently developed a tongue base cancer. By the time he was seen he had developed further difficulty in swallowing and had lost more weight with a current BMI of only 19.

C. Gibb (✉)
Royal Adelaide Hospital, Adelaide, SA, Australia

R. Junckerstorff et al. (eds.), *Beyond Evidence-Based Medicine*,
https://doi.org/10.1007/978-981-99-4440-8_27

His planned surgery was a total glossectomy with prolonged post-operative radiotherapy thereafter. He would be dependent on a feeding tube possibly for ever, and his speech, already poor, would be worse.

Surgery was booked for the following week after extensive discussion with the surgical team.

He was referred for a physician led review to optimise his fitness for surgery given his underlying pulmonary disease.

During the physician led consultation, Graham asked what would happen if he did not have surgery. This led to a discussion about what Graham felt was important and his goals of care.

He revealed that he did not want to spend more time in hospital. Furthermore, he thought the consequences of the planned surgery on his ability to eat, but more importantly to communicate, were unacceptable. To Graham, death was less feared than what he saw as a miserable future.

A shared decision-making process was then undertaken and Graham's treatment plan was changed from radical dual modality therapy with a goal of cure to palliative single modality therapy with radiotherapy as an outpatient, and a referral to the palliative care service to assist in end of life goal setting and planning.

3 Discussion

It is very easy when dealing with cancer to focus on cure. Sometimes however, the consequences of treatment are such that they are incompatible with the patient's wishes.

Some people also have lived the experience of medical interventions which colours their decision making [1].

It is also known that good palliative care, which can include surgery, improves overall outcome both in quality of life and mood [2].

The recognition of the trajectories of death at the end of life are also important in helping people discuss 'what is important to them'. For Graham, a trajectory of maintaining current quality of life with a short final illness was preferable to a longer life but with a future death from frailty.

The concept of trajectories of decline towards death were first described in 2003 [3].

There were four trajectories of death outlined in this original work.

- Sudden death, such as occurs with a major myocardial infarction or stroke.
- Terminal illness, with death occurring in a few short months after diagnosis, such as an aggressive cancer.
- Organ failure, as might be seen with a chronic disease such as heart failure. In this case the end-of-life period may last months to years but is characterised by stepwise declines, where a period of illness or hospitalisation results in a worsened functional outcome until the final illness is not survived.

– Frailty, where the functional decline may last many years without a formal life ending event. In the trajectory of frailty, the end point that may need to be considered is needing long term institutional care, not death.

Being able to articulate these trajectories can help inform discussions with patients who are exploring their own personal wishes for end-of-life care.

4 Other Gems

- Open discussions of patient goals, an understanding of their past health care experience, an openness to discuss trajectories of dying and an understanding of the role of good palliative care can have significant impacts on patient decision making in complex settings.

References

1. Gawande A. Being mortal. London: Profile Books Ltd; 2014.
2. Temel J, Greer J, Muzikansky A, Gallagher E, Admane S, Jackson V, et al. Early palliative care for patients with metastatic non-small-cell lung cancer. N Engl J Med. 2010;363:733–42.
3. Lunney J, Lynn J, Foley D, Lipson S, Guralnik J. Patterns of functional decline at the end of life. JAMA. 2003;289(18):2387–92.

Approaching Goals of Care Discussions at the End of Life

Cathy Corbett

1 Clinical Pearl

> Discussing goals of care is an important communication task, which ideally should happen early and often in the course of illness. In reality, it often takes place in a time of crisis during a hospital admission. Within this context, it is important to recognise dying as it can be helpful to shift the focus to a conversation about dying and how that will be managed.

2 Clinical Case

A 73-year-old female is admitted to the general medical unit with a progressive decline in her conscious state and physical function over the last 3 weeks. She is normally able to mobilise with a gait aid but has been bed bound for the last 2 days. This is on the background of frontotemporal dementia, for which she has required care in a nursing home for the last 4 years. She occasionally recognises her children and has minimal verbal communication at baseline. Investigations do not reveal any infective source and a CT brain has no new pathology. Bloods show a sodium of 162 mmol/L (normal 135–145 mmol/L), urea 15 mmol/L (normal 3–8 mmol/L) and creatinine 130 micromol/L (normal 50–110 micromol/L) from a normal baseline 2 months ago.

A goals of care discussion takes place in the emergency department. The family request that all medical intervention, including intubation and cardiopulmonary resuscitation, be available as their mum was walking only a few days prior. On review the next morning she is minimally responsive and the general medical

C. Corbett (✉)
Department of General Medicine, Alfred Health, Melbourne, VIC, Australia

Department of Palliative Care, Alfred Health, Melbourne, VIC, Australia

R. Junckerstorff et al. (eds.), *Beyond Evidence-Based Medicine*,
https://doi.org/10.1007/978-981-99-4440-8_28

consultant feels that she is dying. The medical registrar has a further conversation regarding goals of care with the family and again they request all available medical intervention.

A family meeting occurs later that day with her two daughters and the medical team led by the consultant. On further exploration, she has lost interest in eating over the last few months, with a resultant loss of weight. Dementia was diagnosed 10 years ago and when the patient's values are explored through her daughters, they state that she had told them that she would not want to live if she could not care for herself and would ideally like to die at home. This presents an opportunity to explain to the daughters that their mum is in fact dying. With this information they are keen to explore how to care for their mother at home at the end-of-her life rather than in her nursing home. The patient is discharged the next day to the care of her daughters supported by the community palliative care team and dies 2 days later.

3 Discussion

Discussing an individual's goals and values for their healthcare should ideally take place outside of a medical crisis. This would happen early and often in the course of a life-limiting diagnosis, allowing time for patients to understand their illness. They could then make informed decisions based on their stated goals, values and preferences and within the context of their illness. This is particularly important for those with a diagnosis of dementia when discussions and documentation of values in an advance care plan are only possible early in the illness.

In reality, goals of care (GOC) discussions often happen in hospital during an acute event or a change in health status. In this setting clinicians often tend to focus solely on preferences for specific interventions such as resuscitation. However, it is still important to use these conversations to explore goals, preferences and values so that we as health professionals can help guide decisions on specific interventions that align with these expressed goals. As illustrated in our case, this can help focus the interaction and bring clarity to the situation.

These conversations always rely on high-quality clinical assessment and good communication skills, and this is even more important when discussing dying [1]. When we identify that a person is in the last days of life, a GOC discussion should focus on preparing the patient and family for this. If there is acceptance that the patient is dying and the goal is for comfort, then a specific discussion about medical interventions such as resuscitation is not beneficial [2]. The focus should instead emphasise the things that can be done to provide a comfortable death, and not on the things that we will not offer. Identifying that a person is imminently dying also allows for discussion of preferences such as place of care and place of death.

4 Other Gems

- Good communication can enhance the quality of care we provide whilst also improving patient and family satisfaction [3].
- Ideally, GOC discussions should be initiated by a health professional that knows the patient well and has had enduring involvement in their care.
- Discussion regarding an individual's goals and preferences, specifically in relation to end-of-life, is linked to a reduction in hospital presentations, decreased interventions at the end-of-life and a greater likelihood of receiving goal concordant care in the preferred location [4].
- GOC discussions often require more than a single conversation and may evolve as the clinical situation changes. It is important to acknowledge that these discussions often evolve and need to be revisited.
- Communication skills can be taught and practised, and we should routinely reflect on our interactions and ask for feedback [5].

References

1. Virdun C, Luckett T, Davidson PM, et al. Dying in the hospital setting: a systematic review of quantitative studies identifying the elements of end-of-life care that patients and their families rank as being most important. Palliat Med. 2014;29(9):774–96.
2. Hayes B. Clinical model for ethical cardiopulmonary resuscitation decision making. Int Med J. 2013;43(1):77–83.
3. Roter DL, Hall JA, Kern LR, et al. Improving physicians' interviewing skills and reducing patients' emotional distress. A randomised clinical trial. Arch Intern Med. 1995;155(17):1877–84.
4. Wright AA, Zang B, Ray A, et al. Associations between end-of-life discussions, patient mental health, medical care near death, and caregiver bereavement adjustment. JAMA. 2008;300:1665–73.
5. VITALtalk. Address goals of care. 2021. https://www.vitaltalk.org/topics/reset-goals-of-care/.

A Multimodal Approach to Managing Chronic Breathlessness

Cathy Corbett

1 Clinical Pearl

Breathlessness is a common and debilitating symptom in both end stage malignancy and chronic disease. A thorough assessment is not only essential to optimise treatment of the underlying condition, but also to tailor an individualised symptom management plan.

2 Clinical Case

A 68-year-old female is seen in the palliative care clinic along with her husband. She has moderate chronic obstructive pulmonary disease (COPD) and is referred by haematology for optimisation of her breathlessness. Recent pulmonary function tests (PFTs) show an FEV1/FVC ratio of 0.47 (normal 0.75–0.85) with an FEV1 of 1 L (57% predicted). Her last CT chest demonstrated severe bilateral emphysema. Of note, is a haemoglobin of 84 g/L (normal 115–165 g/L) in the setting of known multiple myeloma, currently for surveillance. Inhaler technique is good on maximal therapy.

Breathlessness has been present for some years but has progressed in the last 6–12 months. A year ago, she could do some gardening, but now struggles to leave the house. Breathlessness even on dressing is described, equating to a score of 4 on the Modified Medical Research Council dyspnoea scale (see Table 1) [1]. Her husband feels that they are managing and has declined any additional help. There is no breathlessness overnight and no evidence of anxiety or depression. She has not had

C. Corbett (✉)
Department of General Medicine, Alfred Health, Melbourne, VIC, Australia

Department of Palliative Care, Alfred Health, Melbourne, VIC, Australia

R. Junckerstorff et al. (eds.), *Beyond Evidence-Based Medicine*,
https://doi.org/10.1007/978-981-99-4440-8_29

Table 1 Modified Medical Research Council (mMRC) dyspnoea scale [1]

Grade	Description of breathlessness
0	I only get breathless with strenuous exercise
1	I get short of breath when hurrying on level ground or walking up a slight hill
2	On level ground, I walk slower than people of the same age because of breathlessness, or have to stop for breath when walking at my own pace
3	I stop for breath after walking about 100 yards or after a few minutes on level ground
4	I am too breathless to leave the house or I am breathless when dressing

an infective exacerbation of her COPD recently. Completion of pulmonary rehabilitation was within the last 2 years. There is no hypoxia at rest or on exertion.

On review it is felt that the patient has chronic breathlessness related to her COPD, deconditioning and anaemia as a result of her myeloma. A blood transfusion is arranged to optimise her underlying medical issues. An explanation of chronic breathlessness is provided using the 'Breathing, Thinking, Functioning' model [2]. This is complemented with written information regarding non-pharmacological management of breathlessness, including specific postures, breathing techniques and a hand-held fan. A preliminary discussion relating to the use of oral morphine, if needed, once these other factors are optimised also takes place. Ongoing clinic review is arranged for 6 weeks' time.

3 Discussion

Breathlessness can be described as 'an uncomfortable awareness of breathing'. It is a subjective symptom which may not correlate with measurable abnormalities such as hypoxia. Breathlessness is complex with many factors involved, including physiological (increased ventilatory demand and impaired ventilation), psychological, emotional, social, and environmental. Chronic breathlessness is breathlessness that persists beyond 4–8 weeks despite optimal treatment of the underlying pathology. It has a multidimensional impact on the person and family.

Dyspnoea is a common symptom in those with an advanced life-threatening illness and in severe COPD has a prevalence of 90–95% [3]. Effective assessment of dyspnoea is essential and we can measure intensity in the clinical setting using a numeric rating scale (0–10). We can supplement this by using the Modified Medical Research Council (mMRC) Dyspnoea Scale (see Table 1). It is simple to use and allows the patient to indicate the extent to which their breathlessness impacts their mobility.

Our patient has grade 4 symptoms indicating severe impairment which is distressing and debilitating. The Breathing, Thinking, Functioning model can be used as an educational tool to help patients understand their breathlessness (see Fig. 1). The model illustrates emotional and behavioural responses to dyspnoea which can lead to a cycle of worsening symptoms. It can help to conceptualise how a focus on

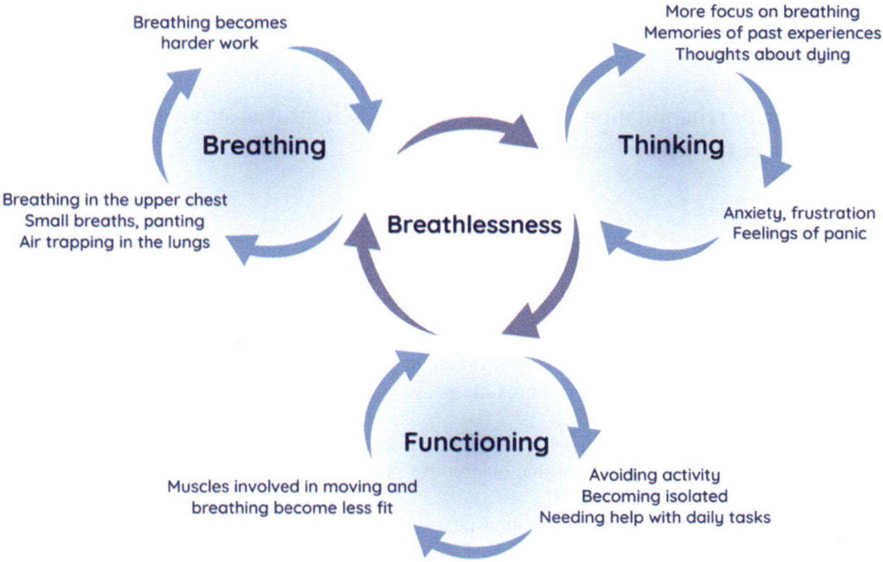

Fig. 1 The Breathing, Thinking, Functioning clinical model [2]

physical activity (including exercise and pacing) and breathing techniques can be useful to break the cycle [4]. Common breathing techniques that can be coached focus on slowing the breathing with breaths in through the nose and out through the mouth, aiming to make the out breath as long as possible [5]. A hand-held fan held about 15 cm from the face and aimed at the cheeks, nose and mouth can also be used during an acute episode.

For those with ongoing high symptom burden despite the measures described opioids can be considered. Sustained-release morphine is the most widely studied drug and at low doses (10–20 mg/day) is shown to reduce breathlessness [6]. It is safest to start during a period of clinical stability with constipation being the main side effect at low doses.

4 Other Gems

- It is important to determine the underlying cause of breathlessness and regularly review its management.
- Anxiety is common in advanced illness, and we should always screen for psychological factors.
- Benzodiazepines have not been shown to improve breathlessness in the absence of anxiety.
- In non-hypoxaemic patients, supplemental oxygen does not improve breathlessness.

- Long term oxygen therapy: 15 hours/day via a concentrator for those that are hypoxaemic, provides a survival benefit but may not improve chronic breathlessness.
- Pulmonary rehabilitation for those with COPD improves survival and improves dyspnoea, fatigue and well-being.

References

1. Mahler DA, Wells CK. Evaluation of clinical methods for rating dyspnea. Chest. 1988;93(3):580.
2. Spathis A, Booth S, Moffat C, et al. The breathing, thinking, functioning clinical model: a proposal to facilitate evidence-based breathlessness management in chronic respiratory disease. Prim Care Resp Med. 2017;27:27.
3. Solano IP, Gomes B, Higginson IJ. A comparison of symptom prevalence in far advanced cancer, AIDS, heart disease, chronic obstructive pulmonary disease and renal disease. J Pain Symptom Manag. 2006;31(1):58.
4. Booth S, Chin C, Spathis A et al. Non-pharmacological interventions for breathlessness in people with cancer. Expert Rev Qual Life Cancer Care. 2018. https://doi.org/10.1080/23809000.2018.1524708.
5. INSPIRE. Managing breathlessness. 2022. https://inspirebreathingbetter.com/managing-breathlessness.
6. Abernethy AP, Currow DC, Frith P, et al. Randomised, double blind, placebo controlled crossover trail of sustained release morphine for the management of refractory dyspnoea. BMJ. 2003;327:523.

Approach to Respiratory Secretions at the End of Life

Jamie Parker-Smith and Cathy Corbett

1 Clinical Pearl

Respiratory secretions at the end of life can be difficult to manage and are often distressing for families; non-pharmacological treatment should be trialled before carefully considering a pharmacological approach.

2 Clinical Case

A 52-year-old woman with metastatic breast cancer, including leptomeningeal disease, is in the terminal phase of her illness. She has been settled with a syringe driver of morphine 30 mg and midazolam 10 mg over 24 hours but has developed noisy breathing. Her husband is distressed by this and asks if it is possible to stop the 'death rattle'. Nursing staff have requested that glycopyrrolate be added to the syringe driver to 'dry up her secretions'.

The palliative care consultant speaks with the husband away from the bedside; she explains the cause of his wife's audible breathing and reassures him that she is deeply asleep and does not look distressed by it. Potential side effects of anti-muscarinic medications are discussed and acknowledgement is made that his wife is nearing the end of her life. The husband agrees to a trial of repositioning, which is carried out shortly after a dose of subcutaneous midazolam 5 mg is given. The

J. Parker-Smith
Department of General Medicine, Alfred Health, Melbourne, VIC, Australia

C. Corbett (✉)
Department of General Medicine, Alfred Health, Melbourne, VIC, Australia

Department of Palliative Care, Alfred Health, Melbourne, VIC, Australia

R. Junckerstorff et al. (eds.), *Beyond Evidence-Based Medicine*,
https://doi.org/10.1007/978-981-99-4440-8_30

patient's secretions drain without the need for medication and her breathing is less audible. She dies peacefully a few hours later with her husband by her side.

3 Discussion

Towards the end of life, many patients are too weak and/or unconscious to swallow their own saliva and/or mucus. There may also be a diminished cough reflex. This can cause noisy or gurgling breathing, commonly referred to as the 'death rattle', when air is drawn through the secretions that have pooled in the upper airway. The death rattle is not usually distressing for the terminal patient [1], however it is often disturbing for family, as well as for some medical staff. Evidence regarding treatment with anti-muscarinic or anti-cholinergic mediations, such as glycopyrrolate bromide or hyoscine hydrobromide is lacking [1–3]. Despite this, they are often started in an attempt to help manage secretions, without consideration of less harmful non-pharmacological options.

In the first instance, it is important to reassure family and carers that the death rattle is a normal part of the dying process. An explanation as to the cause and reassurance that their loved one is unlikely to be distressed is often enough to allay their fears.

A non-pharmacological approach can be effective, although good quality evidence is needed [2]. Techniques include gentle repositioning of the patient into a semi-recumbent position, or a temporary raising of the lower end of the bed to encourage postural drainage [4]. Nursing staff should be encouraged to use analgesia and/or anxiolytic medications, as required, before re-positioning patients.

Anti-muscarinics may be trialled if secretions persist, do not respond to repositioning, or continue to cause distress for patients. Such agents can be administered as needed initially, or via a syringe driver if proven to be effective. Anti-muscarinic drugs do not clear secretions that already exist, instead act to suppress ongoing production of saliva [2], and their use can have significant adverse effects. It is important to consider the side-effects of antimuscarinic medications; they can contribute to delirium, agitation and confusion, and can also cause urinary retention. Placement of an indwelling urinary catheter in such instances will negate potential distress from urinary retention at the end of life. Not all patients respond to the use of anti-muscarinics; it is important to monitor closely for adverse effects as the dying patient may be unable to communicate these, and to discontinue their use if ineffective.

Communication with families and nursing staff as to the cause of noisy respiratory secretions at the end of life is essential. A trial of non-pharmacological techniques should be attempted before considering use of pharmacological agents, which often come with adverse effects as described.

4 Other Gems

- Evidence of superiority of one anti-muscarinic drug over another in the treatment of airway secretions at the end of life is not conclusive [1, 5].
- Attempt to establish, where possible, if the secretions are salivary (thin) or mucous (thick); use of anti-muscarinics are less effective in addressing bronchial secretions and may worsen the clinical picture [5].
- Anti-muscarinic medications are likely to be more effective if given at the beginning of the death rattle, so as to suppress further secretions as early as possible. There is some evidence that prophylactic administration may be effective in preventing the 'death rattle' [6].
- It is important to consider adverse effects of anti-muscarinic medications in patients with renal failure; dose reduction is recommended, and/or consideration of a non-pharmacological approach.
- Suctioning of oropharyngeal secretions can be distressing for patients at the end of life; utilisation should be carefully considered and minimised with avoidance of deep suctioning where possible.
- Glycopyrrolate does not cross the blood brain barrier, and thus causes less adverse effects relating to the central nervous system [4].
- Good mouth care is imperative at the end of life, especially when using anti-muscarinic agents that can cause significant dry mouth.
- The death rattle can have a long-lasting negative impact on caregivers; addressing their perceptions early will limit their distress.

References

1. Lokker ME, van Zuylen L, van der Rijt CC, et al. Prevalence, impact, and treatment of death rattle: a systematic review. J Pain Symptom Manage. 2014;47(1):105–22.
2. Kolb H, Snowden A, Stevens E. Systematic review and narrative summary: treatments for and risk factors associated with respiratory tract secretions (death rattle) in the dying adult. J Adv Nurs. 2018;74(7):1446–62.
3. Campbell ML, Yarandi HN. Death rattle is not associated with patient respiratory distress: is pharmacologic treatment indicated? J Palliat Med. 2014;16(10):1255–9.
4. National Institute for Health and Care Excellence. Palliative care: secretions. 2021. https://www.nice.org.uk/cks-uk-only. Accessed 5 Oct 2022.
5. Bennett M, Lucas V, Brennan M, et al. Using anti-muscarinic drugs in the management of death rattle: evidence-based guidelines for palliative care. Palliat Med. 2002;16(5):369–74.
6. van Esch HJ, van Zuylen L, Geijteman E, et al. Effect of prophylactic subcutaneous scopolamine butylbromide on death rattle in patients at the end of life: the SILENCE Randomized Clinical Trial. JAMA. 2021;326(13):1268–76.

Medication Management in Parkinson's Disease

Jamie Parker-Smith and Cathy Corbett

1 Clinical Pearl

It is important to replace Parkinson's disease medications in those unable to swallow as abrupt withdrawal can cause unpleasant and sometimes severe symptoms.

2 Clinical Case

An 86-year-old gentleman with advanced Parkinson's disease (PD) and related dementia presents with marked functional decline. He has been bed bound for 10 days and his swallowing is impaired. He has had no oral intake for 2 days, nor has he been able to take any of his regular medications including levodopa 100mg and benserazide 25 mg (Madopar), four times daily.

He presents as intermittently agitated, with rigid limbs and occasional dry retching. After discussion with his family, and acknowledgement that he is approaching the end of his life, the decision is made to focus on comfort measures. His Madopar dose is replaced with a transdermal rotigotine patch of 4 mg/24 hrs, and within 12 hours he is more settled and less rigid. He is also given sublingual ondansetron 8 mg for nausea to good effect.

J. Parker-Smith
Department of General Medicine, Alfred Health, Melbourne, VIC, Australia

C. Corbett (✉)
Department of General Medicine, Alfred Health, Melbourne, VIC, Australia

Department of Palliative Care, Alfred Health, Melbourne, VIC, Australia

R. Junckerstorff et al. (eds.), *Beyond Evidence-Based Medicine*,
https://doi.org/10.1007/978-981-99-4440-8_31

3 Discussion

Advanced PD is often complex, with a multitude of symptoms which can be challenging to manage. Dysphagia is a common part of advanced PD, and as such many patients become unable to take their usual treatment.

Sudden cessation of dopaminergic agents can have many consequences, including rigidity and pain, anxiety, agitation and nausea [1, 2]. There is also a rare but significant risk of parkinsonism-hyperpyrexia syndrome [3]. These symptoms can cause significant distress for the both the patient and their carers, particularly at the end of life, as demonstrated with our patient. It is thus important to avoid unnecessary and unpleasant symptoms by replacing oral dopaminergic medications in patients who are unable to swallow for more than 24 hours [4].

Rotigotine transdermal patches can be used as a daily replacement and take 15–17 hours to reach peak plasma concentration [5]. Recommendations for dose conversions can be quite variable depending on which conversion ratio is followed [6, 7]. Administration of too high a dose can also cause symptoms such as confusion and agitation. For our patient we used a more conservative dose to good effect and would advise to start at a lower dose and titrate to symptoms. Using one conversion rate for consistency within teams to avoid confusion is also recommended.

4 Other Gems

- When converting to rotigotine transdermal patches, dose reduction is also necessary in patients with severe liver impairment.
- Care must also be taken when treating nausea and vomiting; it is well established that dopamine receptor antagonist antiemetics, such as metoclopramide and haloperidol, can cause drug-induced parkinsonism and should not be used. Alternatives include oral domperidone, sublingual or intravenous ondansetron, and oral or subcutaneous cyclizine.
- Delirium in advanced PD is often multifactorial. Choice of treatment is important as many anti-psychotic medications may also aggravate parkinsonism. Quetiapine is considered to have the lowest risk.
- Patients with advanced PD at the end of life can suffer with rigidity despite use of levodopa equivalents; in refractory cases midazolam used subcutaneously prn, or via a syringe driver, is often effective in relieving distressing rigidity.
- Prolonged rigidity can be painful, and use of appropriate analgesia should be considered.
- Patients with a nasogastric tube or percutaneous endoscopic gastrostomy tube can utilise dispersible Parkinson medications.
- Carer distress is often significant in advanced PD and must be addressed appropriately.
- Conversion calculators can also be used to convert other PD drugs such as carbidopa and levodopa (Sinamet) and pramiprexole [6].

References

1. Richfield EW, Jones EJ, Alty JE. Palliative care for Parkinson's disease: a summary of the evidence and future directions. Palliat Med. 2013;27(9):805–10.
2. Nirenberg MJ. Dopamine agonist withdrawal syndrome: implications for patient care. Drugs Aging. 2013;30:587–92.
3. Newman EJ, Grosset DG, Kennedy PG. The parkinsonism-hyperpyrexia syndrome. Neurocrit Care. 2009;10(1):136–40.
4. Chung SJ, Asgharnejad M, Bauer L, et al. Switching from an oral dopamine receptor agonist to rotigotine transdermal patch: a review of clinical data with a focus on patient perspective. Expert Rev Neurother. 2017;17(7):737–49.
5. Rotigotine. Aust Prescr. 2008;31:49–55.
6. Northumbria Healthcare NHS Foundation Trust Parkinson's Disease Team PD 'Nil by Mouth' medication dose calculator. 2014. http://pdmedcalc.co.uk/. Accessed 16 Oct 2022.
7. Managing a patient with Parkinson disease who is nil-by-mouth. Melbourne: Therapeutic Guidelines Limited; 2021. https://www.tg.org.au. Accessed 16 Oct 2022.

Liver Disease and Opioid Prescribing

Cathy Corbett

1 Clinical Pearl

While it is important to review all medications a patient is taking, particular attention should be paid to the use of controlled-release oxycodone-with-naloxone (Targin®) in those with liver pathology.

2 Clinical Case

A 59-year-old man is referred to the palliative care clinic for assessment and management of abdominal pain that is not responding to opioids. His past medical history is significant for advanced hepatocellular carcinoma. This occurs on the background of compensated cirrhosis (Child Pugh A) due to past hepatitis C infection. He describes significant right upper quadrant abdominal pain despite escalating doses of controlled-release (CR) oxycodone-with-naloxone (Targin®), currently 40 mg/20 mg bd. He gets no relief from oxycodone immediate release (Endone®) 10 mg. His liver function tests reveal a Bilirubin of 25 μmol/L (normal < 20 μmol/L), ALT 47 units/L (normal < 35 units/L), AST 52 units/L (normal < 40 units/L), GGT 55 units/L (normal < 50 units/L) and ALP 90 units/L (normal 30–110 units/L). His INR is 1.2 (normal 0.8–1.1) and his albumin is 43 g/L (normal 32–45 g/L).

The controlled-release oxycodone-with-naloxone is ceased and controlled-release oxycodone (OxyContin®) 20 mg twice daily is commenced. Although this is a 50% dose reduction, within 2 days the patient's abdominal pain significantly improves.

C. Corbett (✉)
Department of General Medicine, Alfred Health, Melbourne, VIC, Australia

Department of Palliative Care, Alfred Health, Melbourne, VIC, Australia

R. Junckerstorff et al. (eds.), *Beyond Evidence-Based Medicine*,
https://doi.org/10.1007/978-981-99-4440-8_32

3 Discussion

Oxycodone-with-naloxone CR tablets contain a combination of a strong opioid and an opioid antagonist, naloxone, in a CR formulation. The tablets are equivalent in strength to oxycodone CR with the same duration of action of approximately 12 h.

The combination of oxycodone CR with naloxone has been marketed as a strong opioid with a reduced risk of opioid-induced constipation. The tablets deliver a naloxone dose that blocks opioid receptors in the gut, but not elsewhere, and hence reduces gastrointestinal side effects such as constipation [1]. Naloxone undergoes extensive first-pass metabolism in the liver, so negligible amounts reach the systemic circulation and hence it has a minimal effect on analgesia. Its oral bioavailability in healthy people is less than 3% but oxycodone-with-naloxone CR is contraindicated in moderate to severe liver disease (Child-Pugh B-C).

Our patient has mild liver disease, but extensive hepatocellular carcinoma. In clinical practice it has been observed that hepatocellular carcinoma or liver metastases appear to be associated with reduced analgesia when CR oxycodone-with-naloxone is prescribed, even with relatively normal liver function tests. Published cases suggest that reduced first-pass metabolism results in higher concentrations of naloxone reaching the systemic circulation resulting in antagonism of the analgesic effect of the opioid [2, 3]. If a patient is changed from CR oxycodone-with-naloxone to a single opioid formulation, it is imperative to start with a lower equivalent dose (a 50% dose reduction in this case), and monitor closely for opioid toxicity. Failing to do this, can increase the risk of opioid overdose.

4 Other Gems

- Clinical trial data for CR oxycodone-with-naloxone is largely from people with chronic musculoskeletal pain and not those with cancer pain.
- The naloxone component opioid-induced constipation. This is an important consideration in the cancer population, where other factors will contribute to constipation so a laxative must still be prescribed.
- CR formulations are not indicated for acute pain.
- There is no long-term efficacy data regarding the effect on constipation of CR oxycodone-with-naloxone; a key randomised controlled trial only followed patients up for 12 weeks [4].
- The maximum recommended daily dose is oxycodone 80 mg/naloxone 40 mg as higher doses have not been studied.
- For those that are opioid tolerant, CR oxycodone-with-naloxone can initially precipitate withdrawal symptoms or diarrhoea.

- The naloxone component may deter intranasal or injected use as the naloxone will antagonise the acute central nervous system effect of the oxycodone. The tablet may therefore be less appealing for illicit use but there is no trial data to confirm this.
- Reduce the dose of CR oxycodone-with-naloxone and use with caution in those with a creatinine clearance of <60 mL/min.

References

1. Mundipharma Pty Ltd. Targin product information; 12 May 2010.
2. Gelston EA, Coller J, Lopatko O, et al. A cautionary tale of oral naloxone. J Pain Symptom Manag. 2014;47(2):e1–2.
3. Kang JH, Lee GW, Shin SH, et al. Opioid withdrawal syndrome after treatment with low-dose extended-release oxycodone and naloxone in a gastric cancer patient with portal vein thrombosis. J Pain Symptom Manag. 2013;46(2):e15–7.
4. Simpson K, Leyendecker P, Hopp M, et al. Fixed-ratio combination oxycodone/naloxone compared with oxycodone alone for the relief of opioid-induced constipation in moderate-to-severe noncancer pain. Curr Med Res Opin. 2008;24:3503.

A Good Death: Respecting Goals of Care

Joseph Tan, Nicole I. Chan, and Alison M. Mudge

1 Clinical Pearl

Whilst clinicians endeavour to provide therapies that will optimise the clinical outcomes for their patients, it is also an important skill to recognise medical futility and be able to discuss it confidently and sensitively with family members or carers.

2 Clinical Case

An 81-year-old woman is admitted to hospital with rapid atrial flutter, decompensated cardiac failure and acute kidney injury. She is initially admitted under the cardiology team who treat her medically with a frusemide infusion and implant a pacemaker. Her echocardiogram shows moderate to severe aortic stenosis and severe right ventricular dilatation and impairment. The cardiology team considers her too frail for aortic valve implantation. Her exercise tolerance is very poor, and she is transferred to the Geriatric Evaluation and Management unit to titrate her oral diuretic therapy, restore her function and plan for additional support on discharge.

J. Tan
Surgical Treatment and Rehabilitation Services, Metro North Health, Brisbane, QLD, Australia

N. I. Chan
Royal Brisbane and Women's Hospital, Metro North Health, Brisbane, QLD, Australia

A. M. Mudge (✉)
Department of Internal Medicine and Aged Care, Royal Brisbane and Women's Hospital, Metro North Health, Brisbane, QLD, Australia

Medical School, The University of Queensland, Brisbane, QLD, Australia

R. Junckerstorff et al. (eds.), *Beyond Evidence-Based Medicine*,
https://doi.org/10.1007/978-981-99-4440-8_33

However, she develops progressive renal dysfunction, and any reduction in diuretics leads to rapid re-accumulation of pulmonary oedema requiring continuous oxygen therapy, causing dyspnoea and fatigue and a hypoactive delirium which severely limit her mobility and increase her risk of continuing functional decline.

A family meeting is held by the treating team, during which the patient's daughters and her husband (her enduring power of attorney) discuss her previously stated wishes, which have always been to remain independent in her own home for as long as possible and to die peacefully with her family present. In view of poor prognosis for meaningful functional gains, her family express a desire to withdraw active treatment and begin end of life care. As such, medications are commenced for symptom control: fentanyl (in view of her renal failure), midazolam and haloperidol, delivered using a subcutaneous syringe driver and titrated to comfort, maintaining a light slumber. Other medications including the diuretics are ceased and she dies on the ward with her grandchildren around her.

3 Discussion

Caring for the sick and frail comes with many privileges and responsibilities. In times of severe, intractable illness, it can bring sadness and ethical conflict for carers, families as well as health professionals in deciding the best course of action. Often there are situations where further testing or treatments become more burdensome than helpful, creating undue suffering and anguish for the patient and their family [1].

When such a tilting point is recognised, it is vital to have good rapport with patients and family/carers to be able to address this sensitively and meaningfully. Discussion held at the right time, setting and with the right people present is essential. Sometimes the patient (or family) themselves may be the ones initiating the conversation, and clinicians must be attuned to recognise this. Recognising barriers to having conversations around end-of-life (including clinician, patient, or carer factors) and navigating them through open and frank discussions with all those involved can at times be necessary [2].

A good death can be defined as one that is patient-centred and free of pain or distress. It is respectful of one's physical, emotional, and spiritual needs and has its focus on quality of life and dignity [3]. To treat symptoms at the end of life, different classes of medication are often employed (Table 1), and most usual medications are ceased, although some (e.g. antiepileptics) may be continued to reduce burdensome symptoms.

Table 1 Medications frequently used for symptom control at the end of life

Drugs	Purpose
Opiate (e.g. fentanyl, morphine)	Relieve pain or dyspnoea
Benzodiazepine (e.g. midazolam)	Relieve agitation and anxiety
Antipsychotic (e.g. haloperidol)	Relieve agitation and nausea
Anticholinergic (e.g. glycopyrrolate)	Reduce oral secretions

4 Other Gems

- Sensitive, timely communication is an important skill a doctor learns with experience (and often by observing more senior mentors).
- Prognostication around the end of life is difficult even with experienced clinicians. Whilst not precise, families often ask for (and appreciate) an estimated time a patient might have. Phrasing your answer in terms of "short" or "long" days/weeks/months can be another way of conceptualising a patient's prognosis. Tools such as the Supportive and Palliative Care Indicators Tool (SPICT™) [4] can be helpful in recognising patients in the last months of life.

References

1. Ulrich CM. End of life futility conversations: when language matters. Perspect Biol Med. 2017;60(3):433–7.
2. Australian Commission on Quality and Safety in Health Care. National consensus statement: essential elements for safe and high-quality end-of-life care. Sydney: ACSQHC. 2015. www.safetyandquality.gov.au/our-work/comprehensive-care/end-life-care/national-consensus-statement. Accessed 4 Sept 2022.
3. Meier EA, Gallegos JV, Montross-Thomas LP, Depp CA, Irwin SA, Jeste DV. Defining a good death (successful dying): literature review and a call for research and public dialogue. Am J Geriatr Psychiatry. 2016;24(4):261–71.
4. Supportive and palliative care indicators tool. https://www.spict.org.uk/. Accessed 5 Sept 2022.

Part V
Cardiovascular Medicine

Patient Adjusted Brain Natriuretic Peptide Assessment Improves Diagnostic Performance

Harry Gibbs and David Buxton

1 Clinical Pearl

B-type natriuretic peptide (BNP) and N-terminal pro-BNP (NT-proBNP) levels are lower in obesity. Normal levels of BNP and NT-proBNP are less accurate at ruling out heart failure (HF) in patients with obesity.

2 Clinical Case

A 68-year-old man presented to the Emergency Department (ED) with breathlessness on minimal exertion for the previous 2 days on a background of progressive exertional breathlessness for 6 months. He had a history of hypertension for 15 years which was currently well controlled on telmisartan, and type 2 diabetes for 10 years which was managed with metformin with good control. He had been overweight since early adult life and his current body mass index (BMI) was 37.5 kg/m^2. Physical examination demonstrated mild ankle oedema but was otherwise normal. A chest x-ray was normal. NT-proBNP was normal at 120 pg/mL. The patient was reassured that his breathlessness was unlikely to be related to his heart and he was referred to the respiratory clinic. He represented to the ED on the following day with breathlessness at rest and was admitted to hospital. Echocardiography showed normal left ventricular (LV) systolic function, normal valvular function and delayed LV relaxation. Right heart catheterisation was performed and demonstrated an

H. Gibbs (✉)
Department of General Medicine, Alfred Health, Melbourne, Australia

Monash University, Melbourne, Australia

D. Buxton
Department of General Medicine, Alfred Health, Melbourne, Australia

R. Junckerstorff et al. (eds.), *Beyond Evidence-Based Medicine*,
https://doi.org/10.1007/978-981-99-4440-8_34

elevation of the pulmonary capillary wedge pressure indicating elevated left atrial pressure. The final diagnosis was heart failure with preserved ejection fraction and his symptoms improved with therapy.

3 Discussion

Breathlessness is a common presentation and may be due to many conditions. HF is an important differential diagnosis in patients with breathlessness, as it is common and as current therapies are effective at reducing death and hospitalisation due to HF.

Heart failure is a syndrome consisting of symptoms (e.g., breathlessness and ankle swelling) that may be accompanied by signs (e.g. elevated jugular venous pressure, pulmonary crackles, and peripheral oedema) and is due to a structural and/or functional abnormality of the heart with elevated intracardiac pressures and/or inadequate cardiac output.

Natriuretic peptides, such as BNP and NT-proBNP, are released by ventricular myocytes in response to increased filling pressures. The levels of these peptides are usually elevated in HF, although they may also be elevated in other conditions, so their specificity for the diagnosis of HF is not high. The levels of BNP and NT-proBNP are usually normal in patients who do not have HF however, so their sensitivity is high, thus making them useful in ruling out heart failure [1–4]. Generally, in patients with breathlessness who do not have clinical evidence of overt heart failure, a normal BNP or NT-proBNP level makes HF very unlikely [1]. An exception to this is in patients with HF who are obese, as natriuretic peptides may be falsely low in this situation [3, 4]. The exact mechanism by which BNP and NT-proBNP levels are lower in obesity is uncertain but may be related to an increase in their clearance due to increased expression of receptors for these peptides on adipocytes [3, 4]. Conversely, other patient specific factors (such as renal failure, increasing age, atrial fibrillation and inflammation) can increase measured BNP and NT-proBNP levels independent of cardiac failure, leading to the potential misattribution of dyspnoea symptoms to HF [1, 4].

Some authors suggest that the cut-off for the upper limit of normal for BNP and NT-proBNP ranges should vary according to BMI [3] or age [2, 4] but this is not in routine use.

HF remains a clinical diagnosis with supporting laboratory or imaging investigations. A normal BNP or NT-proBNP assay makes HF unlikely but does not exclude it, particularly if obesity is present.

4 Take Home Messages

- In the correct clinical context high BNP or NT-proBNP levels are suggestive of a HF diagnosis, whereas very low levels can be used to rule out HF as a contributor to dyspnoea [1–3]
- Care should be taken to adjust the interpretation of BNP and NT-proBNP thresholds, in particular as obesity reduces circulating BNP and NT-proBNP levels [1, 3, 4].
- Renal failure, atrial fibrillation, increasing age, hyperthyroidism and inflammation are all factors which increase BNP and NT-proBNP levels, independent of HF [4].

References

1. McDonagh TA, Metra M, Adamo M, Gardner RS, Baumbach A, Böhm M, Burri H, Butler J, Čelutkienė J, Chioncel O, Cleland JGF, Coats AJS, Crespo-Leiro MG, Farmakis D, Gilard M, Heymans S, Hoes AW, Jaarsma T, Jankowska EA, Lainscak M, Lam CSP, Lyon AR, McMurray JJV, Mebazaa A, Mindham R, Muneretto C, Piepoli MF, Price S, Rosano GMC, Ruschitzka F, Skibelund AK, ESC Scientific Document Group. 2021 ESC Guidelines for the diagnosis and treatment of acute and chronic heart failure: developed by the Task Force for the diagnosis and treatment of acute and chronic heart failure of the European Society of Cardiology (ESC) With the special contribution of the Heart Failure Association (HFA) of the ESC. Eur Heart J. 2021;42(36):3599–726. https://doi.org/10.1093/eurheartj/ehab368.
2. NHFA CSANZ Heart Failure Guidelines Working Group, Atherton JJ, Sindone A, De Pasquale CG, Driscoll A, PS MD, Hopper I, Kistler PM, Briffa T, Wong J, Abhayaratna W, Thomas L, Audehm R, Newton P, O'Loughlin J, Branagan M, Connell C. National Heart Foundation of Australia and Cardiac Society of Australia and New Zealand: guidelines for the Prevention, Detection, and Management of Heart Failure in Australia 2018. Heart Lung Circ. 2018;27(10):1123–208. https://doi.org/10.1016/j.hlc.2018.06.1042. PMID: 30077227.
3. Kozhuharov N, Martin J, Wussler D, Lopez-Ayala P, Belkin M, Strebel I, Flores D, Diebold M, Shrestha S, Nowak A, Gualandro DM, Michou E, Zimmermann T, Rentsch K, von Eckardstein A, Keller DI, Breidthardt T, Mueller C, BASEL V Investigators. Clinical effect of obesity on N-terminal pro-B-type natriuretic peptide cut-off concentrations for the diagnosis of acute heart failure. Eur J Heart Fail. 2022;24(9):1545–54. https://doi.org/10.1002/ejhf.2618. Epub 2022 Aug 8. PMID: 35851710.
4. Nishikimi T, Nakagawa Y. Potential pitfalls when interpreting plasma BNP levels in heart failure practice. J Cardiol. 2021;78(4):269–74. https://doi.org/10.1016/j.jjcc.2021.05.00.

Heart Failure with Preserved Ejection Fraction: You Don't Know What You Don't Look for

David Buxton and Harry Gibbs

1 Clinical Pearl

Cardiac amyloid is surprisingly common in patients with heart failure with preserved ejection fraction.

2 Clinical Case

76-year-old man was seen in falls clinic, due to recurrent syncope. His past medical history is significant for bilateral total knee replacement, hypertension, heart failure with persevered ejection fraction (HFpEF), and paroxysmal atrial fibrillation (AF). The AF and heart failure were diagnosed 6 months prior after presentation to hospital following a fall with head strike. A permanent pacemaker (PPM) was inserted during that admission for symptomatic pauses identified on telemetry. At this time his troponin was noted to be slightly elevated. Echocardiography demonstrated significant concentric left ventricular remodelling with a hyperdynamic ejection fraction (65%) and a dilated left atrium. There was no significant valvopathy, nor any regional wall motion abnormalities. There was concurrent mild pulmonary hypertension and right ventricular hypertrophy. His documented medications included metoprolol, amlodipine and apixaban.

Despite the insertion of a PPM, the patient continued to experience frequent orthostatic symptoms, reporting dizziness and light-headedness about 1–2 minutes

D. Buxton
Department of General Medicine, Alfred Health, Melbourne, Australia

H. Gibbs (✉)
Department of General Medicine, Alfred Health, Melbourne, Australia

Monash University, Melbourne, Australia

R. Junckerstorff et al. (eds.), *Beyond Evidence-Based Medicine*,
https://doi.org/10.1007/978-981-99-4440-8_35

after standing up, and two episodes of micturition syncope. He reported feeling increasingly fatigued since discharge and had self-ceased amlodipine recently with some improvement in his postural symptoms. Interrogation of the PPM revealed good device function without any significant arrhythmia.

On examination, he was low-normotensive (107/64 mmHg) with a symptomatic 20 mmHg postural drop after 2 minutes. There were no murmurs nor bruits. The jugular venous pressure was elevated and there was mild peripheral oedema, suggestive of right heart failure. The apex beat was not displaced. An electrocardiogram (ECG) demonstrated an intermittently paced rhythm, 68 bpm, with a right bundle brunch block pattern and normal QRS complexes. There were no ischaemic changes.

A neurological examination was negative for features of Parkinsonism; however, a length dependant sensory neuropathy was identified. HbA1c, lipid profile, thyroid function, serum protein electrophoresis, vasculitis screen, and micronutrient deficiency evaluations were all unremarkable.

Autonomic dysfunction was suspected, and a nerve conduction study confirmed a mixed length dependent sensorimotor polyneuropathy. Given the constellation of neuropathy, arrhythmia, and unexplained left ventricular hypertrophy (out of keeping with observed hypotension), a diagnosis of cardiac amyloidosis was suspected. Bone scintigraphy demonstrated grade 3 cardiac uptake and a heart/contralateral chest ratio of 1.9, confirming a diagnosis of transthyretin cardiac amyloidosis (ATTR-CM).

3 Discussion

Cardiac amyloidosis secondary to transthyretin (ATTR-CM) is an under-recognised cause of restrictive cardiomyopathy, and is a distinct clinical entity from AL cardiac amyloidosis (AL-CM), a sequela of light chain deposition secondary to a monoclonal plasma cell dyscrasia.

Transthyretin is a naturally occurring soluble protein responsible for hormone transport. In ATTR-CM structural changes in the transthyretin protein results in misfolding, reducing protein solubility, leading to protein aggregation and deposition of insoluble proteins into affected tissue, resulting in organ failure.

Once considered to be a rare condition, patients with ATTR-CM have heterogenous non-specific presentations, and the diagnosis has previously been limited by the need for a cardiac biopsy. As such, misdiagnosis of ATTR-CM as other types of restrictive heart disease, such hypertrophic or hypertensive cardiomyopathy was common. Prognosis is poor, with an average survival of 2–3 years post diagnosis [1].

Recent improvements in cardiac imaging, namely cardiac scintigraphy, has improved diagnostic sensitivity, and emerging evidence indicates that ATTR-CM accounts for up to 20% of patients presenting with HFpEF on transthoracic echocardiogram (TTE), and up to 16% of patient with degenerative aortic stenosis [2].

In patients with an undifferentiated restrictive cardiomyopathy, features which suggest a possible diagnosis of ATTR-CM include [2]:

- Unexplained AV node block or persistent low-level troponin leak,
- Imaged hypertrophy disproportionate to observed hypertension or ECG voltage,
- Orthostatic hypotension or concurrent peripheral neuropathy,
- Orthopaedic complaints such as carpal tunnel syndrome, or unprovoked tendon rupture.

The majority of cases are sporadic, however three autosomal dominant mutations in the transthyretin gene have been described [3]. Thus, a strong family history of cardiomyopathy should warrant appropriate evaluation and genetic counselling. Importantly, age of onset is not sufficient to discriminate between hereditary and wild-type ATTR-CM.

Traditional imaging modalities such as TTE and cardiac magnetic resonance imaging may be indicative but are non-diagnostic for infiltrative cardiomyopathies such as ATTR-CM. To confirm a diagnosis of ATTR-CM, technetium-based scintigraphy (i.e., heart/rib bone scan) has emerged as a non-invasive alternative to cardiac biopsy [4]. In ATTR-CM technetium uptake in affected myocardium is increased, and two quantitative measures are utilised to assess uptake. Firstly, intensity of cardiac uptake is directly compared to rib uptake, resulting in a grade between 0 (no cardiac uptake, normal rib uptake) and 3 (cardiac uptake greater than rib uptake), with a grade of 2 or 3 being diagnostic of cardiac amyloid. Alternatively, a ratio of cardiac tracer uptake to that of the contra-lateral chest is calculated. In this instance a ratio greater than 1.5 is diagnostic [2, 3]. Concurrent testing for serum light-chains is indicated to delineate between ATTR-CM and AL-CM, as this is not possible to differentiate based on scintigraphy alone [2].

In addition to standard heart failure therapy and arrhythmia management, novel disease modifying agents have been licensed in the treatment of ATTR-CM. These treatments either function to stabilise existing transthyretin proteins, thus preventing aggregation, or silence TTR gene expression, resulting in reduced transthyretin production [2]. The choice of treatment is influenced by the results of genetic testing, as TTR silencers are only approved for hereditary ATTR-CM patients with concurrent peripheral neuropathy.

4 Take Home Messages

- ATTR-CM is an emerging clinical entity in heart failure. ATTR is a common, but under-recognised aetiology of HFpEF, affecting up to 1 in 5 of patients with hypertrophic myocardium.
- Clinicians should suspect ATTR-CM in HFpEF patients, especially if there is an associated (and unexplained): cardiac hypertrophy, persistent troponin leak, orthostatic hypotension, neuropathy, or a strong family history of cardiomyopathy.
- In addition to standard heart failure management, there are additional disease modifying therapeutics which should be considered in patients with confirmed ATTR-CM.

References

1. Lane T, Fontana M, Martinez-Naharro A, Quarta CC, Whelan CJ, Petrie A, Rowczenio DM, Gilbertson JA, Hutt DF, Rezk T, et al. Natural history, quality of life, and outcome in cardiac transthyretin amyloidosis. Circulation. 2019;140:16–26. https://doi.org/10.1161/CIRCULATIONAHA.118.038169.
2. Kittleson MM, Maurer MS, Ambardekar AV, Bullock-Palmer RP, Chang PP, Eisen HJ, Nair AP, Nativi-Nicolau J, Ruberg FL, American Heart Association Heart Failure and Transplantation Committee of the Council on Clinical Cardiology. Cardiac amyloidosis: evolving diagnosis and management: a scientific statement from the American Heart Association. Circulation. 2020;142(1):e7–22.
3. Jain A, Zahra F. Transthyretin amyloid cardiomyopathy (ATTR-CM). In: StatPearls [Internet]. StatPearls Publishing; 2021.
4. Castano A, Haq M, Narotsky DL, Goldsmith J, Weinberg RL, Morgenstern R, Pozniakoff T, Ruberg FL, Miller EJ, Berk JL, et al. Multicenter study of planar technetium 99m pyrophosphate cardiac imaging: predicting survival for patients with ATTR cardiac amyloidosis. JAMA Cardiol. 2016;1:880–9. https://doi.org/10.1001/jamacardio.2016.2839.

Sometimes, the Old Ways Are Best: Cost Effective Bedside Diagnostics for Peripheral Arterial Disease

David Buxton and Harry Gibbs

1 Clinical Pearl

The diagnosis of peripheral artery disease (PAD) should be made by measurement of the ankle brachial index (ABI), not by performing a duplex ultrasound.

2 Clinical Case

A 78-year-old man presented with a 2-week history of acute right leg pain on a background of progressive bilateral exertional leg pain. On examination, the pulses were difficult to elicit. There was subtle hair loss and some distal sensory changes. There were no peripheral ulcerations. Past medical history included previous smoking, hypertension, type 2 diabetes, and stage II chronic kidney disease. An acute right sided deep vein thrombosis (DVT) was suspected with a differential diagnosis of peripheral arterial disease. A referral was made for bilateral arterial and venous duplex ultrasonography of the lower limbs.

Ultrasonography from the femoral to popliteal arteries demonstrated bilateral arterial calcification without any significant focal flow limiting stenosis. Visualisation of the aorta-iliac system was limited by bowel gas. Venous imaging demonstrated a small segment of distal deep vein thrombus in both lower limbs.

The distal DVTs were managed conservatively. Serial ultrasonography demonstrated resolution over a 2-month observation period. Despite the resolution of

D. Buxton
Department of General Medicine, Alfred Health, Melbourne, Australia

H. Gibbs (✉)
Department of General Medicine, Alfred Health, Melbourne, Australia

Monash University, Melbourne, Australia

R. Junckerstorff et al. (eds.), *Beyond Evidence-Based Medicine*,
https://doi.org/10.1007/978-981-99-4440-8_36

thrombus, the pain symptoms were progressive. Nerve conduction studies were obtained, demonstrating a mild length dependent sensory axonal neuropathy. The HbA1c was elevated at 7.4%. Initiation of adjunctive analgesia (duloxetine) for a small fibre neuropathy was ineffective in relieving the pain. After several months the differential of PAD was revisited due to noted reduced capillary refill. Ankle brachial indies were elevated bilaterally (1.4 on left and 1.5 on right), consistent with advanced calcific peripheral arterial disease. The patient was referred to a vascular surgeon. Computed tomography (CT) angiography demonstrated a concurrent modest proximal flow limiting stenosis (~50%) of the iliac systems bilaterally. There were significant improvements in both exertional tolerance and pain post aorto-bifemoral bypass.

3 Discussion

Peripheral arterial disease refers to distal ischemia secondary to blood flow obstruction of any cause. The majority of peripheral arterial disease is secondary to atherosclerotic plaque that results in progressive luminal insufficiency [1]. Atherosclerotic plaque results in either focal areas of flow limiting obstruction, and/or reduced vessel compliance, depending on the morphology and composition of the plaque. These processes can occur in isolation or in sequence, however both processes result in distal ischaemia.

Symptoms arise when oxygen demand outstrips supply, leading to patients reporting predictable ischaemic pain with exertion (claudication), positional changes, or even rest-pain in severe disease [1, 2].

The Ankle Brachial Index (ABI) is an inexpensive, repeatable, and sensitive diagnostic test for PAD. In the reclined patient, brachial blood pressure is compared to ankle blood pressure, utilising a doppler ultrasound probe and a standard blood pressure cuff. The index (ratio) of these measures provides diagnostic insight into both the severity and aetiology of PAD. A normal ABI is between 0.9 and 1.09. Claudication secondary to flow limiting stenosis is associated with an ABI between 0.9 and 0.4, whereas rest pain is typical in patients whose ABIs are less than 0.4 [2]. Tissue loss (ulceration) is expected with ABIs below 0.2 [2]. Conversely, high ABIs (>1.3) suggests diffuse vessel calcification (stiffness) rather than focal stenosis [2]. Vessel calcification inhibits occlusion from the sphygmomanometer, increasing the measured ABI, whilst also increasing peripheral resistance. ABIs greater than 1.4 are commonly painful as the progressive lack of vessel compliance results in flow insufficiency [2]. In these instances, measurement of toe pressures is indicated.

Duplex ultrasound is more expensive and time consuming than ABI measurement [1, 3]. When identified, duplex ultrasound is highly specific for focally occlusive atherosclerotic disease, and in experienced hands, can provide sufficient diagnostic information to guide surgical intervention [3]. However, test performance is reliant on technical factors and expertise, and thus has a lower overall sensitivity than ABI.

In this case the 'convenience' of assessing arterial and venous supply simultaneously and the lack of a visible area of 'higher grade' stenosis led to a false negative test result, and a delay to correct diagnosis. The ABI suggested PAD due to the higher occlusive pressure in the leg (compared with the arm) which is suggestive of a loss of normal vessel compliance and increased arterial stiffness. These stiff vessels are unable to dynamically expand with exertion, thus increasing distal vascular resistance and reducing flow. In this case, reduced perfusion pressure secondary to a modest proximal stenosis (not visible on duplex ultrasound) exacerbated the distal ischemia secondary to diffuse vessel calcification.

4 Take Home Messages

- An abnormal ABI is highly sensitive for peripheral arterial disease, and measurements correlate with disease severity. Normal indices are between 0.9 and 1.09 [2].
- ABI measures below 0.9 are suggest a focal stenosis of at least 50% [3]. ABIs greater than 1.4 are suggestive of more diffuse arterial calcification. Both results are diagnostic of peripheral arterial disease in the appropriately symptomatic patient [2].
- Duplex ultrasound is both more expensive and less sensitive than ABI measurement, and thus should not be used as a screening test of PAD. Duplex ultrasound should be reserved to confirm the site of anatomical obstruction in patients with pathologically low ABIs in order to guide surgical intervention [3].

References

1. Au TB, Golledge J, Walker PJ, Haigh K, Nelson M. Peripheral arterial disease: diagnosis and management in general practice. Aust Fam Physician. 2013;42(6):397–400.
2. Wang JC, Criqui MH, Denenberg JO, McDermott MM, Golomb BA, Fronek A. Exertional leg pain in patients with and without peripheral arterial disease. Circulation. 2005;112(22):3501–8.
3. Koelemay MJ, Den Hartog D, Prins MH, Kromhout JG, Legemate DA, Jacobs MJ. Diagnosis of arterial disease of the lower extremities with duplex ultrasonography. J Br Surg. 1996;83(3):404–9.

Syncope: Keeping the Workup Simple

Chris Cameron

1 Clinical Pearl

Focussed clinical history and examination, and simple investigations can often establish the cause of syncope.

2 Clinical Case

Ms. D, 70yo is brought to hospital by an ambulance from home after an episode of transient loss of consciousness. She had been standing at the kitchen bench preparing lunch, when she felt lightheaded and nauseous briefly, then collapsed to the ground. Her son heard her fall and has accompanied her in the ambulance to hospital.

Ms. D's son tells you that on his arrival she appeared to be unconscious for about 15 seconds, then awoke and was disoriented for a few minutes, before regaining normal cognition. She looked pale and he did not notice any seizure activity.

There have been three similar episodes over the last year, one of which resulted in a head strike, requiring stitches to her scalp.

Ms. D cannot remember much about the episode, only the brief preceding symptoms.

Her past medical history includes hypertension with grade 2 diastolic dysfunction, Type 2 diabetes and a previous knee replacement 5 years prior.

Ms. D's medications are: felodipine 5 mg daily, bendroflumethiazide 2.5 mg daily and metformin 1 g twice daily. There have been no recent changes to this regimen.

C. Cameron (✉)
Wellington Hospital, Wellington, New Zealand

R. Junckerstorff et al. (eds.), *Beyond Evidence-Based Medicine*,
https://doi.org/10.1007/978-981-99-4440-8_37

Ms. D's resting blood pressure is 154/66 mmHg and her heart rate is 68 bpm. On standing, at 1 minute her blood pressure is 94/70 mmHg and her heart rate is 110 bpm. This is consistent with non-neurogenic orthostatic hypotension. There were no cardiac murmurs. Ms. D's ECG did not show any features consistent with a cardiogenic cause of syncope.

On further questioning, Ms. D remembered that she had taken double the dose of felodipine that morning, as she had forgotten yesterday's dose. This resulted in marked non-neurogenic orthostatic hypotension, and she was counselled about what to do if she missed a dose in the future.

3 Discussion

Syncope is transient, self-limited loss of consciousness with an inability to maintain postural tone that is followed by spontaneous recovery. It is caused by reduced cerebral blood flow.

Broadly speaking, the causes of syncope are [1]:

Cardiac arrhythmia
Structural cardiac or pulmonary disease (e.g. valvular disease, pump failure or pulmonary embolus)
Reflex (vasovagal, micturition)
Orthostatic (medications usually)
Autonomic impairment (primary or secondary)

3.1 Key aspects of a focussed history to avoid missing potentially lethal causes of syncope (arrhythmia or structural problems):

A history of ischaemic heart disease makes cardiac arrhythmia more likely. Have a low threshold for admission and telemetry.

Patients do not usually develop reflex/situational syncope in later adulthood—ask regarding childhood syncope e.g. during blood draws, standing in church/assembly etc.

Ask bystanders about the appearance of the patient; pallor/diaphoresis implies activation of the sympathetic nervous system. Patients with autonomic failure may not be able to activate the sympathetic nervous system. If suspecting autonomic failure of any kind ask patient if they still sweat on a hot day, any changes to bowel/bladder or sexual function and any changes in their feet (motor or sensory).

3.2 *Key aspects of a focussed exam:*

Manual blood pressure and heart rate measured in the supine position (resting for 5 minutes first), then on standing at 1 minute and 3 minutes. If there is orthostatic hypotension (systolic blood pressure falls by >20 mmHg), check the increment in heart rate carefully. If the heart rate increment is >50% of the BP decrement then the patient probably has non-neurogenic orthostatic hypotension [2]. For example: if the decrement in BP on standing is 60 mmHg, and the corresponding increment in heart rate is 10 bpm then the patient has neurogenic orthostatic hypotension (suggesting autonomic impairment), if the increment in heart rate is 45 bpm the patient has non-neurogenic orthostatic hypotension, suggesting the problem is probably not related to autonomic impairment. This is a key examination feature that is often forgotten.

Listen carefully for any cardiac murmurs, especially for outflow obstructive murmurs suggestive of haemodynamically relevant aortic stenosis or hypertrophic obstructive cardiomyopathy (HOCM), which can both present with syncope. If a systolic murmur is heard, it is important to perform dynamic manoeuvres to elicit the nature of the murmur. Request an echocardiogram if concerned about an outflow obstruction causing syncope—this is an urgent situation.

If a seizure is part of the differential diagnosis, check for tongue biting. As a general rule, primary seizures result in tongue biting laterally and syncope can occasionally cause biting of the front of the tongue. This is not by any means a hard and fast rule.

Examine the feet for signs of a motor or sensory peripheral neuropathy. Autonomic neuropathy can co-exist with these and cause neurogenic orthostatic hypotension and syncope.

3.3 *Key aspects of the ECG:*

A useful mnemonic for potential cardiogenic causes of syncope is:
"Can Quick BRAD walk home?"

C = Conduction blocks (second or third degree heart block, bi- or trifascicular block, left bundle branch block, left anterior or posterior fascicular block).

Q = Long/ short QT interval.

B = Brugada syndrome (coved ST elevation >2 mm in >1 of V1–V3 followed by a negative T wave).

R = Right Ventricular infarction (ST elevation in V1. If present, check posterior leads).

A = Arrhythmogenic right ventricular dysplasia (ARVD) T wave inversion in right precordial leads V1–3, in the absence of RBBB. Epsilon wave in V1.

D = Dilated Cardiomyopathy (wide variety of ECG changes).

W = Wolff-Parkinson-White Syndrome (PR interval < 120 ms, a Delta wave and QRS > 110 ms).
H = Hypertrophy (HOCM or LVH due to aortic stenosis) (S wave depth in V1 + tallest R wave height in V5–V6 > 35 mm).

Hint: Check V1 closely.

4 Take Home Messages

- If after taking a history, performing an examination and/or based on abnormalities found on the ECG, the differential diagnosis includes syncope due to cardiac arrhythmia or outflow tract obstruction (aortic stenosis, HOCM or PE), the patient requires admission for in-hospital cardiac monitoring (e.g. telemetry) and/or a cardiology consultation.
- If the history suggests reflex syncope, the examination is normal and the ECG does not show any concerning abnormalities, then the patient can be reassured and discharged. History is the gold standard for reflex syncope.
- If the history and examination suggests a primary or secondary autonomic cause, then the patient should be referred for an outpatient work-up. This might include a tilt table test if available.
- Other causes that may directly or indirectly contribute to orthostatic hypotension/dizziness include hypoadrenalism, iron deficiency, hypocalcaemia and Vitamin B12 deficiency.

References

1. 2018 ESC Guidelines for the diagnosis and management of syncope. Eur Heart J. 2018;39:1883–48.
2. Norcliffe-Kaufmann, et al. Orthostatic heart rate changes in patients with autonomic failure caused by neurodegenerative synucleinopathies. Ann Neurol. 2018;83(3):522–31.

Investigation of Syncope

Ian Scott

1 Clinical Pearl

> In patients presenting with syncope, pay particular attention to the details of the presenting history and presence of cardiac risk factors, and avoid needless over-investigation.

2 Clinical Case

A 75-year-old man presents by ambulance to the emergency department (ED) having experienced a sudden transient loss of consciousness while waiting for a bus. He fell to the ground and slowly recovers over the next 5–10 min. He takes medication for mild hypertension but has no other medical history. He recalls feeling lightheaded, sweaty, and nauseated for several minutes prior to the collapse. Eyewitnesses recall him looking pale and staring blankly for some seconds prior to the collapse and then having a short-lived episode of jerking of the hands and feet immediately after falling to the ground. In ED, he feels back to normal although still a little confused about the incident. Physical examination is normal, apart from a mild bruise on his forehead, with normal pulse rate and no postural drop in blood pressure. The electrocardiograph (ECG) on arrival shows sinus rhythm with no conduction abnormalities, and chest X-ray is normal. The medical registrar orders a 24-Holter monitor, echocardiogram, carotid artery ultrasound and electroencephalogram (EEG).

I. Scott (✉)
Internal Medicine and Clinical Epidemiology, Princess Alexandra Hospital, Brisbane, QLD, Australia

Centre for Health Services Research, University of Queensland, Brisbane, QLD, Australia

Faculty of Medicine, Queensland University of Technology, Brisbane, QLD, Australia

R. Junckerstorff et al. (eds.), *Beyond Evidence-Based Medicine*,
https://doi.org/10.1007/978-981-99-4440-8_38

3 Discussion

Holter monitoring, carotid duplex scans, echocardiography, and EEGs have very low diagnostic yield (<5%) in patients with uncomplicated syncope and no clinical features of, or risk factors for, the following [1–5]:

- arrhythmia (e.g. palpitations preceding syncope, exertional syncope, unheralded syncope, history suggestive of heart failure or ischemic heart disease)
- carotid stenosis (transient ischemic attacks do not present as syncope with no focal neurological symptoms or signs),
- cardiac valvular disorders (e.g. definite heart murmurs) or
- seizures (very rarely present as syncope with no post-ictal confusion).

Most syncopal episodes are vasovagal or secondary to orthostatic hypotension. They may be accompanied by short lived jerking of the hands and feet, but this phenomena should not be misinterpreted as seizure activity. A careful minute by minute history from the patient and any eyewitnesses, coupled with lying and standing blood pressure measurements, are the most important diagnostic criteria combined with standard 12-lead ECG [6]. Over-investigation can lead to incidental findings which provoke further testing cascades that, in some cases, may result in patient harm [7].

4 Other Gems

- Syncope is defined as a transient loss of consciousness that is rapid in onset, short in duration, and characterised by spontaneous recovery. Simple (or uncomplicated) syncope is further defined as syncope that is not accompanied by focal neurologic signs or symptoms [4].
- Syncope can be classified as being reflex (neurally mediated or neurocardiogenic or vasovagal) syncope, syncope due to orthostatic hypotension, or cardiogenic syncope. Each syncope class (or phenotype) has distinctive underlying risk factors, environmental triggers and manifestations prior to, during and following the syncopal episode [8].
- Validated risk prediction rules such as the San Francisco Syncope Rule [9] can reliably identify patients presenting with syncope who are at very low risk (<1%) of serious adverse events (such as cardiac arrhythmias, myocardial infarction or stroke) over the following 30 days, and in whom hospital admission and extensive investigations aimed at ruling out underlying cardiovascular causes of syncope can be avoided.

References

1. Johnson P, Ammar H, Zohdy W, et al. Yield of diagnostic tests and its impact on cost in adult patients with syncope presenting to a community hospital. South Med J. 2014;107(11):707–14.
2. Mendu M, McAvay G, Lampertet R, et al. Yield of diagnostic tests in evaluating syncopal episodes in older patients. Arch Intern Med. 2009;169(14):1299–305.
3. Krahn AD, Andrade JG, Deyell MW. Selecting appropriate diagnostic tools for evaluating the patient with syncope/collapse. Prog Cardiovasc Dis. 2013;55(4):402–9.
4. Scott JW, Schwartz AL, Gates JD, et al. Choosing wisely for syncope: low-value carotid ultrasound use. J Am Heart Assoc. 2014;3(4):e001063.
5. Simos P, Scott I. Appropriate use of transthoracic echocardiography in the investigation of general medicine patients presenting with syncope or presyncope. Postgrad Med J. 2023;99:279.
6. Alboni P, Brignole M, Menozzi C, et al. Diagnostic value of history in patients with syncope with or without heart disease. J Am Coll Cardiol. 2001;37:1921–8.
7. Canzoniero JV, Afshar E, Hedian H, et al. Unnecessary hospitalization and related harm for patients with low-risk syncope. JAMA Intern Med. 2015;175(6):1065–7.
8. Albassam OT, Redelmeier RJ, Shadowitz S, et al. Did this patient have cardiac syncope? The rational clinical examination systematic review. JAMA. 2019;321(24):2448–57.
9. Quinn J, McDermott D, Stiell I, et al. Prospective validation of the San Francisco Syncope Rule to predict patients with serious outcomes. Ann Emerg Med. 2006;47(5):448–54.

Atypical Chest Pain: Fact or Fiction?

Jessica Roberts and Luke Phillips

1 Clinical Pearl

Right sided arm and/or neck pain is not atypical chest pain.

2 Clinical Case

A 54-year-old man presents with right arm pain. He works as a carpenter and reports the pain has been present on exertion over the past week. For the past 3 days he has been taking ibuprofen. He attends the emergency department (ED) today as the pain has now been persistent for the past 2 hours. It is dull and aching, he feels sweaty and mildly nauseated. He was triaged to fast track in the ED.

His observations include a heart rate of 90 bpm, blood pressure of 134/90 mmHg and respiratory rate of 16. He has no known personal or family history of cardiovascular disease, smokes 10 cigarettes per day, and drinks approximately 10 standard drinks of alcohol per week. There is no history of any limb trauma. No acute pathology was identified on right upper limb examination.

The ED registrar decides to perform an electrocardiogram (ECG) (Fig. 1) that demonstrates ST segment elevation in leads V2–V5, I and aVL, reciprocal ST

J. Roberts
Western Health, Melbourne, VIC, Australia

L. Phillips (✉)
Alfred Health, Melbourne, VIC, Australia

Department of Epidemiology and Preventative Medicine, Monash University, Melbourne, VIC, Australia

The Mater Misericordiae University Hospital, Dublin, Ireland

R. Junckerstorff et al. (eds.), *Beyond Evidence-Based Medicine*,
https://doi.org/10.1007/978-981-99-4440-8_39

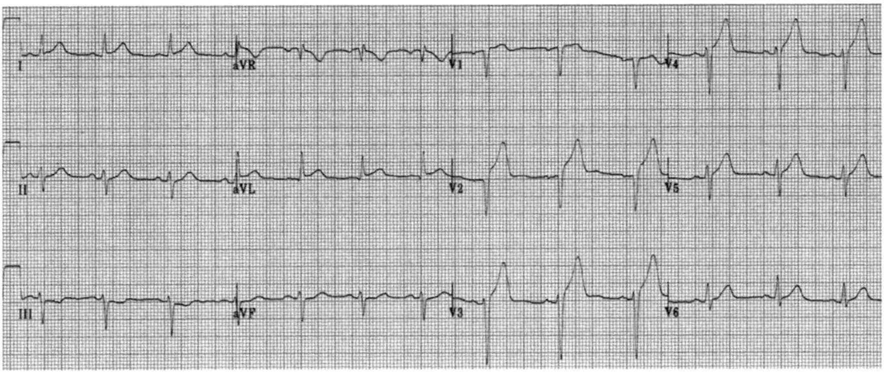

Fig. 1 12 lead ECG showing ST segment elevation in leads V2–V5, V1 and aVL, ST depression in lead III and Q waves in V1–V2. (Reproduced from Life in The Fast Lane 2022) [1]

depression in lead III, and Q waves in V1–2, in keeping with an acute anteroseptal ST segment elevation myocardial infarction (STEMI).

He is moved to a resuscitation bay and is given 300 mg aspirin, 180 mg ticagrelor, 5000 IU of heparin and taken for emergent angiography. This reveals a 100% occlusion of his proximal left anterior descending artery (LAD) within which a drug eluting stent is placed.

3 Discussion

Acute coronary syndromes (ACSs) are one potentially fatal cause of presentation to an emergency department. Their presence is usually heralded by chest pain; however, this is not always the case.

It is often taught that cardiac ischaemia causes chest pain that is central, crushing and radiates down the left arm, and that all other pain is said to be 'atypical'. In practice, the presence of chest pain which radiates to the right arm, or down both arms, carries a higher likelihood ratio for ACS than pain radiating down the left arm [2]. Whilst a higher proportion of patients with ACS present with pain radiating into the left arm, when patients do present with pain radiating into the right arm (Positive likelihood ratio (LR+) 3.78) [3] or both arms (LR+ 2.6), clinicians should still assume that the patient is having an ACS and provide the appropriate workup. Other signs or symptoms that may make an ACS more likely include pain into the neck or jaw (LR+ 1.44), an absence of chest wall tenderness (LR+ 1.4), diaphoresis (LR+ 1.34), vomiting/nausea (LR+ 1.32) [3], pain similar to a previous ACS (LR+ 2.2) and pain associated with dyspnoea (LR+ 1.2) [4].

Previous studies estimated that approximately 2–8% of patients who present to an emergency department with ACS are discharged [5], carrying with them the risk of an adverse event including death. However, this has changed since the advent of high-sensitivity cardiac troponin (hs-cTn) assays. Reassuringly, in patients with two negative troponins, stable observations and no ischaemic changes on their ECG, the rate of probable myocardial ischaemia has been found to be less than 1% [6].

Once cardiac ischaemia is considered, decision algorithms can be used to risk stratify and guide ongoing investigation. Some patients will have an immediately obvious myocardial infarction on ECG with an elevated troponin, whilst others may be suitable for discharge following the return of normal ECGs and hs-cTn levels at 2-hour intervals post presentation [7]. For those with normal initial investigations but ongoing concern for ACS, further objective testing is recommended. The modality chosen depends on several factors including patient suitability, local expertise and available technologies and may require discussion with a cardiologist [7].

To prevent delays to diagnosis and definitive management, clinicians should be attuned to the variety of ways in which a patient with ACS can present, including pain into the right arm or neck.

4 Other Gems

- Do not be reassured by a recent negative stress test. Stress testing looks for the presence of a fixed obstruction. It is not able to identity vulnerable plaques which are at risk of rupture or erosion [8, 9].
- In patients presenting with sudden onset, severe pain which radiates into the back or is associated with a neurological deficit; seek to identify and rule out aortic dissection.
- When attributing chest pain to a musculoskeletal cause, ensure that the pain elicited on palpation of their chest wall is the same pain that the patient has presented with. We would still advocate having a low threshold to investigate for ACS (ECG, hs-cTn).
- Although acute coronary syndrome is more common in patients over 40 years of age, do not dismiss this diagnosis in patients younger than this. In addition to traditional cardiovascular risk factors, younger patients may have additional risk factors such as cocaine use, anomalous coronary arteries and hypercoagulable states [10].
- Silent ischaemia is more likely in patients with diabetes, with a reported prevalence of 10–20% compared to 1–4% in non-diabetic patients [10]. Have a higher index of suspicion for ACS in patients with diabetes who present with non-specific symptoms.
- ACS in women is often due to underlying microvascular disease, and diagnosis can be more challenging [11]. Many studies have demonstrated a delay to reperfusion therapies for women [12]. Be aware that women may present without classical symptoms or ECG changes.
- In young women who present with features suggestive of ACS, but without classical cardiac risk factors, spontaneous coronary artery dissection should be considered [13, 14].

- Clinician gestalt is not sufficient to rule in or rule out ACS. At best you would be correct around 50% of the time. Utilise diagnostics such as a hs-cTn & ECG liberally to diagnose ACS [15].

References

1. Life in the fast lane: anterior myocardial infarction Australia. https://litfl.com/anterior-myocardial-infarction-ecg-library/. Accessed 28 Aug 2022.
2. Body R, Carley S, Wibberley C, McDowell G, Ferguson J, Mackway-Jones K. The value of symptoms and signs in the emergent diagnosis of acute coronary syndromes. Resuscitation. 2010;81(3):281–6.
3. Bruyninckx R, Aertgeerts B, Bruyninckx P, Buntinx F. Signs and symptoms in diagnosing acute myocardial infarction and acute coronary syndrome: a diagnostic meta-analysis. Br J Gen Pract. 2008;58(547):e1–8.
4. Fanaroff AC, Rymer JA, Goldstein SA, Simel DL, Newby LK. Does this patient with chest pain have acute coronary syndrome? the rational clinical examination systematic review. JAMA. 2015;314(18):1955–65.
5. Pope JH, Aufderheide TP, Ruthazer R, Woolard RH, Feldman JA, Beshansky JR, et al. Missed diagnoses of acute cardiac ischemia in the emergency department. N Engl J Med. 2000;342(16):1163–70.
6. Weinstock MB, Weingart S, Orth F, VanFossen D, Kaide C, Anderson J, et al. Risk for clinically relevant adverse cardiac events in patients with chest pain at hospital admission. JAMA Intern Med. 2015;175(7):1207–12.
7. Chew DP, Scott IA, Cullen L, French JK, Briffa TG, Tideman PA, et al. National Heart Foundation of Australia and Cardiac Society of Australia and New Zealand: Australian clinical guidelines for the management of acute coronary syndromes 2016. Med J Aust. 2016;205(3):128–33.
8. Kosowsky JM. Approach to the ED patient with "low-risk" chest pain. Emerg Med Clin. 2011;29(4):721–7.
9. Walker J, Galuska M, Vega D. Coronary disease in emergency department chest pain patients with recent negative stress testing. West J Emerg Med. 2010;11(4):384.
10. Egred M, Viswanathan G, Davis GK. Myocardial infarction in young adults. Postgrad Med J. 2005;81(962):741–5.
11. Mehta LS, Beckie TM, DeVon HA, Grines CL, Krumholz HM, Johnson MN, et al. Acute myocardial infarction in women. Circulation. 2016;133(9):916–47.
12. Vanzetto G, Berger-Coz E, Barone-Rochette G, Chavanon O, Bouvaist H, Hacini R, et al. Prevalence, therapeutic management, and medium-term prognosis of spontaneous coronary artery dissection: results from a database of 11,605 patients. Eur J Cardiothorac Surg. 2009;35(2):250–4.
13. Hayes SN, Kim ESH, Saw J, Adlam D, Arslanian-Engoren C, Economy KE, et al. Spontaneous coronary artery dissection: current state of the science: a scientific statement from the American Heart Association. Circulation. 2018;137(19):e523–e57.
14. Body R, Cook G, Burrows G, et al. Can emergency physicians 'rule in' and 'rule out' acute myocardial infarction with clinical judgement? Emerg Med J. 2014;31:872–6.
15. Janand-Delenne B, Savin B, Habib G, Bory M, Vague P, Lassmann-Vague V. Silent myocardial ischemia in patients with diabetes: who to screen. Diabetes Care. 1999;22(9):1396–400.

Digoxin: Too Much of a Good Thing

Eanna Mac Suibhne and Luke Phillips

1 Clinical Pearl

Digoxin toxicity is one of the most common adverse drug events in elderly patients seen in the Emergency Department (ED).

2 Clinical Case

A 70-year-old lady has presented to the ED following 3 days of vomiting and diarrhoea. Her husband has become concerned as she has become progressively more confused, lethargic and this morning was noted to be drowsy and not responding as per normal. Her past medical history is significant for congestive heart failure and atrial fibrillation which is managed with furosemide, apixaban and digoxin.

On arrival to the ED, her heart rate is 42 bpm with a systolic BP of 70 mmHg. She appears dehydrated and is drowsy and confused to place and time but does respond to voice. There are no localising neurological signs. Her abdomen is soft and non-tender. An Electrocardiogram demonstrates slow atrial fibrillation with

E. Mac Suibhne
Alfred Health, Melbourne, VIC, Australia

Cork University Hospital, Cork, Ireland

L. Phillips (✉)
Alfred Health, Melbourne, VIC, Australia

Department of Epidemiology and Preventative Medicine, Monash University, Melbourne, VIC, Australia

The Mater Misericordiae University Hospital, Dublin, Ireland

R. Junckerstorff et al. (eds.), *Beyond Evidence-Based Medicine*,
https://doi.org/10.1007/978-981-99-4440-8_40

frequent premature ventricular complexes (PVCs) in a pattern of ventricular bigeminy. Blood tests demonstrate an acute kidney injury and a normal potassium level of 3.9 mmol/L. Intravenous rehydration using normal saline is commenced. After some delay her serum digoxin level comes back and is high at 2.3 μg/L (normal 0.5–1.8 μg/L).

3 Discussion

Making a diagnosis of digoxin toxicity can be challenging as presentations can be quite varied, signs quite subtle and symptoms quite vague. Acute toxicity following single ingestion can often be readily identified with the classic toxic features evident on presentation. These can include gastrointestinal symptoms, cardiac arrythmias (increased automaticity and bradyarrhythmias), hyperkalaemia and mental state changes. In terms of chronic overdose, the typical presentation consists of an intercurrent illness over the preceding few days evolving into a mixed clinical picture of culprit illness and toxicity.

As excretion of digoxin is primarily renal (approximately 70%) [1], unchecked steady decline or an acute deterioration in renal function is likely to lead to toxicity. With a narrow therapeutic index, toxicity can easily occur, and the introduction of new medications needs to be carefully considered as multiple potential drug interactions exist. Considered prescribing in elderly patients is important as this population group are particularly prone to toxicity, which can occur at far lower levels in the context of low body weight, advancing age and reduced renal function [2].

Gastrointestinal symptoms are common, as is confusion and lethargy, which reflects central nervous system involvement. Visual changes can include blurry vision, photopsia and colour changes.

Of most relevance, digoxin toxicity may lead to cardiac toxicity. Enhanced automaticity leads to atrial and ventricular tachyarrhythmias, bradyarrhythmias, ultimately contributing to and culminating in hypotension and shock.

Management of chronic toxicity involves treating the underlying cause of the patient's presentation and, in both acute and chronic toxicity, focusing on attending to immediate concerns such as dysrhythmias and hyperkalaemia. Noting that cardiotoxicity originating from digoxin toxicity will most likely not resolve with standard measures, consideration for use of Digoxin-Fab (fragments of anti-digoxin antibody) must be raised early. Indications for immediate use of Digoxin-Fab in chronic toxicity include cardiac arrest scenarios, life threatening dysrhythmias (VF/VT) or bradyarrhythmias with associated hypotension. Administration should be considered in patients with a Digoxin level > 2.0 μg/L with 1 or more of renal impairment, increased automaticity and hyperkalaemia refractory to standard treatment including calcium administration [3, 4]. Dialysis for refractory hyperkalaemia or acute renal failure may be indicated but has no role in the reversal of digoxin toxicity. If in doubt it is important to contact your local toxicology service for further advice.

4 Other Gems

- Serum digoxin levels do not always correlate with toxicity and can be misleading given variable tissue levels and other factors affecting digoxin's toxicodynamic effects.
- Electrolytes require early monitoring to look for hyperkalaemia. Investigation for hypokalaemia and hypomagnesaemia is crucial as they may contribute to cardiac toxicity.
- The 'Stone Heart' Theory, where it is postulated that the administration of IV calcium can result in an irreversible non-contractile state due to impaired diastolic relaxation, is based on case reports in the 1930s and 1950s. This has been contested in the literature [5] and, despite not being evidence-based, controversy still exists. Recommendations are that, in cases of life-threatening hyperkalaemia, IV calcium should not be withheld.
- Hyperkalaemia in the setting of digoxin toxicity does tend to improve with Digoxin-Fab and should be considered early.
- ECG changes associated with digoxin do not indicate toxicity and merely indicate that the patient is taking digoxin. The digoxin effect consists of ST depression, down-sloping in appearance, often described as a 'reverse tick' or 'Salvador Dali' sagging appearance, T waves which can be flattened, inverted or biphasic and a shortened QT interval [6].
- Toxic features found on an ECG arise because of increased automaticity and decreased AV conduction and can manifest as frequent Premature Ventricular Complexes (PVCs), sinus bradycardia, slow atrial fibrillation, any AV blockade and ventricular tachycardia [6].
- Measurement of digoxin levels will be inaccurate for 3 weeks post administration of Digoxin-Fab as serum assays measure digoxin in both free and Digoxin-Fab bound forms.

References

1. Angraal S, Nuti SV, et al. Digoxin use and associated adverse events among older adults. Am J Med. 2019;132(10):1191–8.
2. Pincus M. Digoxin toxicity. Aust Prescr. 2016;39:18–20. https://doi.org/10.18773/austprescr.2016.006.
3. Ip D, Syed H, Cohen M. Digoxin specific antibody fragments (Digibind) in digoxin toxicity. BMJ. 2009;339:b2884.
4. Nickson C. Digibind antidote. Life in the Fast Lane; 11 June 2014. Available from: https://litfl.com/digibind-antidote/.
5. Levine M, Nikkanen H, Pallin DJ. The effects of intravenous calcium in patients with digoxin toxicity. J Emerg Med. 2011;40(1):41–6.
6. Djohan AH, et al. A myriad of electrocardiographic findings associated with digoxin use. Singap Med J. 2020;61(1):9–14. https://doi.org/10.11622/smedj.2020005. PMID: 32043160; PMCID: PMC7900815.

Part VI
Renal Medicine

Acute Kidney Injury Workup

Krita Sridharan and Laila Rotstein

1 Clinical Pearl

During workup of acute kidney injury (AKI) it is important to consider acute tubular necrosis (ATN) and differentiate this from pre-renal AKI.

2 Clinical Case

A 54-year-old man is brought into hospital by ambulance after being found on the floor at home. History suggests collapse secondary to alcohol intoxication. The duration of the collapse is unclear but is thought to have been several hours. Examination reveals a dishevelled, conscious, and oriented gentleman who is clinically dehydrated. Investigations, approximately a month previously, demonstrated normal renal function. Renal function testing on this occasion, reveals an acute kidney injury, with a creatinine of 360 μmol/L (normal range 62–115 μmol/L) and an eGFR of 11 (normal range 90–137 mL/min). Other investigations are demonstrated below:

Hb **128** (normal range 130–180 g/L).
WCC **5.2** (normal range 4–11 × 10^9/L) normal differential count.
Platelets 150 (normal range 150–400 × 10^9/L).
Na 137 (normal range 135–145 mmol/L).
K 4.7 (normal range 3.5–5.2 mmol/L).
HCO_3 22 (normal range 22–32 mmol/L).
Urea **21** (normal range 3–8 mmol/L).
Creatine Kinase (CK) **86,649** (normal range 60–220 units/L).

K. Sridharan (✉) · L. Rotstein
Alfred Health and Monash University, Melbourne, VIC, Australia

R. Junckerstorff et al. (eds.), *Beyond Evidence-Based Medicine*,
https://doi.org/10.1007/978-981-99-4440-8_41

Urine dipstick is positive for blood, but negative for proteinuria, and urine microscopy is negative for red cells, indicating myoglobinuria. Renal tract ultrasound demonstrates normal-sized kidneys with no hydronephrosis. A diagnosis of AKI secondary to rhabdomyolysis and dehydration is made, and the patient treated with aggressive intravenous hydration. However, although serum CK level improves, serum creatinine continues to increase over the next 48 hours and the patient becomes oliguric and fluid overloaded. A diagnosis of acute tubular necrosis is made. He is admitted to intensive care and commenced on renal replacement therapy. He requires renal replacement therapy for 21 days before gradual recovery of renal function.

3 Discussion

ATN is not an uncommon consequence of prolonged pre-renal injury. While pre-renal AKI is rapidly reversible with volume expansion, ATN can take several weeks to resolve and patients with ATN require ongoing support and may, as in this case, require a period of renal replacement therapy. ATN is usually a consequence of three temporally-related events; renal hypoperfusion, sepsis, or nephrotoxin exposure (e.g., aminoglycosides, cisplatin, beta lactams, quinolones, vancomycin, iodinated contrast, heme pigments, among others) [1]. In ATN, there is injury to the renal tubular cells, which leads to these cells being sloughed into the tubular lumen which may then obstruct the lumen [2]. Impairment of the tubular function may result in impaired electrolyte and water reabsorption, loss of urine concentrating mechanisms and acid-base imbalance.

A useful process for evaluating AKI is depicted in the flow chart in Fig. 1. The steps outlined can be considered simultaneously, and this is not an exhaustive list of all possible causes of AKI, however outlines a general approach. The clinical context should always be taken into consideration, and there may be more than one co-existing cause.

3.1 Step 1

Once AKI is identified, urinary tract obstruction should be excluded as this is easy to diagnose and reverse. A bladder scan is a simple bedside test that may exclude bladder neck obstruction. Renal ultrasonography is easy to obtain and non-invasive.

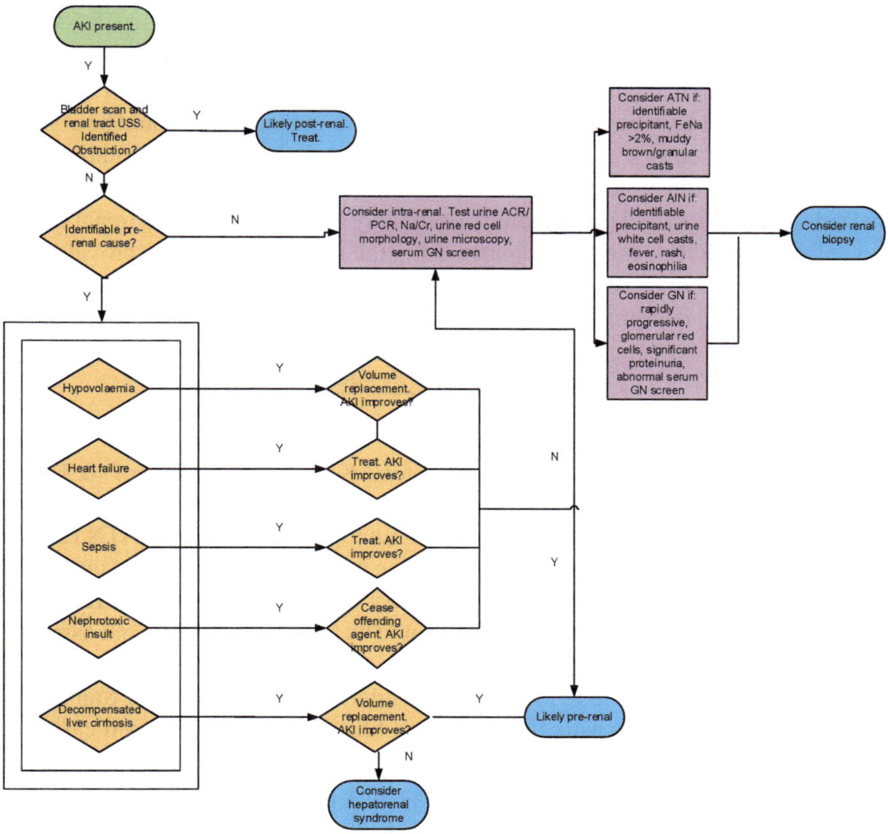

Fig. 1 AKI workup and management flowchart. *AKI* acute kidney injury, *USS* ultrasound, *ACR* albumin-creatinine ratio, *PCR* protein-creatinine ratio, *GN* glomerulonephritis, *ATN* acute tubular necrosis, *FeNa* fractional excretion of sodium, *AIN* acute interstitial nephritis

3.2 Step 2

Pre-renal causes should then be considered, the most common being dehydration. Bed-side assessment of volume status is important. Heart failure is an important cause for pre-renal AKI. Liver cirrhosis can lead to pre-renal AKI, and if unresponsive to volume expansion, then hepatorenal syndrome should be considered [3, 4]. Hepatorenal syndrome is a diagnosis of exclusion. Nephrotoxic agents should be identified and ceased. Receipt of iodinated contrast prior to onset of AKI may be a possible cause. It is useful to check serum creatine kinase to exclude rhabdomyolysis, especially in patients who present after prolonged lie or trauma. Atheroembolic disease should be considered in patients who have undergone recent arterial catheterisation as this is often overlooked or misdiagnosed as contrast nephropathy [5].

3.3 Step 3

If no pre-renal precipitant is identified, or the AKI does not resolve with a trial of fluid replacement or treatment for heart failure, intra-renal causes should be considered. Intra-renal causes can affect the glomeruli, tubules, or interstitium. Urine should be tested for protein-creatinine and albumin-creatinine ratios, microscopy, red cell morphology, and urine sodium, osmolality and creatinine. Fractional excretion of sodium (FeNa) can be calculated using the following formula (provided the patient is not on diuretics or has recently received intravenous saline, as urine sodium cannot be interpreted in this setting):

$$FeNa = 100 \times \frac{Urine\,Na \times Serum\,Cr}{Urine\,Cr \times Serum\,Na}$$

FeNa of <1% suggests a pre-renal cause for AKI, whereas a FeNa of >2% suggests ATN. However, recent evidence suggests that FeNa values may be variable and perhaps serial measurements are more useful [6]. Other features of ATN include elevated urine sodium (>40 mmol/L), low urine osmolality and granular or muddy brown casts on microscopy. Urine biochemistry may help differentiate ATN from pure dehydration where the urine sodium should be low (<20 mmol/L) and osmolality elevated and from the hepatorenal syndrome (urine sodium often ≤10 mmol/L). Subsequent workup can be tailored to the results of the urine studies. Significant proteinuria or haematuria with glomerular red blood cells and/or red cell casts (an active sediment) suggests glomerulonephritis, and serum glomerulonephritis screen should be ordered, and renal biopsy considered. Urine white cell casts or eosinophils, together with peripheral eosinophilia, and clinical features such as fever, rash, or temporal association with known precipitant, may suggest acute interstitial nephritis. In the latter cases, early nephrologist intervention is advisable.

4 Other Gems

- Consider ATN in patients with prolonged dehydration. Although not always reliable, early urine biochemistry may provide clues to the presence of ATN. In such instances, dehydration must be treated. Once euvolaemia is restored, the patient's renal function must be assessed and if ATN is suspected then intravenous fluids should be ceased and depending on the severity of ATN, fluid restriction may be appropriate with supportive measures instituted as necessary [7].
- During recovery from ATN, an excessive diuresis may occur due to loss of tubular concentrating ability. Intravenous hydration should be given to replace salt and water losses during this time [8].
- It is important to dose-reduce renally cleared medications in the presence of AKI, e.g., pregabalin, enoxaparin, certain opioids, and certain antibiotics.

- There is no role for diuretics to treat AKI or enhance urine output in the patient who is not volume overloaded [9].
- Rhabdomyolysis can be identified by urine dipstick, which will be positive for myoglobin but urine microscopy will be negative for erythrocytes.
- Patients can develop uraemic syndromes even with modest urea elevation (this is particularly so in patients with significant nausea and low protein intake). This is because renal failure leads to build up of many toxic solutes other than urea, some of which are, as yet, unidentified [10].

References

1. Ghane Shahrbaf F, Assadi F. Drug-induced renal disorders. J Renal Inj Prev. 2015;4(3):57–60. https://doi.org/10.12861/jrip.2015.12. PMID: 26468475; PMCID: PMC4594214.
2. Erdbruegger U, Okusa M. Etiology and diagnosis of prerenal disease and acute tubular necrosis in acute kidney injury in adults. In: UpToDate, Post, TW (Ed), UpToDate, Waltham, MA, 2023. Accessed 13 March 2022.
3. Russ KB, Stevens TM, Singal AK. Acute kidney injury in patients with cirrhosis. J Clin Transl Hepatol. 2015;3(3):195–204. https://doi.org/10.14218/JCTH.2015.00015. Epub 2015 Sep 15. PMID: 26623266; PMCID: PMC4663201.
4. Ng CK, Chan MH, Tai MH, Lam CW. Hepatorenal syndrome. Clin Biochem Rev. 2007;28(1):11–7. PMID: 17603637; PMCID: PMC1904420.
5. Stratta P, Bozzola C, Quaglia M. Pitfall in nephrology: contrast nephropathy has to be differentiated from renal damage due to atheroembolic disease. J Nephrol. 2012;25(3):282–9. https://doi.org/10.5301/jn.5000093.
6. Ostermann M, Joannidis M. Acute kidney injury 2016: diagnosis and diagnostic workup. Crit Care. 2016;20(1):299. https://doi.org/10.1186/s13054-016-1478-z. PMID: 27670788; PMCID: PMC5037640.
7. Labib M, Khalid R, Khan A, Khan S. Volume management in the critically ill patient with acute kidney injury. Crit Care Res Pract. 2013;2013:792830. https://doi.org/10.1155/2013/792830. Epub 2013 Feb 7. PMID: 23476757; PMCID: PMC3580895.
8. Joseph M, Haniff M, To KC-Y, Ribic CM, Myśliwiec M, Drabczyk R. Acute kidney injury (AKI). In: McMaster textbook of internal medicine. Kraków: Medycyna Praktyczna. https://empendium.com/mcmtextbook/chapter/B31.II.14.1.
9. Khwaja A. KDIGO clinical practice guidelines for acute kidney injury. Nephron Clin Pract. 2012;120(4):c179–84. https://doi.org/10.1159/000339789. Epub 2012 Aug 7. PMID: 22890468.
10. Meyer TW, Hostetter TH. Approaches to uremia. J Am Soc Nephrol. 2014;25(10):2151–8. https://doi.org/10.1681/ASN.2013121264. Epub 2014 May 8. PMID: 24812163; PMCID: PMC4178448.

Beyond the JVP: Overcoming Pitfalls in Fluid Assessment

Kristeen Barker

1 Clinical Pearl

The jugular venous pressure (JVP) should never be regarded in isolation.

2 Clinical Case

A 70-year-old man presented in atrial fibrillation with rapid ventricular rate. He was managed with rate control medications and plans were made for discharge. On the morning of his planned discharge he was dyspnoeic, oedematous and required several more days in hospital to manage his fluid overload. His JVP was difficult to visualise due to his body habitus, but oedema was detected at the level of the sacrum and auscultation of the lung fields revealed coarse bibasal crepitations. His admission weight and current weight were similar, suggesting he had been similarly fluid overloaded at earlier points in the admission.

3 Discussion

The JVP is sought routinely as part of a bedside fluid assessment, yet finding this clinical sign is easier said than done. And when we do find it, we tend to celebrate our clinical skills and label the patient hypervolaemic. However, the JVP does not merely represent the intravascular volume, and indeed may be elevated in

K. Barker (✉)
Department of Renal Medicine, Alfred Hospital, Notre Dame University, Melbourne, VIC, Australia

R. Junckerstorff et al. (eds.), *Beyond Evidence-Based Medicine*,
https://doi.org/10.1007/978-981-99-4440-8_42

euvolaemic patients with underlying cardiac disease [1]. Equally, when the JVP is difficult to visualise we run the risk of mislabelling individuals as euvolaemic when they are fluid overloaded. This represents the trap of the JVP, a clinical sign which may be immensely helpful or lead us astray. And so, the perceived presence or absence of the JVP should not be regarded in isolation. Here, we discuss the global fluid assessment with which to contextualise the JVP, including common pitfalls of fluid assessment and practical tips on how to properly ascertain the fluid status of your patient.

3.1 Oedema Is Not a Binary Sign

A common pitfall in fluid assessment is considering oedema as a binary phenomenon—present or absent—when really we should be asking ourselves what is the level and severity of oedema? This level of how far the oedema ascends and the degree to which oedema pits, provides an estimate of volume excess. For example, in an average sized person, severe pitting oedema to the level of the knee is suggestive of 1–2 L of excess volume, whilst prominent pitting *above* the knee (best appreciated in the posterior thigh) is suggestive of 3–4 L, and sacral oedema in an ambulant patient may represent 5–6 L.

And so, the key to assessing oedema at the bedside, is to venture beyond the ankles.

3.2 Beware of Dependent Oedema

Another trap in fluid assessment is *dependent* oedema. This most commonly occurs in the setting of venous insufficiency in older individuals and is a problem of gravity rather than hypervolaemia. Patients with dependent oedema, classically describe awakening with no oedema, and progressively accumulating oedema throughout the day. On examination there may be additional evidence of venous insufficiency such as haemosiderin deposits, varicosities or spider veins [2]. Dependent oedema alone, does not represent a hypervolaemic state and attempting to correct this with diuretics may lead to dehydration. A more appropriate strategy would be recommending elevation of the lower limbs or venous compression stockings. Thus, the delineation of dependent oedema versus oedema due to hypervolaemic states, is an important distinction to make. That said, pitting oedema only represents fluid within the *extravascular* compartment and says little about the circulating blood volume.

3.3 Intravascular Versus Extravascular Volume

Once we have ascertained the level and severity of oedema, and are satisfied that this oedema represents a hypervolaemic state, as opposed to dependent oedema, the next step is to determine where the excess volume resides—is it intravascular, extravascular or both?

This is important when prescribing diuretics. In a patient with fluid overload and abundant blood volume, we can prescribe diuretics with the confidence that this is unlikely to lead to haemodynamic instability or acute kidney injury. Alternatively, in the patient with fluid overload and a low circulating blood volume, diuresis requires a more cautious approach.

Determining the intravascular volume takes account of two clinical signs, the blood pressure and the JVP. The blood pressure can be particularly helpful when the JVP is difficult to visualise, or the JVP is chronically elevated in the context of another condition such as tricuspid regurgitation. And so, if someone is fluid overloaded and their blood pressure is elevated, this tends to suggest a sufficient intravascular volume for safe diuresis.

Alternatively, as is common in hypoalbuminaemic states such as liver disease or nephrotic syndrome, patients may have excess fluid in the extravascular compartment but have a low circulating blood volume. This would be represented by a reduced JVP, typically at the clavicle, with accompanying low blood pressure.

Once we have ascertained the fluid status of our patient and the degree to which this affects the intravascular volume, we will typically construct a plan to attain negative balance using diuretics, fluid restriction, accurate in/out balance, monitoring biochemical parameters, and requesting daily weighs.

3.4 Daily Weighs and Ascertaining a Dry Weight

One litre of water is equivalent to one kilogram and as such daily weighs are the ultimate clinical tool when managing a patient with fluid overload. The daily weigh conveys progress in attaining a negative balance and allows daily fine tuning of diuretic dose and fluid intake. However, it also serves to increase efficiency when supervising junior doctors on the team. Once a patient's fluid status is established on examination and their current weight is known, we can assign them a target dry weight. We determine this 'dry' weight using the level of oedema as discussed earlier. It is good practice to set the target dry weight at 0.5–1 kg ***above*** what we expect to be euvolaemic for that patient, such that as we approach euvolaemia we can slow diuresis and prevent dehydration.

Having this target weight, unlike fluid assessment itself, is unambiguous and enables the less experienced members of the team to manage hypervolaemic patients with confidence.

3.5 A Holistic Fluid Assessment Is an Accurate Fluid Assessment

Circling back to our clinical case, this patient had atrial fibrillation which was likely triggered by cardiac stretch in the setting of fluid overload. The clinicians caring for this patient addressed the atrial fibrillation but by relying heavily on the JVP for their fluid assessment, the extent of fluid overload was grossly underestimated. Using the approach to fluid assessment we have described here, where clinical signs are considered collectively and which can be applied even if the JVP is difficult to visualise, is likely to enhance our ability to recognise and manage patients with hypervolaemia.

4 Take Home Messages

- Fluid assessment requires a holistic interpretation of multiple clinical signs, none of which can be interpreted in isolation.
- When managing patients with hypervolaemia, estimating a dry weight enables less experienced members of the team to adjust diuretics and fluid restriction with confidence.
- By establishing the severity and extent of oedema we can estimate the dry weight.

References

1. Talley NJ, O'Connor S. Clinical examination : a systematic guide to physical diagnosis. Chatswood: Elsevier Australia; 2018.
2. Bergan JJ, Schmid-Schönbein GW, Smith PDC, Nicolaides AN, Boisseau MR, Eklof B. Chronic venous disease. N Engl J Med. 2006;355(5):488–98.

Magnesium: The Most Forgotten Electrolyte

Kristeen Barker and Peter G. Kerr

1 Clinical Pearl

In order to effectively replace calcium and potassium, magnesium should be replenished.

2 Clinical Case

A 65-year-old female is admitted for management of severe watery diarrhoea and electrolyte disturbance following cisplatin-based chemotherapy for ovarian cancer. Her appetite has been low, with very minimal oral intake although she has not been vomiting. She is commenced on intravenous hydration and electrolyte replacement. Hypokalaemia has responded well to intravenous potassium. However, hypocalcaemia persists despite high dose oral calcium carbonate administered between meals. Her serum magnesium levels are low.

K. Barker (✉)
Department of Renal Medicine, Alfred Hospital, Notre Dame University, Melbourne, VIC, Australia

P. G. Kerr
Department of Renal Medicine, Monash Medical Centre and Monash University, Clayton, VIC, Australia

R. Junckerstorff et al. (eds.), *Beyond Evidence-Based Medicine*, https://doi.org/10.1007/978-981-99-4440-8_43

3 Discussion

Magnesium is an electrolyte with significant physiological importance, serving as a cofactor for over 600 enzymes. Magnesium plays a role in the stabilisation and protection of our DNA and RNA and is essential to the bioavailability of the energy molecule, adenosine triphosphate (ATP). The greatest proportion of our total body magnesium is stored in bone, where it also contributes to healthy mineralisation. Within the nervous and cardiovascular systems, magnesium contributes to normal electrophysiology [1]. And relevant to our clinical case, magnesium is inherently linked to the homeostasis of other electrolytes such as, calcium and potassium.

This concept of optimising magnesium with a view to normalising other electrolytes is well known and tends to be passed down from professor to resident time and again. However, such wisdom is seldom accompanied by an explanation and it is indeed more satisfying to practice medicine equipped with this understanding.

Let us first examine the relationship between calcium and magnesium. These electrolytes share commonalities. They are both divalent cations, and in the loop of Henle they utilise the same reuptake mechanism [2, 3]. Specifically, they use an electrochemical gradient and pores created by claudins to be reabsorbed [4]. However, their uptake here is not proportionate, with far more magnesium being reabsorbed than calcium. Furthermore, at *every* other location in the nephron their reuptake mechanisms are different. In the proximal tubule calcium follows sodium, whilst magnesium is minimally reabsorbed. Within the distal nephron, magnesium and calcium each have their own specialised channels which help to fine tune their reabsorption [2, 5, 6]. As such, the renal handling of calcium and magnesium does not explain their interdependence.

Beyond the nephron, calcium homeostasis is maintained by a dedicated hormone axis. In response to low serum calcium, the parathyroid gland releases parathyroid hormone (PTH) which corrects hypocalcaemia via three mechanisms [3].

Firstly, PTH promotes 1-alpha-hydroxylase in renal tissue to convert inactive vitamin D (25-hydroxycholecalciferol) into activated vitamin D (1,25-dihydroxych olecalciferol). Activated vitamin D increases the calcium channels in the gut such that we can absorb more calcium from out diet. Secondly, PTH promotes the insertion of calcium channels in the distal nephron to reduce calcium losses in our urine. And the final, most potent function of PTH, is promoting the breakdown of bone by osteoclasts, thereby releasing calcium into the circulation. When serum calcium is restored to the normal range, this provides a negative feedback signal to the parathyroid gland [3].

Thus, calcium homeostasis relies on the normal function of this hormone axis and hypocalcaemia will *not* be definitively corrected in the absence of a PTH response. And here we arrive at the true interdependence between magnesium and calcium. Hypomagnesaemia leads to hypoparathyroidism [7] and as such even in the setting of hypocalcaemia the parathyroid gland will be unable to restore calcium balance. In this circumstance normalising the serum magnesium restores parathyroid gland function, thereby facilitating calcium homeostasis.

Potassium homeostasis is also influenced by magnesium. In the collecting ducts we lose potassium in our urine via the ROMK channel. This is the same potassium channel under the influence of aldosterone. When we reabsorb sodium in the collecting ducts, it is exchanged for potassium via the NaK ATPase on the basolateral membrane. The potassium coming into the cell will then be lost in the urine via ROMK [8].

However, magnesium reduces potassium losses in the urine by inhibiting the ROMK channel [9]. Therefore, in the setting of magnesium deficiency we would be expected to lose more potassium in our urine and correcting magnesium deficiency would reduce potassium losses in the nephron.

Overall, magnesium repletion creates a solid physiological foundation on which to optimise calcium and potassium homeostasis and whenever we supplement these electrolytes in clinical practice, we would be wise to consider the role of magnesium in doing so.

4 Take Home Messages

- Hypomagnesaemia impacts calcium homeostasis by blunting the PTH response.
- Hypomagnesaemia promotes loss of potassium in the urine.
- Correcting serum magnesium facilitates correction of hypocalcaemia and hypokalaemia.

References

1. De Baaij JHF, Hoenderop JGJ, Bindels RJM. Magnesium in man: implications for health and disease. Physiol Rev. 2015;95(1):1–46.
2. Moor MB, Bonny O. Ways of calcium reabsorption in the kidney. Am J Physiol Renal Physiol. 2016;310(11):F1337–50.
3. Blaine J, Chonchol M, Levi M. Renal control of calcium, phosphate, and magnesium homeostasis. Clin J Am Soc Nephrol. 2015;10(7):1257–72.
4. Günzel D, Yu ASL. Claudins and the modulation of tight junction permeability. Physiol Rev. 2013;93(2):525–69.
5. Giménez-Mascarell P, Schirrmacher CE, Martínez-Cruz LA, Müller D. Novel aspects of renal magnesium homeostasis. Front Pediatr. 2018;6:77.
6. Quamme GA. Renal magnesium handling: new insights in understanding old problems. Kidney Int. 1997;52(5):1180–95.
7. Rude RK, Oldham SB, Singer FR. Functional hypoparathyroidism and parathyroid hormone end-organ resistance in human magnesium deficiency. Clin Endocrinol (Oxf). 1976;5(3):209–24.
8. Soleimani M, Rastegar A. Pathophysiology of renal tubular acidosis: core curriculum 2016. Am J Kidney Dis. 2016;68(3):488–98.
9. Huang CL, Kuo E. Mechanism of hypokalemia in magnesium deficiency. J Am Soc Nephrol. 2007;18(10):2649–52.

Recognising Renal Tubular Acidosis (RTA)

Kristeen Barker

1 Clinical Pearl

Low serum bicarbonate together with elevated serum chloride (hyperchloraemic acidosis) may represent underlying renal tubular acidosis.

2 Clinical Case

An 80-year-old lady with medullary sponge kidney and recurrent nephrolithiasis attends renal clinic for a routine appointment. She was previously taking potassium citrate three times daily but ceased this medication 6 months ago due to financial difficulties. Her blood tests are shown:

Serum Biochemistry:
sodium 140 mmol/L [135–145]
bicarbonate **15** mmol/L [22–28]
potassium **3.3** mmol/L [3.5–5.5]
chloride **116** mmol/L [98–106]
urea **8.9** [<6.5]
creatinine 88 mmol/L [<120]
eGFR **59** mL/min [>90 mL/min]
calcium 2.20 mmol/L [2.1–2.5]
phosphate 1.08 mmol/L [0.8–1.4]

K. Barker (✉)
Department of Renal Medicine, Alfred Hospital, Notre Dame University, Melbourne, VIC, Australia

R. Junckerstorff et al. (eds.), *Beyond Evidence-Based Medicine*,
https://doi.org/10.1007/978-981-99-4440-8_44

glucose 5.4 mmol/L [3.9–7.1]
Urine Dipstick:
pH 7.0
glucose negative

3 Discussion

Renal Tubular Acidosis (RTA) is a biochemical syndrome caused by impaired urine acidification. This may occur in the setting of impaired bicarbonate reabsorption in the proximal tubule (type II RTA), impaired excretion of hydrogen ions in the distal nephron (Type I RTA), or in the setting of aldosterone deficiency or resistance (Type IV RTA) [1].

Classically, the concept of RTA is learned for exams, but recognising this condition in our clinical practice is easier said than done. Here we discuss the biochemical pattern of hyperchloraemic acidosis, which quickly conveys the presence of a normal anion gap metabolic acidosis [2]. In other words, when you see the combination of low serum bicarbonate and elevated serum chloride, you should consider the possibility of RTA.

To understand this, we must first acknowledge the nature in which acid-base interacts with electrical neutrality. The definition of an acid is a solution in which there are free hydrogen ions. The concentration of free hydrogen ions will determine the strength of the acid which is expressed as the pH. For example, hydrochloric acid is a strong acid because the majority of hydrogen ions are free in solution. Whilst carbonic acid is a weak acid, in which the majority of hydrogen ions remain bound in the form of H_2CO_3, and the concentration of *free* hydrogen is low. And positively charged hydrogen whether bound or unbound is always accompanied by a negatively charged ion (anion), such as lactate or bicarbonate. Thus, when thinking of an acid we can think of this as a solution in which there is an even balance between cations and anions, where the cation is always hydrogen and where the amount of *free* hydrogen will determine the pH of that solution. This concept of electrical neutrality within acidic conditions is key to understanding the anion gap.

3.1 The Serum Anion Gap

When we encounter metabolic acidosis in clinical practice, we next calculate the serum anion gap to guide our further diagnostic work up. And whilst this algorithm is routinely followed, the concept of the anion gap may escape us.

The anion gap is the difference between the sum of the *major* cations and anions in our circulation and is calculated using the following equation [3]:

$$\text{Serum Anion Gap} = \left(Na^+ + K^+\right) - \left(Cl^- + HCO_3^-\right)$$

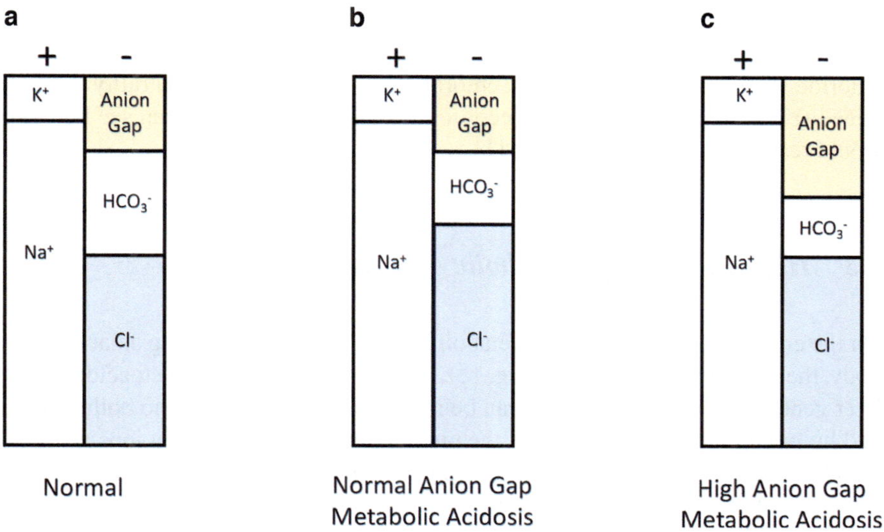

Fig. 1 The anion gap represents the concentration of unmeasured negatively charged ions in our circulation which contribute to electrical neutrality. A normal anion gap is 8–16 mmol/L (**a**). In metabolic acidosis, the anion gap may be normal (**b**) or high (**c**). In normal anion gap metabolic acidosis the chloride will rise as the bicarbonate falls in order to maintain electrical neutrality. In high anion gap metabolic acidosis, the bicarbonate falls but the chloride remains constant because the anions which form part of the acid, have accumulated in the circulation

Throughout our body electrical neutrality is established by maintaining equal amounts of positive and negative ions. If we lose a positive ion, we will gain a positive ion, and if we lose a negative ion, we will gain a negative ion. Because we do not measure every ion routinely, the anion gap equation is used to account for the unmeasured anions in our circulation [3]. In health, the normal anion gap is 8–16 mmol/L [4]. This is the equivalent of saying that with the exception of serum chloride and bicarbonate, the cumulative concentration of negatively charged ions contributing to electrical neutrality is 8–16 mmol/L (Fig. 1a).

Returning to the concept of acids containing anions we begin to appreciate the role of the anion gap in delineating the cause of metabolic acidosis. A high anion gap occurs due to the addition of excessive acid (hydrogen and its respective anion) to the body, whilst a normal anion gap occurs when we lose base (bicarbonate). Each of these scenarios will have different effect on serum chloride. Let us explore this concept in more detail.

3.2 *Normal Anion Gap Metabolic Acidosis*

A normal anion gap metabolic acidosis may be caused by RTA or bicarbonate loss from the gastrointestinal tract. In the example of distal RTA (Type I RTA) there is impaired ability to secrete hydrogen ions into the urine. The excess hydrogen ions in the circulation are buffered by bicarbonate and the serum bicarbonate falls. However, the loss of negatively charged bicarbonate must be balanced by gaining chloride. Thus, as bicarbonate falls, chloride rises, and electrical neutrality is maintained (Fig. 1b). Applying this concept to the equation above, we can see how this would result in a normal anion gap [1].

3.3 High Anion Gap Metabolic Acidosis

On the contrary, in the setting of metabolic acidosis driven by adding an acid to the body, the anion gap will be high (Fig. 1c). For example, in diabetic ketoacidosis, the liver generates more ketones than can be metabolised. In this scenario both ketones and hydrogen ions are increased in the circulation. Excess hydrogen ions are buffered by bicarbonate and the serum bicarbonate falls but the fall in bicarbonate does not threaten electrical neutrality because there are plenty of anions (ketones) in the circulation. Thus, in the setting of an acid being added to the body, serum bicarbonate falls, whilst chloride remains constant [5]. When we apply these parameters to the equation above the anion gap will be high. And so even without measuring specific anions pertaining to an acid, their presence is inferenced by the high anion gap. This finding should prompt us to explore the underlying cause. Causes of a high anion gap metabolic acidosis can be easily remembered with the mnemonic, MUDPILES: **M**ethanol, **U**raemia, **D**iabetic Ketoacidosis, **P**araldehyde, **I**ron & **I**soniazid, **L**actic Acidosis, **E**thylene Glycol, **S**alicylates [6].

3.4 Hyperchloraemic Acidosis = Normal Anion Gap Metabolic Acidosis

Overall, understanding this connection between acid-base and electrical neutrality provides rationale for the anion gap equation itself, but also serves to highlight the varied behaviour of serum chloride concentration in acidotic states. In normal anion gap acidosis, the chloride increases as the bicarbonate falls and indeed 'hyperchloraemic acidosis' and 'normal anion gap metabolic acidosis' can be interchangeable terms which hold the same meaning. Of course there are clinical scenarios where hyperchloraemia and *high* anion gap acidosis may coexist, such as the shocked patient with severe dehydration [7] but in a relatively well patient such as our case, this biochemical pattern is suggestive of an underlying normal anion gap acidosis and this can be helpful in clinical practice.

Arguably the pattern of hyperchloraemic acidosis is appreciated more quickly than the anion gap itself. Detection of this pattern with a mere glance at the serum biochemistry results should prompt us to formally calculate the anion gap and align our further evaluation with the result. Indeed, if the anion gap is normal, in the absence of diarrhoeal illness, this is suggestive of an underlying renal tubular acidosis. As such being able to detect hyperchloraemic acidosis can help us to recognise RTA when we encounter this condition in our clinical practice.

4 Take Home Messages

- The combination of low serum bicarbonate and elevated serum chloride should prompt calculation of the anion gap and consideration of underlying RTA
- 'Hyperchloraemic acidosis' and 'normal anion gap metabolic acidosis' are interchangeable terms

References

1. Soleimani M, Rastegar A. Pathophysiology of renal tubular acidosis: core curriculum 2016. Am J Kidney Dis. 2016;68(3):488–98.
2. Berend K, de Vries APJ, Gans ROB. Physiological approach to assessment of acid–base disturbances. N Engl J Med. 2014;371(15):1434–45.
3. Sirker AA, Rhodes A, Grounds RM, Bennett ED. Acid−base physiology: the 'traditional' and the 'modern' approaches: acid−base physiology. Anaesthesia. 2002;57(4):348–56.
4. Kraut JA, Madias NE. Serum anion gap: its uses and limitations in clinical medicine. Clin J Am Soc Nephrol. 2007;2(1):162–74.
5. Fenves AZ, Emmett M. Approach to patients with high anion gap metabolic acidosis: core curriculum 2021. Am J Kidney Dis. 2021;78(4):590–600.
6. Seifter JL. Integration of acid–base and electrolyte disorders. N Engl J Med. 2014;371(19):1821–31.
7. Berend K. Review of the diagnostic evaluation of normal anion gap metabolic acidosis. Kidney Dis. 2017;3(4):149–59.

Acute Kidney Injury and Cancer

Benjamin Lazarus and Peter G. Kerr

1 Clinical Pearl

While acute kidney injury caused by tumour lysis syndrome (TLS) is often considered among patients being treated for an aggressive malignancy, TLS can also occur in patients with an aggressive de novo haematological malignancy that may not yet have been diagnosed.

2 Clinical Case

A 74-year-old previously independent male from a regional town with a past medical history of hypertension, ischemic heart disease, benign prostatic hypertrophy, and chronic obstructive pulmonary disease (COPD) was transferred to a tertiary hospital with confusion and acute kidney injury of unclear cause. A Computed Tomography-Kidney Ureter Bladder (CT-KUB) revealed two normal size kidneys without evidence of obstruction, but incidentally identified mild intra-abdominal lymphadenopathy. Urine sediment was bland, and no other precipitants of confusion or acute kidney injury were identified. The patient was volume replete and his blood pressure was maintained at 130/80 mmHg. His kidney function continued to deteriorate and he became anuric over the subsequent 2 days.

On presentation his blood tests were as follows: creatinine 280 μmol/L (Reference 60–110 μmol/L), potassium 5.3 mmol/L (Reference 3.5–5.2 mmol/L), phosphate 2.2 mmol/L (Reference 0.75–1.50 mmol/L) and calcium 2.1 mmol/L (Reference 2.1–2.6 mmol/L). Serum uric acid was markedly elevated at 1200 μmol/L (Reference <430 μmol/L) and LDH was 950 U/L (Reference 120–250 U/L). The patient's white

B. Lazarus · P. G. Kerr (✉)
Monash Health and Monash University, Clayton, VIC, Australia

R. Junckerstorff et al. (eds.), *Beyond Evidence-Based Medicine*,
https://doi.org/10.1007/978-981-99-4440-8_45

cell count increased from 9×10^9/L (Reference 4–11 × 10^9/L) on arrival to 15×10^9/L three days later. Abnormal leukocytes of unclear origin appeared in the peripheral blood film. Further investigations confirmed a diagnosis of an aggressive diffuse large B-cell lymphoma (DLBCL) with prominent circulating disease. The patient received rasburicase, commenced haemodialysis and further management for tumour lysis syndrome and DLBCL, but unfortunately died 2 weeks later.

3 Discussion

Acute kidney injury (AKI) is common among hospitalised patients and multiple coexisting factors may contribute to its onset. A systematic framework to clinically evaluate AKI, considering pre-renal, renal, and post-renal causes, and their temporal relationship to the trajectory of kidney function decline is important in identifying the aetiology, initiating appropriate treatment, and preventing future complications. Common causes of AKI in hospitalised patients include urinary tract obstruction, heart failure, volume depletion, sepsis, shock, and nephrotoxins including medications, contrast, recreational drugs, and pigment nephropathies [1]. A careful history, examination, urinalysis and kidney imaging will generally suggest a likely cause. There are limited treatments to reverse AKI, and comprehensive measures to treat the underlying causes are the best way to achieve favourable outcomes. Early referral to nephrology is strongly recommended.

Tumour lysis syndrome (TLS) occurs when large numbers of malignant cells undergo lysis, and the cell contents, including nucleic acid, are released into the peripheral circulation [2]. Metabolic breakdown of the nucleic acids into uric acid leads to marked hyperuricaemia, which can precipitate in and obstruct kidney tubules and induce kidney vascular dysregulation, culminating in acute kidney injury [3]. TLS is often a concern among patients undergoing treatment of an aggressive malignancy, however it is also possible for TLS to occur in patients with a de novo malignancy that has not yet been diagnosed. The characteristic abnormalities of TLS: hyperuricaemia, hyperkalaemia, hyperphosphatemia and hypocalcaemia, can also be seen in other causes of kidney failure, so identifying TLS in someone without a known malignancy can be challenging. The disproportionately high uric acid, markedly elevated LDH, and rising white cell count are important clues to the diagnosis in the above vignette. Early diagnosis and involvement of nephrology and haematology teams is essential.

Rasburicase is a recombinant enzyme that rapidly metabolises uric acid into allantoin, which is more water soluble, and is a first-line treatment for established tumour lysis syndrome. Close monitoring and management of electrolyte abnormalities is a top priority [2]. Hyperkalaemia requires urgent treatment and may require medical therapy and haemodialysis. Administering IV calcium gluconate, either for treatment of symptomatic hypocalcaemia or cardiac membrane stabilisation, is challenging in the setting of hyperphosphataemia because of the risk of precipitation of calcium phosphate. As a result, smaller doses of calcium are generally recommended. Aggressive hydration and phosphate binders are also important considerations.

Tumour lysis syndrome from an undiagnosed haematological malignancy is an uncommon cause of AKI but should be considered in the differential of an otherwise unexplained AKI. Serum uric acid, LDH and blood film are useful tests to evaluate this possibility.

4 Other Gems

- Detailed history, examination, renal tract ultrasound and urine microscopy and Urinary Protein:Creatinine Ratio/Urinary Albumin:Creatinine Ratio will identify most causes of AKI among hospitalised patients [1]
- Early detection and management of the causes of AKI is key to minimising the severity of kidney failure and optimising patient outcomes
- The risk of cardiac arrest in hyperkalaemia is strongly related to the magnitude of the potassium and the rate of rise [4]. In true acute hyperkalaemia, even in the absence of symptoms or ECG changes, calcium gluconate should be considered to stabilise the cardiac membrane if the serum potassium is greater than 7 mmol/L, or if the rate of increase is expected to be rapid [4, 5].

References

1. Moore PK, Hsu RK, Liu KD. Management of acute kidney injury: core curriculum 2018. Am J Kidney Dis. 2018;72:136–48.
2. Larson RA, Pui CH. Tumour lysis syndrome: prevention and treatment. UpToDate. 2022.
3. Howard SC, Jones DP, Pui CH. The tumor lysis syndrome. N Engl J Med. 2011;364:1844–54.
4. Palmer BF, Carrero JJ, et al. Clinical management of hyperkalemia. Mayo Clinic Proc. 2021;96:744–62.
5. Sterns RH, Grieff M, Bernstein PL. Treatment of hyperkalemia: something old, something new. Kidney Int. 2016;89:546–54.

It's Not Always Essential Hypertension

Benjamin Lazarus and Peter G. Kerr

1 Clinical Pearl

Consider secondary causes of hypertension, especially among young adults or patients that have severe or resistant hypertension.

2 Clinical Case

A 42-year-old man presented for routine review after an insurance health check found that his blood pressure was 165/86 mmHg. He was asymptomatic and only suffered from infrequent gout attacks, which he managed with ibuprofen. On examination his repeat blood pressure was 152/88 mmHg and was overweight with body mass index of 27.8 kg/m^2 (weight 85 kg, height 175 cm). His serum creatinine was 93 µmol/L (eGFR 87 mL/min/1.73 m^2) and potassium was 3.5 mmol/L (reference 3.5–5.2 mmol/L). A dipstick of urine showed 1 + blood and 1 + protein and his urine albumin to creatinine ratio was 50 mg/mmol (reference <2.5 mg/mmol). An ultrasound of the renal arteries did not detect any stenosis. An aldosterone-renin ratio was within normal limits. An exercise and diet program targeting 8 kg of weight loss and less than 2 g/day of salt intake was instituted, low dose perindopril was prescribed, and the patient was referred to a nephrologist. Subsequent workup revealed that the patient had IgA nephropathy.

B. Lazarus · P. G. Kerr (✉)
Monash Health and Monash University, Clayton, VIC, Australia

R. Junckerstorff et al. (eds.), *Beyond Evidence-Based Medicine*,
https://doi.org/10.1007/978-981-99-4440-8_46

3 Discussion

Hypertension is common and a major risk factor for cardiovascular events, particularly stroke. There are detailed guidelines on the management of essential hypertension, however secondary causes are often overlooked and represent an important opportunity for effective and directed therapy.

It is estimated that between 5% and 10% of the general hypertensive population have an identifiable cause for their hypertension [1]. Common causes of secondary hypertension include parenchymal kidney disease, renal artery disease, hyperaldosteronism, and obstructive sleep apnoea (OSA). Less common causes include Cushing's syndrome, phaeochromocytoma, thyroid disease, hyperparathyroidism, and aortic coarctation.

In adults, after excluding OSA, parenchymal and vascular kidney disease are the most common causes of hypertension. Each has a prevalence of between 2% and 8% among general hypertensive population, and of up to 10–20% in a population with resistant hypertension [1]. An annual kidney health check, including a blood test for serum creatinine, and urine test for microalbuminuria, is recommended for all adult patients with hypertension [2]. A dipstick test of the urine also offers valuable information, and is a sensitive test for microscopic haematuria [3]. In the clinical vignette, proteinuria, haematuria, and mildly abnormal serum creatinine were important clues to a possible underlying glomerulonephritis.

Primary hyperaldosteronism is one of the most common endocrine causes of secondary hypertension [1]. Useful additional clues of primary hyperaldosteronism include hypokalaemia and a family history of early onset hypertension or cerebrovascular accident at a young age (<40 years). A plasma aldosterone-renin ratio (ARR) is recommended as the first test for detecting primary hyperaldosteronism [4]. This test can be affected by many antihypertensive medications. Verapamil, hydralazine, and prazosin have a relatively small effect on the ARR.

4 Other Gems

- Accurate blood pressure measurement technique [5] includes
  - Avoiding measurement within 30 min of coffee, smoking or food
  - Appropriate positioning, including being seated for 3–5 min with back supported, both feet flat on the floor, and arm resting at chest height
  - Removal of clothing covering the location of cuff placement
  - An appropriately sized cuff [5]
- Clues to the presence of a secondary cause and some simple screening tests are included in the following Table 1:

Table 1 Common and important secondary causes of hypertension

Secondary cause	Prevalence[a] [1]	Clues	Screening test
Obstructive sleep apnoea	5–15%	Daytime sleepiness, snoring, overweight, large neck circumference	Sleepiness questionnaire
Parenchymal kidney disease	1.6–8%	Haematuria, oedema	eGFR, urinary albumin:creatinine ratio, urine dipstick
Kidney artery stenosis	1–8%	Cardiovascular risk factors	Renal artery duplex ultrasound
		Flash pulmonary oedema	
Primary hyperaldosteronism	1.4–10%	Hypokalaemia	Plasma aldosterone-renin ratio
Thyroid disease	1–2%	Palpitations, anxiety, heat intolerance	Serum thyroid stimulating hormone (TSH)
Cushing's syndrome	0.5%	Skin changes, hirsutism	Midnight salivary cortisol
Phaeochromocytoma	0.2–0.5%	Paroxysmal hypertension with headache, sweating and palpitations	Plasma metanephrines
Aortic coarctation	<1%	Radio-femoral delay	Echocardiogram

[a] Prevalence is calculated among patients with hypertension

References

1. Rimoldi S, Scherrer U, et al. Secondary arterial hypertension: when, who, and how to screen. Eur Heart J. 2014;35:1245–54. https://academic.oup.com/eurheartj/article/35/19/1245/661916.
2. Kidney Health Australia. Chronic kidney disease management in primary care. 4th ed. 2020. https://kidney.org.au/uploads/resources/CKD-Management-in-Primary-Care_handbook_2020.1.pdf.
3. Cohen R, Brown R. Clinical practice: microscopic hematuria. N Engl J Med. 2003;348:2330–8. https://www.nejm.org/doi/full/10.1056/NEJMcp012694.
4. Funder J, Carey R, et al. The management of primary aldosteronism: case detection, diagnosis, and treatment: an Endocrine Society Clinical Practice Guideline. J Clin Endocrinol Metab. 2016;101:1889–916.
5. Muntner P, Shimbo D, et al. Measurement of blood pressure in humans: a scientific statement from the American Heart Association. Hypertension. 2019;73:e35–66.

Swollen Legs

Benjamin Lazarus and Peter G. Kerr

1 Clinical Pearl

Nephrotic syndrome should be considered in patients with unexplained peripheral oedema, and urinary protein should be quantified.

2 Clinical Case

A 52-year-old woman presented to her GP with postural dizziness, progressive leg oedema and 8 kg weight gain over the last 6 weeks. Her past medical history included asthma and dyslipidaemia for which she was taking a regular budesonide/formoterol inhaler and atorvastatin. On examination, her blood pressure was 101/50 mmHg and her Body Mass Index was 24 kg/m^2. She had severe pitting oedema to her mid shin and her jugular venous pressure was elevated to 4 cm above the sternal angle. Her examination was otherwise unremarkable; her apex beat was not displaced, and she did not display any stigmata of chronic liver disease. A urine dipstick showed 3+ protein and trace blood. Her serum creatinine was 62 μmol/L (reference 60–110 μmol/L), albumin was 27 mmol/L (reference 32–47 g/L) and HbA1c was 4.5%. Subsequent early morning Urine Protein: Creatinine Ratio was 530 mg/mmol (reference <30 mg/mmol) indicating nephrotic range proteinuria. She was referred to nephrology and found to have a 4 g/L IgG lambda paraprotein (reference undetectable), kappa:lambda ratio of 0.1 (reference 0.26–1.65), and a detectable urine Bence Jones Protein. Further investigations confirmed the diagnosis of systemic AL amyloidosis with kidney and heart involvement.

B. Lazarus · P. G. Kerr (✉)
Monash Health and Monash University, Clayton, VIC, Australia

R. Junckerstorff et al. (eds.), *Beyond Evidence-Based Medicine*,
https://doi.org/10.1007/978-981-99-4440-8_47

3 Discussion

The possibility of nephrotic syndrome should be considered in the evaluation of unexplained peripheral oedema and urinary protein should be quantified. Normally less than 150 mg of protein is excreted in the urine over 24 hours [1]. A practical test to estimate the quantity of urinary protein excretion is the urine protein creatinine ratio (UPCR). An average person excretes approximately 10 mmol of creatinine in the urine over 24 hours, so the daily urine protein can be conveniently estimated from the UPCR. For example, a urine protein creatinine ratio of 15 mg/mmol, approximates to 150 mg of protein in the urine over 24 hours [1]. The accuracy of a spot urine protein creatinine ratio is improved if the time over which the urine is collected is longer. As a result, a spot test in the early morning, after urine has accumulated overnight, or a formal 12- or 24-hour urine collection, is more accurate [2].

Nephrotic syndrome is characterised by oedema, proteinuria of greater than 3.5 g/day, hypoalbuminaemia, and hyperlipidaemia. The mechanism of oedema in nephrotic syndrome is likely multifactorial, with sodium retention due to activation of tubular epithelial sodium channels activated by protease enzymes in the glomerular filtrate being an important contributor [3]. Patients with nephrotic syndrome are also at risk of venous thromboembolism, with a risk that is thought to be proportional to the severity of the hypoalbuminaemia [2].

Urgent evaluation and management by a specialty nephrology service is recommended for patients with nephrotic syndrome or nephrotic range proteinuria. While several conditions can cause nephrotic syndrome, it is important to consider the possibility of AL amyloidosis, because earlier diagnosis and treatment can substantially improve long-term outcomes [4]. Other possible causes of nephrotic syndrome include glomerulopathies, such as minimal change disease, focal-segmental glomerulosclerosis, membranous nephropathy, membranoproliferative glomerulopathy, and other systemic disorders such as infection-related glomerulonephritis and lupus nephritis. Blood tests that can provide clues to the aetiology of a nephrotic syndrome include serum protein electrophoresis, serum free light chains, Phospholipase A2 Receptor (PLA2R) antibody, Anti Nuclear Antibody (ANA), C3 and C4, Hepatitis B, C and HIV serology. Urine Bence Jones proteins can also be useful, and coagulation studies may help facilitate an urgent kidney biopsy.

4 Other Gems

- Severe proteinuria can manifest with the presence of frothy urine.
- An early morning urine protein creatinine ratio provides a practical and reasonable estimate of 24-hour urinary protein.
- The urine dipstick detects albumin [5], and may miss Bence Jones proteins [6].

- Serum paraproteins and monoclonal light chains can cause a wide variety of kidney diseases and should be included in the workup of proteinuria or an unexplained decline in kidney function.
- As opposed to monoclonal gammopathy of unknown significance (MGUS) and myeloma, light chains in AL amyloidosis are more commonly lambda, rather than kappa (4:1) [4].
- Monoclonal gammopathy is prevalent in 3% of the general adult population over the age of 50 years [7]. Detecting a paraprotein in a patient with amyloidosis does not mean that the paraprotein is the culprit protein. If there is evidence of kidney involvement, a kidney biopsy and other investigations are often required.
- Patients diagnosed with amyloidosis should be referred to a centre with expertise in management and a specialised comprehensive multidisciplinary team.

References

1. Beetham R, Cattell WR. Proteinuria: pathophysiology, significance and recommendations for measurement in clinical practice. Ann Clin Biochem. 1993;30:425–34. https://www.rcpa.edu.au/Manuals/RCPA-Manual/Pathology-Tests/P/Protein-urine.
2. Kidney Disease: Improving Global Outcomes (KDIGO) Glomerular Diseases Work Group. KDIGO 2021 clinical practice guideline for the management of glomerular diseases. Kidney Int Suppl. 2021;100:S1–276.
3. Siddall EC, Radhakrishnan J. The pathophysiology of edema formation in the nephrotic syndrome. Kidney Int. 2012;82:635–42.
4. Wechalekar AD, Gillmore JD, Hawkins PN. Systemic amyloidosis. Lancet. 2016;387:2641–54.
5. White SL, Yu R, Craig JC, et al. Diagnostic accuracy of urine dipsticks for detection of albuminuria in the general community. Am J Kidney Dis. 2011;58:19–28.
6. Beetham R. Detection of Bence-Jones protein in practice. Ann Clin Biochem. 2000;37:563–70.
7. Go RS, Rajkumar V. How I manage monoclonal gammopathy of undetermined significance. Blood. 2018;131:163–73.

Haematuria and Acute Kidney Injury

Benjamin Lazarus and Peter G. Kerr

1 Clinical Pearl

Rapidly worsening kidney function plus macroscopic haematuria suggests acute nephritic syndrome, and requires urgent evaluation by nephrology.

2 Clinical Case

A 55-year-old male stonemason presented to his General Practitioner with recurrent "Coca-Cola" coloured urine over the past 2 weeks, associated with malaise, anorexia, leg oedema and a subjective reduction in urine output. A blood test showed that his serum creatinine had risen from 90 to 450 μmol/L (reference 60–110 μmol/L) over the last 2 months.

On examination his blood pressure was 160/95 mmHg and his Body Mass Index was 31 kg/m^2 (weight 95 kg, height 168 cm). There was no rash. Urinalysis showed 4+ blood and 2+ protein.

He was referred to the Emergency Department and nephrology was consulted. A pulse dose of methylprednisolone was empirically commenced for treatment of a possible small vessel vasculitis, and a serum anti-neutrophil cytoplasmic antibody (ANCA) titre was requested urgently. Within 6 hours, the serum antibody titre for myeloperoxidase-antineutrophil cytoplasmic antibody (MPO-ANCA) was found to be markedly elevated. A subsequent kidney biopsy showed crescents in 90% of glomeruli and confirmed the diagnosis of MPO-ANCA vasculitis with kidney involvement. Further evaluation with a chest x-ray demonstrated patchy lung infiltrates, which in the clinical context, were suspicious for alveolar haemorrhage.

B. Lazarus · P. G. Kerr (✉)
Monash Health and Monash University, Clayton, VIC, Australia

R. Junckerstorff et al. (eds.), *Beyond Evidence-Based Medicine*,
https://doi.org/10.1007/978-981-99-4440-8_48

Specific therapies for systemic MPO-ANCA vasculitis with lung and kidney involvement were commenced.

3 Discussion

Blood in the urine may come from anywhere in the urinary tract; from the glomerulus to external genitalia. Macroscopic haematuria may be due to glomerular or urological disease, and certain features on history, examination and investigations can help to distinguish its origin. The appearance of the urine as "Coca-Cola" coloured, the absence of clots, and the emergence of new hypertension or oedema may suggest a glomerular origin [1]. Red to brown "Coca-cola" coloured urine occurs in glomerular bleeding because the blood has a longer transit time through the urinary tract and haemoglobin, in the presence of acidic urine, changes into methaemoglobin, which has a more brownish-red colour [2]. Concurrent proteinuria, red cell casts seen on urine microscopy, or dysmorphic red cells on phase contrast microscopy strongly suggest a glomerular cause. Therapeutic anticoagulation does not significantly increase the frequency of macroscopic haematuria in the general population and therefore haematuria should be investigated even in patients taking anticoagulation [3].

Glomerular haematuria and rapidly worsening kidney function are features of rapidly progressive glomerulonephritis (RPGN) and requires urgent nephrology evaluation for prompt diagnosis and treatment. Major causes of RPGN include ANCA vasculitis, anti-Glomerular Basement Membrane (GBM) disease, crescentic IgA nephropathy or vasculitis, lupus nephritis, infection-related glomerulonephritis and cryoglobulinaemic vasculitis. ANCA and IgA vasculitis are more common in elderly patients, whereas lupus nephritis is more common in young women [4]. Testing the blood for ANCA antibodies, anti-GBM antibodies, complement levels (C3 and C4), and biomarkers of lupus and cryoglobulins can be helpful to identify the most likely cause. Ultimately a kidney biopsy is required for definitive diagnosis.

Treatment of RPGN should involve the nephrology team. Empirical treatment is often commenced concurrently with the diagnostic evaluation because delays can result in substantial loss of kidney function. Infection needs to be carefully excluded, as infection related glomerulonephritis can closely mimic other causes of RPGN. In the absence of clinical infection, pulse methylprednisolone may be commenced followed by targeted immunosuppressive regimens depending on the disease aetiology.

RPGN is uncommon, but an important clinical emergency because early referral to a nephrologist for rapid diagnostic evaluation and concurrent treatment can save lives and kidneys.

4 Other Gems

- Macroscopic haematuria with blood clots suggests a urological cause, because a focal point of bleeding into the urinary tract allows sufficient leakage of procoagulant factors into the urine, which are required for clots to form. In glomerular bleeding, on the other hand, smaller amounts of clotting factors enter the urinary tract, leaked blood is spaced out across a larger filtrate volume, and the presence of urokinase in the glomeruli and tubules inhibits clot formation.
- Rapidly worsening kidney function + macroscopic haematuria = vasculitis until proven otherwise.
- Consider small vessel vasculitis in patients with worsening kidney function with unexplained patchy changes on chest x-ray.
- Infection-related GN can often mimic vasculitis.
- RPGN with low complement levels of C3 and C4 is characteristic of lupus nephritis and post-infectious GN. Other causes of low C3 and C4 include membranoproliferative GN, cryoglobulinaemic GN, and atheroembolic kidney disease.

References

1. Perazella MA, O'Leary MP. Etiology and evaluation of hematuria in adults. UpToDate updated through to June 2022.
2. Pimstone NR. Renal degradation of hemoglobin. Semin Hematol. 1972;9:31–42.
3. Yeoh M, Lai NK, Anderson D, Appadurai V. Macroscopic haematuria. Aust Fam Physician. 2013;42:123–6. https://www.racgp.org.au/afp/2013/march/macroscopic-haematuria#ref-3.
4. Kidney Disease: Improving Global Outcomes (KDIGO) Glomerular Diseases Work Group. KDIGO 2021 clinical practice guideline for the management of glomerular diseases. Kidney Int Suppl. 2021;100:S1–276.

Part VII
Emergency and Critical Care Medicine

Beware Intravenous Fluids in the Management of Pulmonary Embolism

Luke Phillips

1 Clinical Pearl

> Early identification and nuanced management are required in the treatment of patients with pulmonary embolism (PE) with signs of right ventricle (RV) dysfunction.

2 Clinical Case

A 55-year-old female who underwent a trans-abdominal hysterectomy for uterine fibroids 1 week ago presents to the emergency department (ED). She states that she woke up this morning feeling short of breath, lightheaded and dizzy, and has some pain in her left chest. She has a history of hypertension.

Her vital signs include a heart rate of 120 beats per minute, blood pressure of 85/60 mmHg, oxygen saturations of 96% on supplemental oxygen 2 L/min delivered via nasal prongs and a respiratory rate of 24. She is afebrile. On examination she looks unwell and is pale and diaphoretic. She feels most comfortable sitting up. She has no murmurs, and her chest is clear. She has no leg swelling or calf tenderness.

The patient is initially managed in the resuscitation bay and is given 1 L of intravenous normal saline, after which she becomes more hypotensive and tachycardic. She is too unstable to move to the Computed Tomography (CT) scanner to confirm

---

L. Phillips (✉)
Alfred Health, Melbourne, VIC, Australia

Department of Epidemiology and Preventative Medicine, Monash University, Melbourne, VIC, Australia

The Mater Misericordiae University Hospital, Dublin, Ireland

R. Junckerstorff et al. (eds.), *Beyond Evidence-Based Medicine*,
https://doi.org/10.1007/978-981-99-4440-8_49

the diagnosis of a suspected massive PE and is also struggling to lie flat. What are the key principles to prevent further deterioration in this patient and could this deterioration have been prevented?

3 Discussion

Most patients who die from PE's do so not from hypoxia but from circulatory collapse. Nuanced treatment of the right heart dysfunction associated with PE is imperative to prevent deterioration both from the disease and iatrogenic causes. Stabilisation of these patients should focus primarily on haemodynamic support whilst also preventing hypoxia and hypercarbia which can also increase pulmonary vasoconstriction.

In patients with no pre-existing conditions the right ventricle will continue to function normally until 25–30% of the pulmonary vasculature is obstructed by thrombus. As the clot burden increases beyond 50% the RV will begin to dilate increasing wall tension and O_2 demand leading to decreased RV output through both obstruction (afterload) and ischemia [1].

Ventricular interdependence is an important concept where the function of one ventricle is altered by the filling of the other ventricle as both structures are contained within the pericardium. A dilated, poorly functioning RV together with paradoxical intraventricular septal movement leads to an overall decrease in cardiac output in the systemic circulation [1]. As the RV function worsens, patients enter a spiral of negative feedback which eventually leads to cardiogenic shock and death. This is outlined in Fig. 1 below.

Utilising point of care ultrasound (POCUS) early to help confirm the diagnosis of PE or discover alternative pathologies is extremely useful especially in patients unable to tolerate CT Pulmonary Angiography due to respiratory distress or haemodynamic instability. It is also helpful for risk stratification as patients with evidence of RV dysfunction and haemodynamic instability have a high 30-day mortality risk [2]. Key findings on echocardiography include a RV approaching an 1:1 ratio with the left ventricle (LV), a D-shaped septum and encroachment of the RV into the LV, RV dysfunction which can be characterised by an abnormal Tricuspid annular plane systolic excursion (TAPSE) (<16 mm) and a dilated and non-collapsible inferior vena cava (IVC). You may also be able to identify a clot in transit or a positive McConnell's sign (RV hypokinesis with apical sparing) [3].

Key treatments that may need to be instituted in the ED alongside the gold standard of care that is anticoagulation, include:

1. Consideration of an extremely judicious fluid bolus of no more than 250–500 mL, noting that this may increase RV pressure [4]. Administer this with caution in patients who already have signs of RV strain on echo or CT scan and perform a point of care echo prior to giving fluid where possible to assess for signs of RV dysfunction.

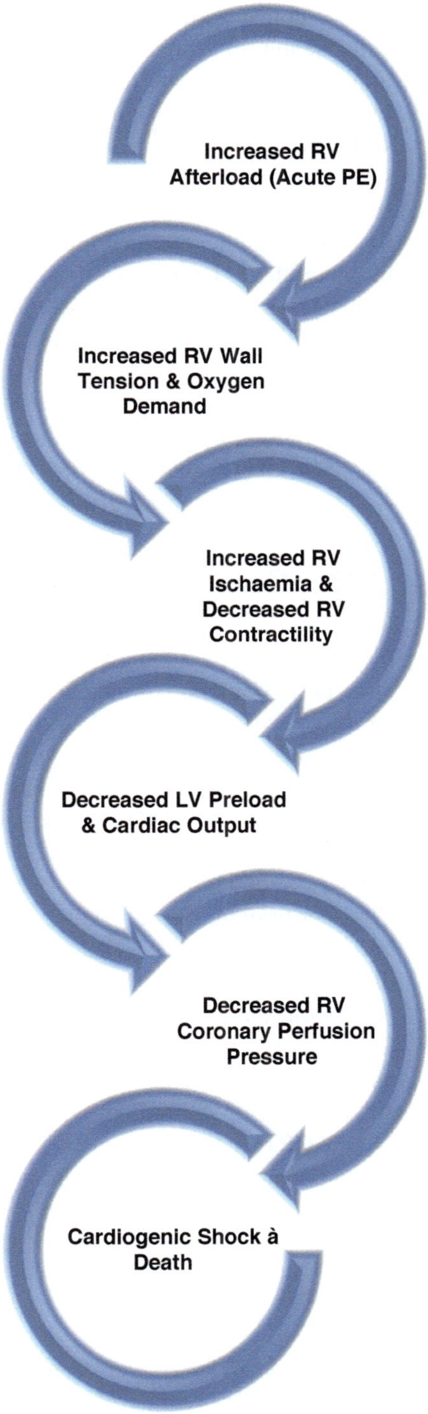

Fig. 1 Pathophysiology of haemodynamic collapse and death in acute pulmonary embolism [2]

2. Early commencement of inotropes. In most cases this would be noradrenaline with the aim of increasing pre-load and RV inotropy. It may also be useful in improving coronary perfusion [2].
3. Systemic thrombolysis should be considered and prioritised for patients with sustained hypotension (systolic BP <90 mmHg for 15 min or requiring inotropic support or pulselessness/cardiac arrest or sustained HR <40 beats/min with signs/symptoms of shock) [5]. Deciding whether to perform thrombolysis is time critical; other interventions merely act as temporising measures. It may also be helpful to involve your local Intensive Care Unit (ICU)/Respiratory/Haematology teams in this decision-making process. Ensure that any heparin is ceased if thrombolysis is given due to the increased risk of catastrophic haemorrhage [6].
4. Consider mechanical interventions such as catheter directed thrombolysis, surgical thrombectomy or extracorporeal membrane oxygenation (ECMO) if thrombolysis is contraindicated or the patient continues to deteriorate [2, 5].

4 Other Gems

- In patients with a submassive pulmonary embolism consider thrombolysis or other invasive therapy if there is a very high thrombus burden, poor cardiorespiratory reserve and low bleeding risk. Whilst no overall mortality benefit, thrombolysis has been associated with a significant decrease in haemodynamic compromise. This needs to be balanced with the risk of bleeding [7].
- Intubation should be avoided if possible as the negative effects on haemodynamics of both the induction drugs and subsequent venous return from the positive pressure ventilation can lead to haemodynamic collapse and cardiac arrest. Consider bridging therapy with high flow nasal oxygen or non-invasive ventilation whilst you are resuscitating the patient and waiting for your thrombolytic therapy to work. These may also help with recruitment of lung tissue and improve ventilation and oxygen exchange.
- In the event of a cardiac arrest, patients with proven or suspected pulmonary embolism should be considered for thrombolysis with a bolus dose of 50 mg of Alteplase. The Australian and New Zealand Committee on Resuscitation (ANZCOR) recommends that CPR should continue for at least 60 min before termination of resuscitation attempts [8].

References

1. Price LC, Wort SJ, Finney SJ, Marino PS, Brett SJ. Pulmonary vascular and right ventricular dysfunction in adult critical care: current and emerging options for management: a systematic literature review. Crit Care. 2010;14(5):R169.

2. Konstantinides SV, Meyer G, Becattini C, Bueno H, Geersing GJ, Harjola VP, et al. 2019 ESC Guidelines for the diagnosis and management of acute pulmonary embolism developed in collaboration with the European Respiratory Society (ERS). Eur Heart J. 2020;41(4):543–603.
3. Kennedy Hall M, Coffey EC, Herbst M, Liu R, Pare JR, Andrew Taylor R, et al. The "5Es" of emergency physician-performed focused cardiac ultrasound: a protocol for rapid identification of effusion, ejection, equality, exit, and entrance. Acad Emerg Med. 2015;22(5):583–93.
4. Mercat A, Diehl JL, Meyer G, Teboul JL, Sors H. Hemodynamic effects of fluid loading in acute massive pulmonary embolism: critical care medicine. 1999;27(3):540–4.
5. Tran HA, Gibbs H, Merriman E, Curnow JL, Young L, Bennett A, et al. New guidelines from the Thrombosis and Haemostasis Society of Australia and New Zealand for the diagnosis and management of venous thromboembolism. Med J Aust. 2019;210(5):227–35.
6. Castillo C, Tapson VF. Right ventricular responses to massive and submassive pulmonary embolism. Cardiol Clin. 2012;30(2):233–41.
7. Meyer G, Vicaut E, Danays T, Agnelli G, Becattini C, Beyer-Westendorf J, et al. Fibrinolysis for patients with intermediate-risk pulmonary embolism. N Engl J Med. 2014;370(15):1402–11.
8. ANZCOR guideline 11.5 – medications in adult cardiac arrest. 2016;13.

Fall Injuries in the Elderly

Laura Scott and Luke Phillips

1 Clinical Pearl

Never underestimate the potential for major injuries in a low height fall in older adult patients.

2 Clinical Case

An 88-year-old lady, from home, presents to the Emergency Department (ED) after tripping over her slippers and landing on her right side. She reports hitting her head on the wall but denies loss of consciousness and has some right sided hip and wrist pain. A Computerised Tomography (CT) scan of her brain and cervical spine and X-ray of her chest (CXR), pelvis and right wrist are performed, all of which are reported as normal.

Due to ongoing pain and difficulty mobilising, the patient is admitted under general medicine for analgesia and physiotherapy.

Three days into her admission, she develops shortness of breath and mild tachypnoea. A CXR reveals a right sided pneumonia but due to increasing pain, a CT scan of her chest is performed. This reveals multiple, un-displaced right sided rib fractures and a right scapula body fracture. On advice from the trauma team, completion imaging, comprising CT scan of abdomen, pelvis and thoraco-lumbar spine, is

L. Scott
Alfred Health, Melbourne, VIC, Australia

L. Phillips (✉)
Alfred Health, Melbourne, VIC, Australia

Department of Epidemiology and Preventative Medicine, Monash University, Melbourne, VIC, Australia

R. Junckerstorff et al. (eds.), *Beyond Evidence-Based Medicine*, https://doi.org/10.1007/978-981-99-4440-8_50

performed revealing a L2 compression fracture which requires an anteflexion brace. The patient spends a further 2 weeks in hospital prior to being discharged to rehabilitation.

3 Discussion

Falls are Australia's largest contributor to injuries requiring hospitalisation and are a leading cause of injury deaths, with the very oldest most at risk of a serious fall injury [1]. Fractures are by far the most common injury after a fall in patients over 65 years old [1]. It is imperative that these patients are thoroughly assessed for injury after any seemingly benign fall from standing height, as well as for any potential causes of the fall.

Cognitive impairment, in the form of delirium or dementia, may render a patient unable to communicate their history, why they fell, or the site of their pain. If the fall has been unwitnessed, it may not even be a feature of the history. A full trauma secondary survey to look for occult injuries is vital. This requires adequate exposure of the patient, including systematic gentle palpation of all limbs, movement of all joints and examination of the spine. Immediately after the secondary survey, ensure the patient is kept warm by redressing them and providing them with a warm blanket.

Older adult patients are more likely to have impaired renal function and ordering trauma scans may generate concern about precipitating contrast nephropathy. Considering which scan is most appropriate for the patient involves careful clinical examination and consideration, weighing up the balance of risks versus benefits. If your clinical concern pertains primarily towards fractures of the ribs, spine or pelvis, a non-contrast scan will likely suffice. Persistent unexplained haemodynamic instability should lead to concern for bleeding or underlying vascular injuries, in which case the benefits of a contrast scan may outweigh the risks [2, 3].

3.1 Ribs

Older adult patients with rib fractures have a much higher morbidity, mortality rate and length of hospital stay when compared to adults under 65 with similar injuries [4, 5]. Pneumonia is a dangerous complication. Early and regular analgesia that enables the patient to deep breathe and cough will assist in preventing deterioration. An ultrasound guided serratus anterior plane block or erector spinae plane block is a helpful analgesic adjunct to minimise opioid use [6, 7]. Patients at particular risk or those with four or more rib fractures should be considered for admission to a high dependency unit and referred to an acute pain service. A rolled towel to brace against their chest wall can assist patients in their ability to deep breathe and cough.

Older adult patients with rib fractures require early chest physiotherapy and must be promptly treated with antibiotics if any signs of pneumonia develop.

3.2 Spine

Spinal fractures are common in older adult patients after a low level fall [8]. All older adult patients who fall must be log rolled and have their spine examined. They should be placed in spinal precautions lying flat until the thoracolumbar spine is clinically and/or radiologically cleared. In most cases, patients can then sit up to 30°.

It is imperative to clear the spine of older adult patients both clinically and radiologically as soon as is reasonably possible to assist with avoiding delirium, pressure sores and distress.

Cervical spine CT imaging must be closely reviewed and clinically correlated, with the patient examined for any ongoing midline neck tenderness or neurological findings. Elderly patients who fall and hyper-extend their neck must be checked for signs of central cord syndrome. These can be subtle and easily overlooked typically including motor weakness with the upper limbs being more affected than the lower limbs and the distal limb more than proximal [9].

Magnetic Resonance Imaging (MRI) of the cervical spine should be performed when there is any ongoing concern for cervical spine injury.

3.3 Pelvis

Older adult patients commonly fracture their femoral neck or pubic rami from a fall. Patients with a fractured neck of femur should receive an ultrasound guided femoral nerve or fascia iliaca block within 90 min of arrival to hospital.

3.4 Analgesia

Older adult patients may under-report their pain for a variety of reasons; being stoic or not wanting to 'bother the staff', to try and avoid admission to hospital or if they are confused. Patients should be prescribed analgesia in keeping with the analgesic ladder and, where appropriate, the utilisation of regional blocks should be facilitated. In this cohort, Non Steroidal Anti Inflammatory Drugs (NSAID) should be avoided, and the use of opiates minimised. Ensure early and proactive use of laxatives when opiates have been prescribed.

4 Other Gems

- Patients over 65 will benefit from early review by a geriatrician, especially if they have fallen because of a syncopal episode. In emergency departments where geriatricians are rostered, this review can commence in ED to ensure optimal care.
- Older adult patients may require assistance with feeding, especially if they have injured their upper limbs/torso or have cognitive impairment.
- Consider screening for osteoporosis in any patient over the age of 65 with a fracture, especially when minimal impact, e.g. Colles fracture.

References

1. Australian Institute of Health Welfare. Falls. Australian Institute of Health and Welfare; 2022. Available from: https://www.aihw.gov.au/reports/injury/falls.
2. Hinson JS, Ehmann MR, Fine DM, Fishman EK, Toerper MF, Rothman RE, et al. Risk of acute kidney injury after intravenous contrast media administration. Ann Emerg Med. 2017;69(5):577–86.e4.
3. Aycock RD, Westafer LM, Boxen JL, Majlesi N, Schoenfeld EM, Bannuru RR. Acute kidney injury after computed tomography: a meta-analysis. Ann Emerg Med. 2018;71(1):44–53.e4.
4. Peek J, Beks RB, Hietbrink F, De Jong MB, Heng M, Beeres FJP, et al. Epidemiology and outcome of rib fractures: a nationwide study in the Netherlands. Eur J Trauma Emerg Surg. 2022;48(1):265–71.
5. Bulger EM, Arneson MA, Mock CN, Jurkovich GJ. Rib fractures in the elderly. J Trauma. 2000;48(6):1040–6; discussion 6–7.
6. Schultz C, Yang E, Mantuani D, Miraflor E, Victorino G, Nagdev A. Single injection, ultrasound-guided planar nerve blocks: an essential skill for any clinician caring for patients with rib fractures. Trauma Case Rep. 2022;41:100680.
7. Tekşen Ş, Öksüz G, Öksüz H, Sayan M, Arslan M, Urfalıoğlu A, et al. Analgesic efficacy of the serratus anterior plane block in rib fractures pain: a randomized controlled trial. Am J Emerg Med. 2021;41:16–20.
8. Jawa RS, Singer AJ, Rutigliano DN, McCormack JE, Huang EC, Shapiro MJ, et al. Spinal fractures in older adult patients admitted after low-level falls: 10-year incidence and outcomes. J Am Geriatr Soc. 2017;65(5):909–15.
9. Nickson, C. Spinal Cord Anatomy and Syndromes. Life in the Fast Lane; Nov 3 2020. Available from: https://litfl.com/spinalcord-anatomy-and-syndromes/

Injecting Drug Use and Sepsis

Tom Bourne and Luke Phillips

1 Clinical Pearl

Have a high level of suspicion for occult sepsis in persons who inject drugs (PWID).

2 Clinical Case

A 28-year-old male PWID is brought into the Emergency Department (ED) by ambulance after being found in an altered conscious state by a member of the public. His initial observations reveal mild hypothermia, tachycardia and tachypnoea. The patient is difficult to assess due to non-compliance with physical examination and initial investigations. He is managed expectantly in a low stimulus environment. After a period of observation, he deteriorates and is noted to be hypotensive and initial investigations reveal raised inflammatory markers and an elevated lactate. The patient is diagnosed with sepsis and broad-spectrum antibiotics are commenced. Subsequently, he is admitted to the Intensive Care Unit due to inotropic requirements. A transoesophageal echocardiogram shows a vegetation on the tricuspid valve and infective endocarditis is diagnosed.

T. Bourne
Alfred Health, Melbourne, VIC, Australia

L. Phillips (✉)
Alfred Health, Melbourne, VIC, Australia

Department of Epidemiology and Preventative Medicine, Monash University, Melbourne, VIC, Australia

The Mater Misericordiae University Hospital, Dublin, Ireland

R. Junckerstorff et al. (eds.), *Beyond Evidence-Based Medicine*,
https://doi.org/10.1007/978-981-99-4440-8_51

3 Discussion

Persons who inject drugs often have poor engagement in primary health care and seek much of their acute care via the ED (Table 1). They have a 22-times higher mortality than the age-adjusted population and are at a higher risk of sepsis secondary to pneumonia and skin infections, but also from more uncommon sources such as endocarditis, osteomyelitis, discitis or epidural abscesses [1].

The assessment of PWID can be complicated by concomitant recreational drug use, psychiatric history, and non-specific symptomatology. The tachycardia and even fever can easily be discounted as part of a toxidrome. This non-specific and clouded presentation places the clinician at risk of anchoring bias and failing to fully consider sepsis as an underlying aetiology.

Infective endocarditis has an incidence of 1–20 cases per 10,000 PWID every year and accounts for 5–20% of hospital admissions in this population. Of PWID admitted with fever, 20% will have infective endocarditis. It has a mortality rate of 5–10% and is associated with significant complications and morbidity [2]. Infective endocarditis, in this population, tends to be due to Staphylococcal infection, which less commonly provides the diagnostic clues of the extra-cardiac manifestations [3]. Infective endocarditis in PWID commonly affects the tricuspid valve but the mitral and aortic valves can also be involved [4]. PWID are at significantly higher risk of relapses of infective endocarditis and may not volunteer this as part of their past medical history. Interrogation of the patient's health record and previous microbiology is imperative to ensure appropriate antimicrobial choice [5].

Blood cultures form a key part of the investigative strategy for endocarditis. Most guidelines recommend three separate sets from distinct sites [6]. In the PWID this can be challenging and leads to delays in antibiotic administration. In the stable patient with suspected infective endocarditis, this is undoubtedly the correct strategy. However, in the patient with septic shock, a risk-benefit analysis needs to be made at the bedside as to the value of the additional diagnostic yield of further blood cultures against the potential mortality benefit of early antibiotics. The clinician should set a time limit during which they will try and achieve the blood cultures and if unsuccessful they should proceed with antibiotic administration regardless of blood culture acquisition.

Table 1 Standardised admission ratio for severe bacterial infections in PWID [1]

Primary diagnosis	Standardised admission ratio[a]
Pneumonia	10
Osteomyelitis and septic arthritis	174
Endocarditis	44
Cellulitis	36
Necrotising fasciitis	600

[a] Compared to general population X times more likely to be admitted

4 Other Gems

- Invariably clinicians aim to provide equitable care to all patients. However, several studies show that clinicians demonstrate prejudice and stereotyping towards stigmatised patients which can impact on their judgement [7]. Clinicians should reflect on these conscious or unconscious biases and take extra care when assessing these patient populations. Establishing an open therapeutic and collaborative relationship involving the patient and identifying their needs to address them will likely lead to better engagement in their care.
- 1 in 5 patients with sepsis in PWID discharge against medical advice compared to 3% of the general hospital population. This most commonly occurs in the first 48 h of admission [8].
- Clinicians should make an early assessment of established withdrawal symptoms and to the risk of withdrawal. Prevention and alleviation of these withdrawal symptoms is imperative to reducing risk of discharge against medical advice. Nicotine replacement therapy with both a longer acting patch and a shorter acting modality such as inhaler or gum should be offered to the patient and prescribed as part of this risk assessment.
- Clear boundaries of acceptable behaviour should also be established and communicated early in the patient presentation, and these should be consistently adhered to.

References

1. Lewer D, Hope VD, Harris M, Kelleher M, Jewell A, Pritchard M, Strang J, Morley KI. Incidence and treatment costs of severe bacterial infections among people who inject heroin: a cohort study in South London, England. Drug Alcohol Depend. 2020;212:108057. https://doi.org/10.1016/j.drugalcdep.2020.108057. Epub 2020 May 6. PMID: 32422537; PMCID: PMC7301433.
2. Chung-Esaki H, Rodriguez RM, Alter H, Cisse B. Validation of a prediction rule for endocarditis in febrile injection drug users. Am J Emerg Med. 2014;32(5):412–6. https://doi.org/10.1016/j.ajem.2014.01.008. Epub 2014 Jan 18. PMID: 24560394.
3. Bayer AS, Bolger AF, Taubert KA, Wilson W, Steckelberg J, Karchmer AW, Levison M, Chambers HF, Dajani AS, Gewitz MH, Newburger JW, Gerber MA, Shulman ST, Pallasch TJ, Gage TW, Ferrieri P. Diagnosis and management of infective endocarditis and its complications. Circulation. 1998;98(25):2936–48. https://doi.org/10.1161/01.cir.98.25.2936. PMID: 9860802.
4. Akinosoglou K, Apostolakis E, Marangos M, Pasvol G. Native valve right sided infective endocarditis. Eur J Intern Med. 2013;24(6):510–9. https://doi.org/10.1016/j.ejim.2013.01.010. Epub 2013 Jan 28. PMID: 23369408.
5. Scheggi V, Del Pace S, Ceschia N, et al. Infective endocarditis in intravenous drug abusers: clinical challenges emerging from a single-centre experience. BMC Infect Dis. 2021;21:1010. https://doi.org/10.1186/s12879-021-06697-1.
6. Baddour LM, Wilson WR, Bayer AS, Fowler VG Jr, Tleyjeh IM, Rybak MJ, Barsic B, Lockhart PB, Gewitz MH, Levison ME, Bolger AF, Steckelberg JM, Baltimore RS, Fink AM, O'Gara P, Taubert KA; American Heart Association Committee on Rheumatic Fever, Endocarditis, and

Kawasaki Disease of the Council on Cardiovascular Disease in the Young, Council on Clinical Cardiology, Council on Cardiovascular Surgery and Anesthesia, and Stroke Council. Infective endocarditis in adults: diagnosis, antimicrobial therapy, and management of complications: a scientific statement for healthcare professionals from the American Heart Association. Circulation. 2015;132(15):1435–86. https://doi.org/10.1161/CIR.0000000000000296. Epub 2015 Sep 15. Erratum in: Circulation. 2015;132(17):e215. Erratum in: Circulation. 2016;134(8):e113. Erratum in: Circulation. 2018;138(5):e78–9. PMID: 26373316.

7. Chapman EN, Kaatz A, Carnes M. Physicians and implicit bias: how doctors may unwittingly perpetuate health care disparities. J Gen Intern Med. 2013;28:1504–10. https://doi.org/10.1007/s11606-013-2441-1.
8. Kimmel SD, Kim JH, Kalesan B, Samet JH, Walley AY, Larochelle MR. Against medical advice discharges in injection and non-injection drug use-associated infective endocarditis: a nationwide cohort study. Clin Infect Dis. 2021;73(9):e2484–92. https://doi.org/10.1093/cid/ciaa1126. PMID: 32756935; PMCID: PMC8563193.

Arterial Blood Gas Interpretation

Krita Sridharan and Laila Rotstein

1 Clinical Pearl

When interpreting an arterial blood gas, it is important to calculate the alveolar-arterial gradient.

2 Clinical Case

A 28-year-old female presents to the emergency department with shortness of breath. She has an elevated respiratory rate. Her oxygen saturation is 96% on room air (normal range >95%). Her chest is clear to auscultation, and chest X-ray is clear.

Her arterial blood gas is demonstrated below:

pH **7.48** (normal range 7.35–7.45)
paO2 91 (normal range 80–100 mmHg)
paCO2 **27** (normal range 35–45 mmHg)
HCO3 **20** (normal range 22–30 mmol/L)

The treating doctor is reassured by the patient's investigations, in particular the oxygen saturation and partial pressure of oxygen and makes a diagnosis of anxiety disorder with hyperventilation. The patient is observed in the short stay unit. During her stay she develops pleuritic chest pain. This prompts the treating doctor to refer the patient for a CT pulmonary angiogram, which demonstrates a large pulmonary embolus. She is then admitted to hospital and commenced on appropriate treatment.

K. Sridharan (✉) · L. Rotstein
Alfred Health and Monash University, Melbourne, VIC, Australia

R. Junckerstorff et al. (eds.), *Beyond Evidence-Based Medicine*,
https://doi.org/10.1007/978-981-99-4440-8_52

3 Discussion

It is important to calculate the alveolar-arterial (A-a) gradient in the interpretation of arterial blood gases. The A-a gradient measures the difference in oxygen concentration between the alveoli and the arterial system. It has an important role in differentiating the cause for hypoxaemia, distinguishing alveolar hypoventilation from other causes of hypoxia (e.g., V/Q mismatch). If the A-a gradient is elevated, this suggests dysfunction of the alveolar-capillary unit as the cause for hypoxaemia. Such examples include asthma, chronic obstructive pulmonary disease, pneumonia, pulmonary oedema, pulmonary embolism, interstitial lung disease, etc. If the A-a gradient is normal, this suggests that the alveolar-capillary unit is preserved. Causes for hypoxaemia with a normal A-a gradient include hypoventilation such as neuromuscular disease, depression of the respiratory centre e.g., from opioid over-use, obesity hypoventilation, or kyphoscoliosis. A-a gradient will also be preserved if hypoxaemia is due to low atmospheric oxygen concentration, such as with high altitude.

The formula to calculate A-a gradient is below:

$$A - a\,gradient = PAO_2 - PaO_2$$

PaO_2 is arterial oxygen partial pressure and can be assessed on arterial blood gas.

PAO_2 is alveolar oxygen partial pressure and can be estimated using the alveolar gas equation [1]:

$$PAO_2 = FiO_2\left(Patm - pH_2O\right) - \frac{PaCO_2}{RQ}$$

Patm is atmospheric pressure, at sea level this is approximately 760 mmHg.

FiO_2 is fraction of inspired oxygen, at sea level and breathing room air this is 0.21 (this value should be altered if the patient is on supplementary oxygen).

pH_2O is partial pressure of water, which is approximately 47 mmHg.

RQ is the respiratory quotient, defined as the volume of CO_2 released over the volume of O_2 absorbed during respiration, which is approximately 0.8 at rest.

Using these numbers in the equation, achieves a PAO_2 value of approximately 150—$PaCO_2$/RQ for a person at sea level breathing room air.

Now we can proceed to calculate our patient's A-a gradient in our patient.

$$A - a\,gradient = \left[150 - \frac{PaCO_2}{0.8}\right] - PaO_2$$

$$A - a\,gradient = \left[150 - \frac{27}{0.8}\right] - 91$$

$$A - a\,gradient = 25.25$$

Expected A-a gradient can be roughly calculated with the following formula [2]:

$$A - a\,gradient = \frac{Age}{4} + 4$$

In this 28-year-old patient the expected A-a gradient would be 11. Therefore, her A-a gradient is clearly elevated. Calculation of A-a gradient as part of interpreting the arterial blood gas in this scenario would have led to earlier identification of a problem in the alveolar-capillary unit and earlier diagnosis of pulmonary embolism.

4 Other Gems

- Calculation of the A-a gradient gives an important clue to the presence of gas exchange pathology. It should be part of routine ABG interpretation.
- A VBG cannot be used as a substitute for an ABG when assessing respiratory failure. Although the pH and to a lesser extent $PaCO_2$, correlate well with arterial values, the PaO_2 does not [3].
- A VBG can be used to screen for hypercapnia. $PaCO_2$ <45 mmHg has been shown to have excellent negative predictive value to rule out hypercapnia [4, 5].
- A normal A-a gradient should not preclude further diagnostic procedures if there is a high index of suspicion for pulmonary embolus.
- An important limitation is that the A-a gradient increases with higher FiO_2. When a patient receives a high FiO_2, the PAO_2 increases disproportionately to the PaO_2, causing the A-a gradient to increase [6].

References

1. Sharma S, Hashmi MF, Burns B. Alveolar gas equation. StatPearls. Treasure Island, FL: StatPearls Publishing; 2021.
2. McFarlane MJ, Imperiale TF. Use of the alveolar-arterial oxygen gradient in the diagnosis of pulmonary embolism. Am J Med. 1994;96(1):57–62. https://doi.org/10.1016/0002-9343(94)90116-3. PMID: 8304364.
3. Byrne AL, Bennett M, Chatterji R, Symons R, Pace NL, Thomas PS. Peripheral venous and arterial blood gas analysis in adults: are they comparable? A systematic review and meta-analysis. Respirology. 2014;19(2):168–75. https://doi.org/10.1111/resp.12225. Epub 2014 Jan 3. PMID: 24383789.
4. Kelly AM, Kerr D, Middleton P. Validation of venous pCO2 to screen for arterial hypercarbia in patients with chronic obstructive airways disease. J Emerg Med. 2005;28(4):377–9. https://doi.org/10.1016/j.jemermed.2004.10.017. PMID: 15837016.
5. McCanny P, Bennett K, Staunton P, McMahon G. Venous vs arterial blood gases in the assessment of patients presenting with an exacerbation of chronic obstructive pulmonary disease. Am J Emerg Med. 2012;30(6):896–900. https://doi.org/10.1016/j.ajem.2011.06.011. Epub 2011 Sep 9. PMID: 21908141.
6. Kanber GJ, King FW, Eshchar YR, Sharp JT. The alveolar-arterial oxygen gradient in young and elderly men during air and oxygen breathing. Am Rev Respir Dis. 1968;97(3):376–81. https://doi.org/10.1164/arrd.1968.97.3.376. PMID: 5638492.

Will a Venous Blood Gas Suffice?

Stephen Gilmartin and Luke Phillips

1 Clinical Pearl

In most cases a venous blood gas will be sufficient to manage your patient and usually has good correlation with the arterial blood gas.

2 Clinical Case

A 68-year-old lady is brought to the Emergency Department (ED) by ambulance with acute shortness of breath. She has a history of Chronic Obstructive Pulmonary Disease (COPD), hypertension and hypothyroidism. On arrival, she is in respiratory distress, her heart rate is 126 bpm (regular), respiratory rate 32 breaths/min and O_2 Saturations 92% on 15 L of O_2 by non-rebreather mask. You meet her in the resuscitation area and start her on salbutamol inhalers and intravenous corticosteroids. The patient has had previous COPD exacerbations and knows what they entail, she asks 'will you be doing that painful test at my wrist?'

Her venous blood gas (VBG) is below. Usual reference ranges are displayed in brackets

S. Gilmartin
Sligo University Hospital, Sligo, Ireland

L. Phillips (✉)
Alfred Health, Melbourne, VIC, Australia

Department of Epidemiology and Preventative Medicine, Monash University, Melbourne, VIC, Australia

Mater Misericordiae University Hospital, Dublin, Ireland

R. Junckerstorff et al. (eds.), *Beyond Evidence-Based Medicine*,
https://doi.org/10.1007/978-981-99-4440-8_53

pH	7.36	(7.35–7.45)
PCO_2	42 mmHg	(35–45)
PO_2	**51** mmHg	(80–100)
HCO_3	25 mmol/L	(22–26)
BE	**2.8** mmol/L	(−2 to +2)
K+	4.3 mmol/L	(3.5–5.2)
Na+	138 mmol/L	(135–145)
Cl−	98 mmol/L	(96–106)
Lactate	**2.1** mmol/L	(<1.8)

3 Discussion

Blood gases are frequently performed in the Emergency Department (ED). Common indications are Diabetic Ketoacidosis (DKA), COPD exacerbations, septic and peri-arrest patients. Arterial blood gases (ABG) are more accurate than VBGs when comparing pH, PO_2 and PCO_2, however ABGs are more painful and have an increased risk of significant vascular and neurological injury when compared with VBGs [1]. In what situations may the less invasive approach of using a VBG be sufficient?

As per the GOLD guidelines for COPD [2], once a patient with an acute exacerbation is started on oxygen, they should have blood gases performed frequently in order to assess oxygenation and monitor trends in CO_2 and pH. This helps determine if the patient is responding to therapy and if they require or need adjustment to their non-invasive ventilation (NIV). The 2023 report states that VBG is accurate when comparing pH and bicarbonate levels to ABG but additional data is required to establish the full utility of VBG analysis in patients with respiratory distress.

A meta-analysis of 18 studies found that pH is comparable between ABG and VBG samples with venous pH being usually 0.03 higher than arterial [3]. Not surprisingly, PO_2 results were on average 36.9 mmHg lower in VBG samples. The venous and arterial PCO_2 values were found not to be comparable. These findings have been replicated by a prospective study published in 2016 [4].

Although venous PCO_2 is not reliably predictive of arterial PCO_2, perhaps a more pertinent question is whether hypercapnia can be excluded with purely a VBG? This is one of the clinically relevant questions we need to ask when assessing a patient with acute respiratory distress to determine if they are in type 2 respiratory failure and require NIV. Multiple studies have looked at this question [5, 6] and the evidence suggests that hypercapnia can safely be ruled out in patients with a normal venous PCO_2. In fact in one study, using VBG's to assess for hypercapnia led to reduction of ABG's by 29% [5]. If a VBG has a normal PCO_2 and a normal pH and HCO_3, it is very likely that the patient is not hypercapnic.

Table 1 Correlation of VBG with ABG

	Correlation with ABG
pH	– Good correlation
	– Venous sample 0.03 higher than arterial (95% confidence interval 0.029–0.038) [3]
PCO_2	– Poor correlation
	– Mean difference for PCO_2 5.92 mmHg [7]
	– 95% prediction interval unacceptably wide (−10.7 to +2.4 mmHg) [3]
	– 100% sensitive in detecting arterial hypercarbia in COPD exacerbations using cut off of PCO_2 45 mmHg [6]
HCO_3	– Good correlation
	– 95% limits of agreement 0 (−0.5 to 0.5) [8]
Lactate	– Strong correlation at low/normal levels, less accurate at higher values [10, 11]
	– If VBG lactate <2 mmol/L this is 100% for ABG lactate <2 mmol/L [11]

ABG's may be the gold standard investigation, however there is a role for the use of VBG's without a concomitant ABG and this strategy may be a more patient centred approach. The correlation between VBG and ABG is summarised in Table 1.

A reasonable approach to our patient would be to use her O_2 saturations along with her PCO_2 and pH values from her VBG to determine her initial treatment and monitor for response. If there is a clinical deterioration and/or her oxygen saturations drop then an ABG would be indicated.

4 Other Gems

- **PCO_2trend:** Venous PCO_2 has wide and unpredictable variations depending on when and where samples are taken. This means it cannot be used to accurately trend PCO_2 levels. If PCO_2 >45 mmHg is identified on VBG an ABG should be considered.
- **DKA:** There is good evidence showing agreement between VBG and ABG samples when analysing pH, bicarbonate and potassium levels in DKA patients [4, 9, 10].
- **Electrolytes:** There is a statistical difference in mean values between VBG and lab-based assays looking at sodium, potassium and creatinine. These have not been found to be clinically significant, apart from potassium readings in acidotic states. It is acceptable to use blood gas electrolyte values in time critical situations [9, 11].

References

1. Rowling SC, Fløjstrup M, Henriksen DP, Viberg B, Hallenberg C, Lindholt JS, et al. Arterial blood gas analysis: as safe as we think? A multicentre historical cohort study. ERJ Open Res. 2022;8(1):535–2021. http://openres.ersjournals.com/content/8/1/00535-2021.abstract.
2. 2022-2023 G scientific committee members. Global strategy for prevention, diagnosis and management of COPD, report 2023. 2023. https://goldcopd.org/2023-gold-report-2/.
3. Byrne AL, Bennett M, Chatterji R, Symons R, Pace NL, Thomas PS. Peripheral venous and arterial blood gas analysis in adults: are they comparable? A systematic review and meta-analysis. Respirology. 2014;19(2):168–75.
4. McKeever TM, Hearson G, Housley G, Reynolds C, Kinnear W, Harrison TW, et al. Using venous blood gas analysis in the assessment of COPD exacerbations: a prospective cohort study. Thorax. 2016;71(3):210–5.
5. Kelly A-M, Kerr D, Middleton P. Validation of venous pCO2 to screen for arterial hypercarbia in patients with chronic obstructive airways disease. J Emerg Med. 2005;28(4):377–9.
6. McCanny P, Bennett K, Staunton P, McMahon G. Venous vs arterial blood gases in the assessment of patients presenting with an exacerbation of chronic obstructive pulmonary disease. Am J Emerg Med. 2012;30(6):896–900.
7. Lim BL, Kelly A-M. A meta-analysis on the utility of peripheral venous blood gas analyses in exacerbations of chronic obstructive pulmonary disease in the emergency department. Eur J Emerg Med. 2010;17(5):246–8.
8. Zeserson E, Goodgame B, Hess JD, Schultz K, Hoon C, Lamb K, et al. Correlation of venous blood gas and pulse oximetry with arterial blood gas in the undifferentiated critically ill patient. J Intensive Care Med. 2018;33(3):176–81.
9. Herrington WG, Nye HJ, Hammersley MS, Watkinson PJ. Are arterial and venous samples clinically equivalent for the estimation of pH, serum bicarbonate and potassium concentration in critically ill patients? Diabetes Med. 2012;29(1):32–5.
10. Kelly A-M. The case for venous rather than arterial blood gases in diabetic ketoacidosis. Emerg Med Australas. 2006;18(1):64–7.
11. Pouryahya P, Tan L, Lin ZC, Meyer A. Reliability of venous blood gas sodium, potassium and creatinine. N Z Med J. 2018;131(1487):38–43.

Danger of Intrahospital Transfer

Edward T. H. Fysh

1 Clinical Pearl

Transportation of critically ill patients entails significant risk and complexity. Transport teams should be prepared to be able to provide all necessary care throughout the journey.

2 Clinical Case

A 68-year-old man was admitted to an intensive care unit with severe type 2 respiratory failure secondary to an exacerbation of chronic obstructive pulmonary disease. He required non-invasive ventilation and oxygen supplementation. He developed a pneumothorax, required a chest drain and was stabilised in the intensive care unit. However, the position of the drain was unclear on portable chest radiograph, so a decision was made to obtain a Computed Tomography (CT) scan of his chest. Whilst being transported, his Bilevel Positive Airway Pressure (BiPAP) mask slipped and was difficult to refit in the tight confines of an elevator. Oxygen desaturation prompted the escorting doctor to increase his oxygen flow rate from 4 to 15 L/min. There was then further delay getting the patient into the CT scanner, (where wall oxygen was available), because the patient had missed their scheduled time. The patient desaturated again in the corridor and the transport team realised the portable oxygen cylinder was empty. By the time the patient was able to be connected to wall oxygen, he was in cardiorespiratory arrest. Despite successful resuscitation and a protracted intensive care admission, the patient did not survive.

E. T. H. Fysh (✉)
Curtin University and St John of God Midland Hospital, Perth, WA, Australia

R. Junckerstorff et al. (eds.), *Beyond Evidence-Based Medicine*,
https://doi.org/10.1007/978-981-99-4440-8_54

3 Discussion

Critically ill patients suffer from severe, life-threatening illness or trauma and have limited physiological reserves. Deterioration can therefore be rapid, unpredictable, and potentially deadly even in a fully resourced intensive care unit. Transportation of such patients is inherently complex and risky, however it is frequently necessary when the needs of the patient cannot be met where the patient is located. As a guiding principle, the level of care of a critically ill patient throughout transportation should be equal to the level of care provided at the referral point [1].

As illustrated above, even a relatively short, intrahospital transfer can result in adverse outcomes and the benefits of transport should be weighed against the risks to the patient. A recent systematic review found that 26% of intrahospital transportations are associated with adverse events, 1.5% of which were life-threatening [2].

Equipment is one of the key factors to consider before transportation. In this case, insufficient oxygen was brought with the patient. It should be assumed any critically ill patient may deteriorate during transport and enough oxygen should be brought to be able to provide as high a flow rate as could be required, for the longest potential transport duration. A full "E size" oxygen cylinder holds approximately 660 L, adequate for just over 40 min at 15 L/min. However, delays during transport should be expected and leaks can occur, so generally a second, back-up cylinder should be included, even for shorter journeys.

Communication is another key element to safe patient transport. Before leaving a safe area, the receiving team must be aware of the estimated time of arrival and provisions should be made to receive the patient before the expected time of arrival. As outlined in Table 1, staff seniority and specific training in the transportation of critically ill patients are further key considerations.

Table 1 Summary of key elements to safe transportation of critically ill patients

Key transport factors	Important elements
Staff	Clear team leader; sufficient training/experience; familiarity with equipment and environment
Communication	Clear communication between senior referring and receiving clinicians regarding patient details and requirements, confirmed at time of departure; formal handover to transporting team and then to receiving team; estimated time of arrival with updates as required; consider out of hours access difficulties at receiving location
Equipment: monitoring	Continue the basic monitoring the patient was requiring pre-transport; consider size of equipment/space, ability to secure in transport vehicle in case of accident, mode of transport etc.
Equipment: resuscitation	Respiratory support including airway equipment, circulatory support including defibrillator and intravenous access equipment
Equipment: medications/oxygen	Ensure quantities in excess of expected and sufficient pump battery life for maximum transport duration; include resuscitation drugs and sedatives
Equipment: other	Specific equipment that may be required, e.g. chest drain, nasogastric tube, drainage bags etc.
Documentation	Predeparture records; monitoring and events during transport; handover summary

Whilst the errors illustrated in this case may appear basic, in a comprehensive prospective study, failure to communicate with radiology, equipment malfunction and empty oxygen tanks were three of the top ten most common intrahospital transportation related adverse events [3]. Preparation and attention to these key elements is advised, no matter how apparently simple or routine the patient transfer.

References

1. CICM, ACEM and FANZCA guideline for transport of critically-ill patients. 2015. https://www.cicm.org.au. Accessed Aug 2022.
2. Murata M, Nakagawa N, Kawasaki T, et al. Adverse events during intrahospital transport of critically ill patients: a systematic review and meta-analysis. Am J Emerg Med. 2022;52:13–9.
3. Brunsveld-Reinders AH, Arbous MS, Kuiper SG, de Jonge E. A comprehensive method to develop a checklist to increase safety of intra-hospital transport of critically ill patients. Crit Care. 2015;19(1):214.

Post-operative Drowsiness

Edward T. H. Fysh

1 Clinical Pearl

Opioid toxicity is common in hospitalised patients and all administration sources should be considered in a medical emergency.

2 Clinical Case

An 82-year-old lady was transferred to a rehabilitation ward following a total hip replacement for a fractured femur sustained in a fall at home 6 days previously. The day after transfer, a medical emergency call was put out for reduced conscious level. Initial assessment revealed partially obstructed breathing, that improved with jaw thrust manoeuvre and suction of secretions. Her respiratory rate was 8 breaths/min and her oxygen saturations were 90% on 8 L/min of oxygen via a Hudson mask. There was mild hypotension (95/50 mmHg) and hypoperfusion (peripheral capillary refill time 4 s). Her Glasgow Coma Scale score was 8 (E1, V3, M4). Her pupils were equal and reactive at 2 mm and there were no obvious localising signs on neurological examination or new signs of trauma beyond some old bruising from the original fall. Review of her medication chart, that had been newly rewritten on arrival to the rehabilitation ward, revealed that she had been given 5 mg of oxycodone in the preceding 24 h, with a regular dose of 10/5 mg of oxycodone Slow Release (SR) and naloxone twice daily. Blood tests revealed mild acute kidney injury, (urea of 17 mmol/L and creatinine of 160 μmol/L), normal electrolytes and glucose. There was acute type 2 respiratory failure on arterial blood gas, with mild respiratory acidosis (pH 7.28, pCO_2 71 mmHg, pO_2 71 mmHg, HCO_3 27 mmol/L).

E. T. H. Fysh (✉)
Curtin University and St John of God Midland Hospital, Perth, WA, Australia

R. Junckerstorff et al. (eds.), *Beyond Evidence-Based Medicine*,
https://doi.org/10.1007/978-981-99-4440-8_55

She had a marked improvement in conscious level and respiratory rate in response to 200 μg of intravenous naloxone, but required repeat doses after 20 min and was therefore admitted to a high dependency unit (HDU) for monitoring and administration of a naloxone infusion. After several hours in HDU, and an ongoing requirement for the naloxone infusion to manage her opioid toxicity, a 10 μg/h buprenorphine patch applied over the left scapula was discovered. This was removed and by the next day she was able to be discharged back to the rehabilitation ward. The buprenorphine patch had been charted on a previous medication chart and discontinued, but the patch had not been removed.

3 Discussion

Reduced conscious level is one of the most common reasons for medical emergency team calls. Stabilisation focusing on an Airway, Breathing, Circulation, Disability and Exposure (ABCDE) approach should be combined with urgent assessment and treatment of the underlying cause. In the absence of focal neurological deficit, head trauma or meningism, metabolic, toxic and hypoxia/hypoperfusion insults are likely [1]. Indeed, in one study of all emergency presentations with a GCS of 10 or lower, 38% were found to have suffered poisoning [2]. A recent systematic review of the literature found that 0.6–2.5% of all medical and surgical patients admitted to hospital suffer from opioid overdose [3]. Risk factors for opioid overdose were extremes of age, medical comorbidity, diagnosis of substance misuse and combining opioids with other sedatives.

Naloxone is a competitive inhibitor of opioids at the opioid receptor and is an effective treatment for overdosage. However, it must be remembered that it's duration of action is short (approximately 30–120 min depending on route of administration). This is much shorter that the duration of most opioids, especially long-acting oral preparations and close monitoring or naloxone infusions are often necessary to prevent repeat toxicity. The dosage and preparation of the opioids given to the patient need to be carefully sought to inform management. It should be remembered that drug errors can be made, and also patients may be able to access non-prescribed medication from visitors or even other patients.

In this instance, when transitioning from intravenous perioperative analgesia to oral analgesia, the patient had also been prescribed transdermal buprenorphine, as there had initially been some concern about her ability to take and absorb oral medication. Whilst the patch had been prescribed correctly (with a prescribed date of removal/changing of the patch), when the chart was rewritten, this item was omitted and nursing staff on the new ward were not aware that the patch remained in place. Strict adherence to local prescribing guidelines should be encouraged and prescription of multiple formulations of opioids and other sedatives at once should be avoided.

References

1. Sprigings D, Chambers JB, editors. Acute medicine: a practical guide to the management of medical emergencies. 5th ed. New York: Wiley; 2018.
2. Forsberg S, Höjer J, Enander C, Ludwigs U. Coma and impaired consciousness in the emergency room: characteristics of poisoning versus other causes. Emerg Med J. 2009;26(2):100–2.
3. Danovitch I, Vanle B, Van Groningen N, Ishak W, Nuckols T. Opioid overdose in the hospital setting: a systematic review. J Addict Med. 2020;14(1):39–47.

Part VIII
Respiratory Medicine

Pneumomediastinum in Acute Asthma Exacerbation

Carrie-Anne Wagner and Matthew T. Naughton

1 Clinical Pearl

Chest pain in asthma may indicate the presence of pneumomediastinum.

2 Clinical Case

A woman in her early 20s presented to the emergency department with chest pain associated with the sensation of fullness and bubbling underneath the skin in her neck. Her only past medical history was of eosinophilic asthma treated with medium dose preventer (budesonide/formoterol) and salbutamol reliever therapy. Her asthma had been well controlled over the past 6 months, but she had previous infective exacerbations requiring intubation. For 48 h prior to presentation, she was experiencing a severe acute attack and was using 4–6 puffs of salbutamol every 2–3 h during the day and night. In the emergency department her chest X-ray demonstrated pneumomediastinum with significant subcutaneous emphysema and pan viral polymerase chain reaction (PCR) was positive for picornavirus.

C.-A. Wagner
Department of Respiratory Medicine, Alfred Hospital, Melbourne, VIC, Australia

M. T. Naughton (✉)
Department of Respiratory Medicine, Alfred Hospital and Monash University, Melbourne, VIC, Australia

R. Junckerstorff et al. (eds.), *Beyond Evidence-Based Medicine*,
https://doi.org/10.1007/978-981-99-4440-8_56

3 Discussion

Asthma is a chronic disease that results in inflammation of the airway causing variable respiratory symptoms of wheeze, shortness of breath, chest tightness or cough associated with fluctuating expiratory airflow limitation. Exacerbations of asthma are frequently triggered by exercise, environmental exposures to allergens or irritants, or viral respiratory infections [1]. Risk factors associated with increased risk of asthma exacerbations are poor asthma control, any exacerbation during the previous 12 months, poor lung function and smoking [2].

Pneumomediastinum is a condition causing extraluminal gas in the mediastinum following alveolar rupture and air leak into the bronchovascular sheath. This air can then track towards the mediastinum (see diagram Fig. 1) [3].

The most common cause of pneumomediastinum is secondary to barotrauma from mechanical ventilation. In spontaneously breathing unventilated patients, common causes include diving (due to rapid gas expansion), traumatic injury (post bronchoscopic biopsy), Valsalva manoeuvre (e.g. child birth and smoking illicit drugs) or diseases causing local airway obstruction with gas trapping such as asthma [3]. Oesophageal rupture due to repeated vomiting is an important but rare cause (known as Boerhaave syndrome). COVID-19 related pneumonia in non-mechanically ventilated patients is also associated with pneumomediastinum [4].

The most common symptom of pneumomediastinum is chest pain, most likely due to mechanical stretching in the mediastinum as the air dissects through tissue planes [5]. The pain may be associated with subcutaneous swelling, crepitations or

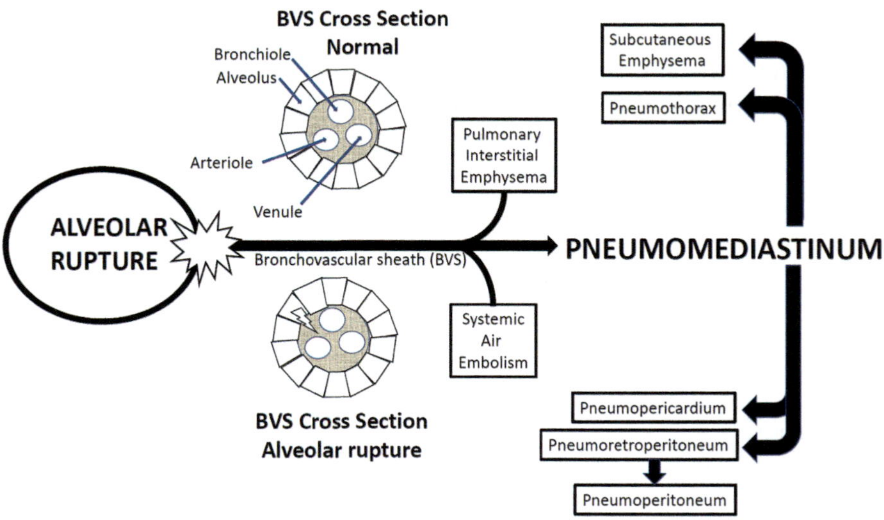

Fig. 1 Pathogenesis of the various downstream effects following alveolar rupture into the bronchovascular sheath (BVS). (Adapted from Murray and Nadel [3])

dysphonia [3]. The most notable clinical examination finding is palpable subcutaneous emphysema. Chest X-ray may detect pneumomediastinum [5] as gas forming linear lucencies highlighting mediastinal structures. If subcutaneous emphysema is present without apparent pneumothorax or clinical suspicion is high, computed tomography (CT) imaging should be considered.

Pneumomediastinum in isolation is generally considered a benign diagnosis (with exception of oesophageal rupture) and should be treated conservatively with analgesia and observation [5]. In asthma, pneumomediastinum may indicate a more severe exacerbation. Pneumomediastinum is a rare complicating factor for asthma exacerbations in adults but has been reported to occur in up to 5% of children with severe asthma requiring a chest X-ray [3].

Most patients with acute exacerbations of asthma presenting to hospital do not require basic blood examination or medical imaging. Additional diagnostic testing with imaging should be considered in the setting of a severe exacerbation or to investigate unusual findings such as chest pain or subcutaneous emphysema on presentation. Patients requiring admission should be screened for viral triggers with PCR testing including COVID-19.

Post-acute exacerbation care is vital in the management of asthma. It is important to emphasise that the use of regular inhaled corticosteroids should be maintained for 2–4 weeks following symptom improvement [1]. In the setting of pneumomediastinum, diving should be avoided lifelong and flying avoided for 6 weeks. At outpatient clinic review asthma control should be reassessed and lung function quantified by spirometry testing. Patients with severe or difficult to treat asthma should be referred for specialist review and considered for monoclonal antibody therapies [2].

4 Take Home Messages

- Pneumomediastinum usually occurs as a result of alveolar rupture and usually precursor for pneumothorax or subcutaneous emphysema.
- Chest X-ray has low sensitivity and specificity for isolated pneumomediastinum, hence a CT scan may be required.
- In isolation, pneumomediastinum is benign and should be managed conservatively.
- An important exception is pneumomediastinum due to a ruptured oesophagus often related to vomiting. This carries a high mortality and morbidity.
- Atypical symptoms of asthma (e.g. pain) should be further investigated with medical imaging.
- Personalised written asthma management plans are important guides for patients. They should detail what to do it their asthma symptoms are worsening, when to initiate oral corticosteroids and when to seek help [2].

References

1. Global Initiative for Asthma. Global strategy for asthma management and prevention. GINA. 2022. https://ginasthma.org. Accessed Sep 2022.
2. National Asthma Council Australia. Australian asthma handbook, Version 2.2. Melbourne: National Asthma Council Australia; 2022. https://www.asthmahandbook.org.au. Accessed Sep 2022.
3. Murray JF, Nadel JA. Textbook of respiratory medicine. 2nd ed. Philadelphia: WB Saunders Company; 1994.
4. Manna S, Maron SZ, Cedillo MA, Voutsinas N, Toussie D, Finkelstein M, Steinberger S, Chung M, Bernheim A, Eber C, Gupta YS, Concepcion J, Libes R, Jacobi A. Spontaneous subcutaneous emphysema and pneumomediastinum in non-intubated patients with COVID-19. Clin Imaging. 2020;67:207–13.
5. Kouritas VK, Papagiannopoulos K, Lazaridis G, Baka S, Mpoukovinas I, Karavasilis V, Lampaki S, Kioumis I, Pitsiou G, Papaiwannou A, Karavergou A, Kipourou M, Lada M, Organtzis J, Katsikogiannis N, Tsakiridis K, Zarogoulidis K, Zarogoulidis P. Pneumomediastinum. J Thorac Dis. 2015;7(Suppl 1):S44–9.

Cough Induced Carotid Artery Dissection

Miloš Nikolić and Matthew T. Naughton

1 Clinical Pearl

Prolonged or severe coughing can lead to carotid artery dissection and a constellation of neurological symptoms, including Horner's syndrome. A comprehensive respiratory system examination should always include a thorough examination of the peripheries.

2 Clinical Case

A male manual labourer in his early 50s with no past medical history had an episode of bronchitis associated with severe coughing. Two weeks into his respiratory illness he developed a feeling of fullness behind his eyes. Several days later he developed neck pain, worsening of his headache, dysphagia, dysarthria, and left posterior tongue paraesthesia. He was initially treated for migraine, however, thorough neurological examination showed left eye ptosis and miosis, dysarthria and tongue deviation to the left. Cranial imaging confirmed the presence of a long segment of dissection of the extracranial portion of the left internal carotid artery (ICA) (Figs. 1 and 2), with mass effect from the expanded ICA wall affecting the hypoglossal nerve and sympathetic fibres accompanying the ICA (Fig. 3), thereby causing an ipsilateral Horner's syndrome and hypoglossal nerve palsy.

M. Nikolić
Department of Respiratory Medicine, Alfred Hospital, Melbourne, VIC, Australia

M. T. Naughton (✉)
Department of Respiratory Medicine, Alfred Hospital and Monash University, Melbourne, VIC, Australia

R. Junckerstorff et al. (eds.), *Beyond Evidence-Based Medicine*,
https://doi.org/10.1007/978-981-99-4440-8_57

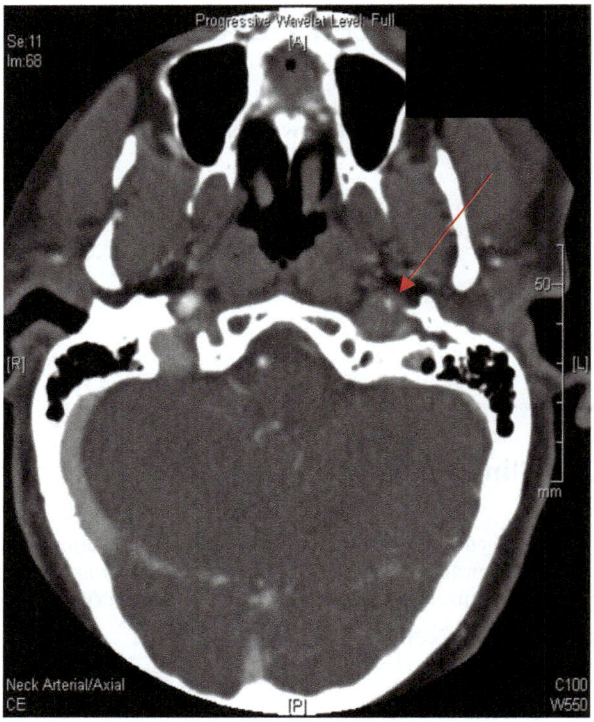

Fig. 1 Axial CT-angiogram showing left extracranial ICA dissection (arrow) with resultant thrombosis and 80% narrowing in vessel calibre

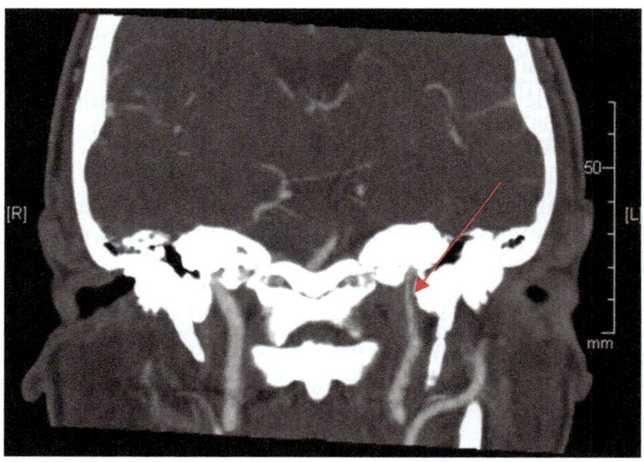

Fig. 2 Coronal CT-angiogram showing left extracranial ICA dissection (arrow) with resultant thrombosis and 80% narrowing in vessel calibre

He was commenced on antiplatelet therapy and made a good recovery of his Horner's syndrome when followed up as an outpatient, but still had mild hypoglossal nerve palsy at follow up 6 months later.

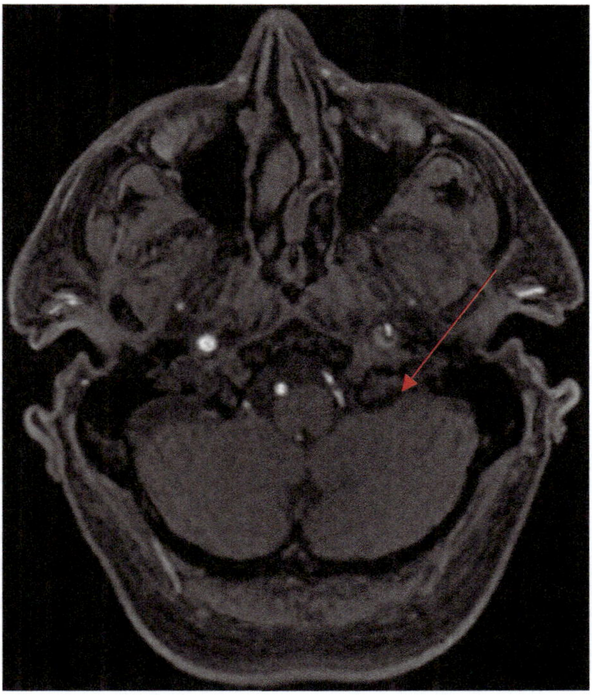

Fig. 3 Sagittal MRA demonstrating left ICA dissection and thrombosis (arrow). Note expansion of false lumen causing mass effect

3 Discussion

While rare, cough induced carotid artery dissection has been reported in over 80 cases in the literature to date [1].

Carotid or vertebral artery dissection can occur either spontaneously or secondary to trauma and may result in cerebral ischemia or transient neurological symptoms. Dissection leads to formation of intramural haematoma, which can cause stenosis of the lumen and/or aneurysmal dilatation of the artery. Cerebral ischaemia can occur due to interruption of flow at the level of the dissection but can also occur due to distal embolisation of thrombus.

The mechanism of injury in a traumatic dissection can be readily identified, for example manipulation of the neck, however the causes for spontaneous dissection are less well understood. While spontaneous dissection is more common in those with classic vascular risk factors, it is an important cause of stroke in younger patients without vasculopathy. They are estimated to account for 20% of strokes in younger patients [2]. Of these, approximately 80% are due to extracranial carotid artery dissections, and 20% due to vertebral artery dissections [2].

It is estimated that about 5% of patients with spontaneous dissections have an underlying connective tissue disease or fibromuscular dysplasia [3]. In addition, environmental and inflammatory factors may also be at play. Infection, and in particular, respiratory tract infection, appears to be associated with spontaneous dissection. Two case series have shown an increased prevalence of recent infection in those with spontaneous dissection compared to other causes of cerebral ischaemia, with an odds ratio of 2.4 [4, 5]. There was a further association with an increased prevalence in the "cold season", where respiratory infections are more common, compared to other times of the year [4]. Recent infection may also be a risk factor for multiple rather than single vessel dissection [5].

Vigorous coughing can generate impressive intrathoracic pressures, in excess of 300 mmHg [6]. These large pressures can exert strong shearing force on vascular walls, substantial enough to cause vessel dissection. Apart from carotid artery dissection, many other rare and serious sequalae of vigorous coughing have been reported, including coronary artery dissection, oesophageal rupture and diaphragmatic rupture [7].

Whilst cough induced carotid artery dissection is a rare complication, it is important to recognise the possibility as it is treatable. In addition to mechanical forces generated by severe coughing, inflammation, infection and underlying connective tissue disease all add to the cumulative risk.

4 Take Home Messages

- Repeated and forceful coughing can result in neurological impairment.
- A respiratory assessment should always include an examination of pupil size and reactivity. It takes <5 seconds and follows upper airway (i.e. oro-nasal) examination nicely.

References

1. Tai ML, Sia SF, Kadir KA, Idris MI, Tan KS. Cough-induced extracranial internal carotid artery dissection. Case Rep Neurol. 2020;12(1):149–55.
2. Bogousslavsky J, Pierre P. Ischemic stroke in patients under age 45. Neurol Clin. 1992;10(1):113–24.
3. Schievink WI, Wijdicks EF, Michels VV, Vockley J, Godfrey M. Heritable connective tissue disorders in cervical artery dissections: a prospective study. Neurology. 1998;50(4):1166–9.
4. Grau AJ, Brandt T, Buggle F, Orberk E, Mytilineos J, Werle E, Conradt C, Krause M, Winter R, Hacke W. Association of cervical artery dissection with recent infection. Arch Neurol. 1999;56(7):851–6.
5. Guillon B, Berthet K, Benslamia L, Bertrand M, Bousser MG, Tzourio C. Infection and the risk of spontaneous cervical artery dissection: a case-control study. Stroke. 2003;34(7):e79–81.
6. Sharpey-Schafer EP. The mechanism of syncope after coughing. Br Med J. 1953;2(4841):860.
7. Irwin RS, Dudiki N, French CL, Altman KW, Azoulay E, Barker AF, Birring SS, Bolser DC, Boulet LP, Braman SS, Brightling C. Life-threatening and non-life-threatening complications associated with coughing: a scoping review. Chest. 2020;158(5):2058–73.

Cough Syncope

Suzy Guo and Matthew T. Naughton

1 Clinical Pearl

Cough syncope is a rare condition and a diagnosis of exclusion. Often used as a medico-legal defence, with serious ramifications, the diagnosis of cough syncope should be subject to rigorous and standardised criteria.

2 Clinical Case

A 55-year-old man is involved in a serious single vehicle collision. At around 5:50 pm, he drove across a central median strip, across a dual lane road and across a footpath before impacting a block wall. Immediately prior to the accident, the patient described drinking water from a bottle, possible aspiration and difficulty breathing. There is a vague self-report of altered consciousness ("I thought I went to sleep"). He began his work shift at 4:30 am. His past medical history is significant for obesity (body mass index 38 kg/m^2), dyslipidaemia, hypertension, and diet-controlled type 2 diabetes mellitus. There is no history of respiratory, cardiac or neurological disease. There is no medication history of sedative or analgesic. He has been a commercial driver for more than 30 years, is an active smoker, and urinary drug screen immediately post-accident is negative. When the patient is taken to hospital, a preliminary diagnosis of cough syncope is made.

S. Guo
Department of Respiratory Medicine, Alfred Hospital, Melbourne, VIC, Australia

M. T. Naughton (✉)
Department of Respiratory Medicine, Alfred Hospital and Monash University, Melbourne, VIC, Australia

R. Junckerstorff et al. (eds.), *Beyond Evidence-Based Medicine*,
https://doi.org/10.1007/978-981-99-4440-8_58

Two months later, severe obstructive sleep apnoea is diagnosed (apnoea-hypoapnoea index 45 events/h; minimum SpO2 65%) and the patient is commenced on continuous positive airway pressure therapy.

3 Discussion

Cough syncope (CS) is rare and poorly understood. Clinical descriptions of CS patients typically characterise obese middle-aged males who experience syncope after prolonged coughing [1].

The proposed mechanisms of transient cerebral hypoperfusion in CS include an increase in intra-thoracic pressure causing reduced cardiac output; rapid alterations in intra-thoracic pressure causing peripheral vasodilation; increased intracranial pressure causing reduced cerebral perfusion; and reduced carotid blood flow [2]. Currently, the diagnosis of CS relies heavily on self-report and the exclusion of other causes of loss of consciousness.

This is especially troubling given the medico-legal ramifications of using cough syncope as a legal defence in serious motor vehicle accidents. Contrasting with CS, sleepiness [3] related to sleep deprivation or sleep disorder and distraction [4], both potential legal offences, are common causes of road accidents.

Based on the current understanding of CS pathophysiology [5], we present a diagnostic approach (Table 1).

4 Take Home Messages

- Drivers who suffer blackouts whilst driving need to have limitations placed upon their driving according to the local driving authority guidelines
- Drivers involved in motor vehicle crashes due to blackouts need formal cardiac, neurological, endocrine and sleep assessment
- Considerable ambiguity exists between descriptions of blackouts, excessive sleepiness and fatigue
- Although untreated obstructive sleep apnoea more than doubles one's lifetime risk of crash, sleep deprivation is a more powerful cause.
- Cough syncope is a rare cause of blackout, and should only be considered if it meets the criteria above.

Table 1 A diagnostic approach to the suspected CS patient

(a) Patient:
Condition predisposing to cough and/or cerebral hypoperfusion (e.g. chronic lung and/or vascular disease)
(b) Situation:
Syncope, induced by coughing, which is
Immediately recognised
Witnessed
Reproducible
Lasting <5 s
(c) Exclusion of other causes of syncope:
Cardiac
Arrhythmia (e.g. heart block, sick sinus syndrome)
Valvular (e.g. aortic stenosis)
Endocrine
Hypoglycaemia, hyponatremia, hypothyroidism
Carcinoid syndrome
Phaeochromocytoma
Neurological
Cerebral tumours (e.g. meningioma, glioblastoma)
Herniation of cerebellar tonsils
Hydrocephalus
Carotid and vertebral arterial occlusive disease
Basilar invagination
Autosomal dominant hereditary sensory neuropathy
Medullary infarction
Psychiatric
Pseudo-seizures
Suicide
Sleep related
Sleep deprivation (<5 h of sleep)
Diagnosis of circadian rhythm disorder, sleep disordered breathing, narcolepsy
Inattention (e.g. using mobile phone)
Drugs Prescribed
Social
Illicit

References

1. Skolnick JL, Dines DE. Tussive syncope. Minn Med. 1969;52(10):1609–13.
2. Dicpinigaitis PV, Lim L, Farmakidis C. Cough syncope. Respir Med. 2014;108:244–51.
3. Howard ME, Desai AV, Grunstein RR, Hukins C, Armstrong JG, Joffe D, et al. Sleepiness, sleep-disordered breathing, and accident risk factors in commercial vehicle drivers. Am J Respir Crit Care Med. 2004;170(9):1014–21.
4. Neale VL, Dingus TA, Klauer SG, Sudweeks JD, Goodman MJ. An overview of the 100-car naturalistic study and findings; 2005.
5. Guo H, Naughton CW, Naughton MT. Cough syncope as a cause of motor vehicle crash: fatal distraction. Int Med J. 2022;52:139–45. https://doi.org/10.1111/imj.15641.

Unilateral Diaphragm Palsy

Duncan J. Sweeney and Matthew T. Naughton

1 Clinical Pearl

Although classically associated with heart failure, orthopnoea is commonly seen in diseases impacting respiratory muscle mechanics, including neuromuscular disorders.

2 Clinical Case

A 70-year-old woman presented with neck pain following a fall, in the setting of morbid obesity (body mass index 38.1 kg/m^2). Initial neck x-ray demonstrated advanced spondylotic change at C4–5, with prominent osteophyte formation from C3 to 7, without acute fracture. Multiple weeks following presentation, the patient complained of worsening orthopnoea. Further questioning revealed unrefreshing sleep and morning headache. Clinical examination revealed dullness at the left base, and arterial blood gases demonstrated compensated hypercapnia (pH 7.39, $PaCO_2$ 59 mmHg, HCO_3 38 mmol/L). Re-review of initially performed chest X-ray from presentation suggested an elevated left hemidiaphragm; diaphragmatic palsy was later demonstrated on a fluoroscopic sniff test. Diagnostic sleep study confirmed the presence of nocturnal hypoventilation, and nocturnal non-invasive ventilation was commenced. At long-term follow-up the patient noted marked improvement in their symptoms of sleep disordered breathing, and daytime hypoventilation had resolved ($PaCO_2$ 44 mmHg).

D. J. Sweeney
Department of Respiratory Medicine, Alfred Hospital, Melbourne, VIC, Australia

M. T. Naughton (✉)
Department of Respiratory Medicine, Alfred Hospital and Monash University, Melbourne, VIC, Australia

R. Junckerstorff et al. (eds.), *Beyond Evidence-Based Medicine*,
https://doi.org/10.1007/978-981-99-4440-8_59

3 Discussion

In this case, a patient complained of orthopnoea as a result of a traumatic unilateral cervical nerve root injury leading to nocturnal hypoventilation in setting of concurrent obesity.

Orthopnoea is a common clinical symptom, and often readily attributed to heart failure. Due to changes in respiratory muscle and ventilatory mechanics in the supine position, a number of other conditions can also lead to orthopnoea. Prominent amongst these are diseases impacting diaphragmatic function, including diaphragmatic palsy and neuromuscular disorders (e.g. motor neuron disease, muscular dystrophies).

The diaphragm, the major muscle of respiration, is supplied bilaterally by spinal cord segments C3–5 via the phrenic nerves. Damage to the phrenic nerve, or spinal cord at or above the C3–5 level, will lead to a variable degree of diaphragmatic dysfunction, depending on the level and completeness of injury [1]. While bilaterally phrenic nerve injury has been described, typically diaphragm palsy is unilateral [2]. There are numerous causes of diaphragm palsy, including trauma (neck and shoulder), post cardiac surgery, iatrogenic (e.g. nerve block), compression (e.g. lung cancer, cervical spondylosis), and neuropathy [2]. Despite thorough investigation, a large number remain idiopathic.

Diagnosis of diaphragmatic palsy is challenging, and requires awareness of suggestive symptoms and clinical scenarios in which it can occur. The degree and magnitude of symptoms can be highly variable. Not infrequently patients will be asymptomatic, and the diagnosis is first entertained in the setting of an incidental finding of an elevated hemidiaphragm on chest X-ray. Outside of orthopnoea, patients can variably experience exertional dyspnoea and symptoms of nocturnal hypoventilation (sleep fragmentation, morning headache, unrefreshing sleep, and daytime sleepiness) [3].

Confirmation of diaphragm palsy is equally challenging. Historically fluoroscopic diaphragmatic screening has been utilised, particularly the sniff test looking for paradoxical ascent of the diaphragm on inspiration. Due to the insensitivity of diaphragm screening, however, more sensitive radiologic assessment with diaphragmatic ultrasound is increasingly employed which assesses both diaphragmatic movement and contraction. While lung function can assist in demonstrating the physiologic consequences of diaphragm palsy by quantifying the degree of associated restrictive defect on spirometry, or magnitude or inspiratory muscle weakness on maximal respiratory pressure testing, these studies are not specific for diaphragm palsy. Definitive diagnosis with electromyographic studies is very rarely performed due to the invasive and specialised nature of the procedure. Imaging studies can be useful in helping assess for an underlying structural cause along the course of the phrenic nerve.

For the majority of patients with unilateral diaphragm palsy, management is expectant. A small number of cases are secondary to a clear structural abnormality that requires specific intervention (e.g. malignancy causing compression on the adjacent phrenic nerve). Many consequences of neuropathy and traumatic injury are self-limiting, and see return of nerve function with time. It is not uncommon for diaphragm function to return 1–2 years after initial diagnosis.

While isolated unilateral diaphragm palsy does not typically cause significant nocturnal hypoventilation, those with pre-existing sleep disordered breathing or a co-existent cause of hypoventilation (e.g. obesity, COPD) can be symptomatic [4]. In these patients, nocturnal non-invasive ventilation is infrequently required, and typically instituted after polysomnography and arterial blood gases [5]. In highly symptomatic individuals with persistent diaphragm palsy, diaphragm fundoplication can be considered; while case series describing improvement in symptoms and physiologic parameters have been published, it is unclear which patients are likely to derive most benefit from this invasive intervention.

4 Take Home Messages

- Orthopnoea is commonly due to heart failure but can also occur with diaphragm weakness.
- A unilateral diaphragm palsy can be easily mistaken for an effusion, or lung lower lobe collapse.
- Classically, patients with a unilateral diaphragm weakness prefer to sleep with pathological diaphragm prone.
- Diagnosis of a diaphragm palsy is best done with a sniff test during fluoroscopy, although other techniques include pleural ultrasound and EMG.
- Functional assessment of diaphragm paralysis (or weakness) should include lung function and arterial blood gas (awake) and polysomnography with SpO_2, respiratory rate, position and transcutaneous CO_2 monitoring.

References

1. Berlowitz D, Wadsworth B, Ross J. Respiratory problems and management in people with spinal cord injury. Breathe (Sheff). 2016;12(4):328–40.
2. Jijatnur L, Rudrappa M. Diaphragm palsy. Diseases. 6(1):16.
3. Aboussouan LS. Sleep-disordered breathing in neuro-muscular disease. Am J Respir Crit Care Med. 2015;191(9):979.
4. Ambrosino N, Carpene N, Gherardi M. Chronic respiratory care for neuromuscular diseases in adults. Eur Respir J. 2009;34(2):444–51.
5. Pfeffer G, Povitz M. Respiratory management of patients with neuromuscular disease: current perspectives. Degener Neurol Neuromuscul Dis. 2016;6:111.

Oxygen in OSA: Swim Between the Flags

Freya Breyeni and Matthew T. Naughton

1 Clinical Pearl

Hyperoxia is an important iatrogenic cause of deterioration in patients with chronic hypercapnic respiratory failure. It should be recognised and managed carefully in the post-operative setting, especially in patients with obstructive sleep apnoea and obesity hypoventilation syndrome.

2 Clinical Case

A 54-year-old female is admitted with multiple skeletal injuries after a car accident. She is obese, with a body mass index of 43 kg/m^2. Her other past medical history includes hypertension, hyperlipidaemia, atrial fibrillation and diet-controlled Type 2 Diabetes. On admission she is commenced on multiple analgesic medications, including long and short-acting opioids. She requires emergency surgery for her multiple injuries. Following the operation, her oxygen levels are 88%. She is alert. An arterial blood gas completed shows a pH of 7.37 (range 7.35–7.45), $PaCO_2$ 58 (range 35–45 mmHg), PaO_2 61 (range 80–100 mmHg) and HCO_3 38 (range 22–32 mmol/l). She is commenced on supplemental oxygen therapy, which is continued overnight. A morning blood gas is completed, which demonstrates a pH of 7.24 and a pCO_2 of 81 mmHg.

F. Breyeni
Department of Respiratory Medicine, Alfred Hospital, Melbourne, VIC, Australia

M. T. Naughton (✉)
Department of Respiratory Medicine, Alfred Hospital and Monash University, Melbourne, VIC, Australia

R. Junckerstorff et al. (eds.), *Beyond Evidence-Based Medicine*,
https://doi.org/10.1007/978-981-99-4440-8_60

3 Discussion

Both under-oxygenation and over-oxygenation can be detrimental. Australia and New Zealand Thoracic Guidelines recommend targeting oxygen therapy to a specific range, so-called "swimming between the flags" of 92–96% in most patients and lower targets of 88–92% in those with certain underlying respiratory conditions, such as chronic obstructive pulmonary disease (COPD) [1]. Problems associated with over-oxygenation include increased risk of hypercapnia, direct pulmonary toxicity, cardiovascular effects (such as increased systemic vascular resistance and reduced cardiac output) and reduced cerebral blood flow [1]. Having an upper limit of oxygen therapy is intended to prevent over-oxygenation and enables recognition of clinical improvement. In some circumstances, provision of supplemental oxygen when not required may mask the development of respiratory failure until it has progressed to a critical point [2]. The changes in oxygen saturation may not reflect the extent of the underlying changes of pH and carbon dioxide (CO_2).

Obstructive sleep apnoea (OSA) is common and underdiagnosed in the Australian population. OSA involves the repeated collapse of the upper airways, despite persistent effort to breathe. The obstructive episode is terminated by a micro-arousal, which wakes the person, causing an increase in the respiratory drive and release of CO_2. The rapid change in CO_2 triggers the central chemoreceptors, resulting in hypoventilation.

Obesity hypoventilation syndrome (OHS) is defined by elevated arterial pressure of CO_2 ($PaCO_2$), in an obese patient where alternative causes of hypercapnia have been excluded. Further clues to diagnosis include daytime low baseline oxygen levels, elevated serum bicarbonate (>27 mmol/l) and daytime hypercapnia (>45 mmHg). Adiposity over the chest wall in obese patients alters the chest wall mechanics, with resultant hypoventilation and hypercapnia. The chronic respiratory acidosis with hypercapnia results in bicarbonate retention by the kidneys. The bicarbonate causes the central chemoreceptors to be less sensitive to changes in CO_2, resulting in persistent hypercapnia.

There are multiple contributing factors for the development of acute and chronic hypercapnic respiratory failure. This includes reduced ventilatory drive, changes in ventilation and perfusion mismatch and the Haldane effect. Due to the Haldane effect, provision of supplemental oxygen causes a shift right of the CO_2 dissociation curve, increasing levels of CO_2. Opioid medications cause respiratory depression, which can result in hypercapnia, which may increase baseline hypercapnia. Within the first 12 to 24 h following the post operative period, systemic opioids significantly increase the risk of respiratory depression. Other risk factors include female sex, other medical comorbidities and OSA with an elevated arousal threshold. To avoid CO_2 narcosis, multi-modal analgesia is recommended. This is particularly important in the post operative setting and includes the use of paracetamol, non-steroidal anti-inflammatories and use of regional anaesthesia.

In a healthy adult, the mean oxygen saturations during sleep can be around 90%. In a patient with OSA or OHS, the baseline oxygen saturations may be lower, with further severe oxygen desaturations with obstructive events [3]. Exposure to prolonged hypoxia during sleep has significant negative impacts upon the cardiovascular system, as well as adversely affecting associated comorbidities, such as increased insulin resistance [3]. However, the initiation of supplemental oxygen during these hypoxic events can result in hyperoxia and subsequent hypercapnia overnight. This can result in acute type 2 respiratory failure. The recommended treatment is application of continuous positive airway pressure (CPAP).

To reduce the risk of iatrogenic contribution to type 2 respiratory failure in high-risk patients, such as those with OSA, CPAP should be used in the immediate post-operative period. Prior to procedures, all patients should be screened with questionnaires, such as Epworth Sleepiness Scale and the STOP BANG questionnaire to identify the high-risk patients. Ensuring the availability and application of CPAP therapy post procedure reduces the risk of morbidity and mortality for this patient cohort.

4 Other Gems

- Oxygen therapy can disguise type 2 respiratory failure.
- Oxygen therapy should be used cautiously.
- Oxygen therapy can induce hypercapnia and heart failure.
- OHS is worse than OSA in terms of post operative outcomes.
- Questionnaires (such as the Stop Bang Questionnaire) and blood gases (identifying elevated bicarbonate and carbon dioxide) are useful in identifying high risk OSA and OHS patients.
- Sleepiness as a cause of motor vehicle accident should be considered before returning to drive.

References

1. Beasley R, Chien J, Douglas J, Eastlake L, Farah C, King G, Moore R, Pilcher J, Richards M, Smith S, Walters H. Thoracic Society of Australia and New Zealand oxygen guidelines for acute oxygen use in adults: ‘Swimming between the flags’. Respirology. 2015;20(8):1182–91.
2. Lynn LA, Curry JP. Patterns of unexpected in-hospital deaths: a root cause analysis. Patient Saf Surg. 2011;5(1):1–25.
3. Ryan S, Cummins EP, Farre R, Gileles-Hillel A, Jun JC, Oster H, Pepin JL, Ray DW, Reutrakul S, Sanchez-De-La-Torre M, Tamisier R. Understanding the pathophysiological mechanisms of cardiometabolic complications in obstructive sleep apnoea: towards personalised treatment approaches. Eur Respir J. 2020;56(2):1902295.

Adenocarcinoma Presenting as Lobar Consolidation

Ashleigh Witt and Alistair Miller

1 Clinical Pearl

Adenocarcinoma with lepidic spread can present radiologically as lobar consolidation and must be considered in a patient with consolidation and normal inflammatory markers.

2 Clinical Case

A 67 year-old receptionist is referred to the emergency department by her general practitioner with 3 weeks of productive cough, dyspnoea and lethargy. A chest X-ray performed by the referring doctor shows dense lobar consolidation in the right middle and lower lobes. She is afebrile, normoxic on room air and not in respiratory distress. Laboratory investigations demonstrate a total white cell count of 6.0 × 10^9/L (normal range 4.0–12.0 × 10^9/L), and a C-Reactive Protein of 2.1 mg/L (normal range < 5 mg/L).

She is an ex-smoker of 40 pack years, having given up 12 months prior to this illness. She has no other significant past medical history or exposures. She is

A. Witt
Department of Respiratory and Sleep Medicine, Royal Melbourne Hospital, Melbourne, VIC, Australia

A. Miller (✉)
Department of Respiratory and Sleep Medicine, Royal Melbourne Hospital, Melbourne, VIC, Australia

Department of Internal Medicine, Peter MacCallum Cancer Centre, Melbourne, VIC, Australia

Department of Medicine—RMH, Faculty of Medicine, Dentistry and Health Services, The University of Melbourne, Melbourne, VIC, Australia

R. Junckerstorff et al. (eds.), *Beyond Evidence-Based Medicine*,
https://doi.org/10.1007/978-981-99-4440-8_61

admitted to the Respiratory unit and treated with intravenous antibiotics for community acquired pneumonia. After 48 h she feels subjectively improved and is discharged home on oral antibiotics.

A repeat chest X-ray is performed at a 6-week review and demonstrates no change to the dense consolidation. She describes an ongoing productive cough. She proceeds to computed tomography which shows lobar consolidation and then to bronchoscopy. Cytology from the bronchoalveolar lavage fluid and histology from transbronchial biopsies return as adenocarcinoma.

3 Discussion

While conventional bacterial infection is the commonest cause of consolidation, the absence of infective symptoms or elevation of inflammatory markers, and the persistence over time must raise the possibility of alternative diagnoses. While the differential is broad (see Table 1 below), malignancy must be considered and appropriately investigated for.

Lung cancer is the commonest cause of cancer death worldwide [2], but has a broad range of clinical presentations and prognoses. It is divided into two groups, Non-Small Cell Lung Cancer (NSCLC) which accounts for the majority of lung cancer (~80%) and Small Cell Lung Cancer (SCLC). NSCLC has been divided according to histological appearance for many years but is increasingly further delineated by mutational analysis and evaluation of cell-surface marker expression. Over the past 50 years, adenocarcinoma has become the predominant NSCLC

Table 1 Differential diagnosis of consolidation seen on X-ray or CT of the chest. (Adapted from [1])

Cause	Examples
Malignant	Lung adenocarcinoma—AIS; MIA Pulmonary lymphoma Metastases particularly from GI source
Inflammatory	Sarcoidosis Organising pneumonia Eosinophilic pneumonia Vasculitis (e.g. EGPA; GPA) Drug-induced
Infective	Fungal infection Mycobacterial infection Pneumocystis jirovecii
Other	Lipoid pneumonia Alveolar haemorrhage Pulmonary alveolar proteinosis

AIS adenocarcinoma in-situ, *MIA* minimally invasive adenocarcinoma, *EGPA* eosinophilic granulomatosis with polyangiitis, *GPA* granulomatosis with polyangiitis

diagnosed, and while it remains more common in smokers than non-smokers, particularly in men, it is the most common lung cancer diagnosed in non-smokers [3].

A rare form of adenocarcinoma arises from the epithelial cells of the terminal bronchioles and grows along the alveolar septa, in a 'scale like' (or lepidic) pattern [4–6]. Due to this growth pattern along the walls of the lung, without destroying the lung parenchyma, it may not appear mass-like, but may present as lobar consolidation radiologically [6].

This entity was previously known as bronchioalveolar carcinoma but was reclassified by the International Association for the Study of Lung Cancer (IASLC) in 2011 into five histologic categories: adenocarcinoma in situ (AIS); minimally invasive adenocarcinoma, lipidic predominant adenocarcinoma, adenocarcinoma predominantly invasive with some lepidic component and invasive mucinous adenocarcinoma [7].

Of note, Positron Emission Tomography (PET) scans are frequently negative in this disease [8] and often a definitive histologic diagnosis can only be made with a surgical specimen [5]. Treatment options are similar to other forms of non-small cell lung carcinoma, with surgical resection standard of care for early-stage disease [6].

4 Other Gems

- Bronchorrhoea (sputum production >100 mL/day) is a symptom that is unusual for pneumonia and should prompt consideration of invasive mucinous adenocarcinoma.
- Lobar consolidation has a broad range of differentials including infection, carcinoma, granulomatous disease and interstitial lung disease.
- Repeat chest X-ray at 6 weeks following an acute lobar pneumonia is recommended by the National Institute for Care and Health Excellence (NICE) for patients with ongoing symptoms or risk factors for malignancy (age over 50 or smoking history) [9].

References

1. Ansari-Gilani K, Chalian H, Rassouli N, Bedayat A, Kalisz K. Chronic airspace disease: review of the causes and key computed tomography findings. World J Radiol. 2020;12(4):29–47.
2. Collaboration GBoDC. Cancer incidence, mortality, years of life lost, years lived with disability, and disability-adjusted life years for 29 cancer groups from 2010 to 2019: a systematic analysis for the global burden of disease study 2019. JAMA Oncol. 2022;8(3):420–44.
3. Dubin S, Griffin D. Lung cancer in non-smokers. Mo Med. 2020;117(4):375–9.
4. Garfield DH, Cadranel JL, Wislez M, Franklin WA, Hirsch FR. The bronchioloalveolar carcinoma and peripheral adenocarcinoma spectrum of diseases. J Thorac Oncol. 2006;1(4):344–59.

5. Thompson WH. Bronchioloalveolar carcinoma masquerading as pneumonia. Respir Care. 2004;49(11):1349–53.
6. Alshati MH, Yaktien MM, Katchy KC. Former mucinous bronchioloalveolar carcinoma revisited. Case Rep Med. 2013;2013:284323.
7. Zugazagoitia J, Enguita AB, Nunez JA, Iglesias L, Ponce S. The new IASLC/ATS/ERS lung adenocarcinoma classification from a clinical perspective: current concepts and future prospects. J Thorac Dis. 2014;6(Suppl 5):S526–36.
8. Heyneman LE, Patz EF. PET imaging in patients with bronchioloalveolar cell carcinoma. Lung Cancer. 2002;38(3):261–6.
9. NICE. Pneumonia in adults: diagnosis and management: National Institute of Clinical Excellence; 2014; https://www.nice.org.uk/guidance/cg191.

Neuromuscular Disease as a Cause of Hypercapnic Respiratory Failure

Ashleigh Witt and Alistair Miller

1 Clinical Pearl

New hypercapnic respiratory failure in the absence of severe lung disease should raise the suspicion of neuromuscular disease.

2 Clinical Case

A 68 year-old man presents with a 6-week history of generalised weakness and fatigue, on a background of hypertension and gastro-oesophageal reflux disease. He is a never smoker. On arrival to the emergency triage, he is noted to have saturations of 91% on room air and is commenced on supplemental oxygen at a rate of 2 L/min via nasal prongs. Several hours later he becomes drowsy and obtunded and undergoes rapid sequence intubation.

Arterial blood gas demonstrates a pH of 7.14 (normal range 7.35–7.45), $paCO_2$ of 105 mmHg (normal range 35–45 mmHg), paO_2 of 100 mmHg (normal range 80–100 mmHg) and bicarbonate of 38 mmol/L (normal range 22–30 mmol/L). He

A. Witt
Department of Respiratory and Sleep Medicine, Royal Melbourne Hospital, Melbourne, VIC, Australia

A. Miller (✉)
Department of Respiratory and Sleep Medicine, Royal Melbourne Hospital, Melbourne, VIC, Australia

Department of Internal Medicine, Peter MacCallum Cancer Centre, Melbourne, VIC, Australia

Department of Medicine—RMH, Faculty of Medicine, Dentistry and Health Services, The University of Melbourne, Melbourne, VIC, Australia

R. Junckerstorff et al. (eds.), *Beyond Evidence-Based Medicine*,
https://doi.org/10.1007/978-981-99-4440-8_62

is managed as an exacerbation of previously undiagnosed COPD with steroids, bronchodilators and antibiotics. The hypercapnia corrects rapidly with invasive ventilation and after 48 h the patient is extubated. In the 24 h following extubation the pCO_2 slowly rises and he is reintubated.

An MRI brain is performed and is within normal limits. His medication history prior to admission consisted of perindopril and pantoprazole, with no recreational drug use. His BMI is 27 and he has no features of obstructive sleep apnoea on collateral history from his wife.

He is extubated again, this time onto bilevel non-invasive ventilation. Respiratory functional testing is performed demonstrating an apparent restrictive deficit on spirometry which is confirmed on total body plethysmography. Maximal inspiratory and expiratory pressures are reduced. He proceeds to needle electromyography which confirms a diagnosis of amyotrophic lateral sclerosis.

3 Discussion

Respiratory failure is commonly differentiated into hypoxic (type 1) and hypercapnic (type 2) respiratory failure. Hypercapnic respiratory failure is distinguished by a partial pressure of carbon dioxide of >45 mmHg and a pH of <7.35 [1]. The partial pressure of oxygen may be normal or low depending on the cause of the respiratory failure. The predominant aetiology for hypercapnic respiratory failure is hypoventilation, however increased production of carbon dioxide due to states of oxidative metabolism such as sepsis can occur [2].

Hypercapnic respiratory failure is commonly encountered in hospital practice, with a prevalence of 163 cases per 100,000 population [3]. The differential diagnoses are broad and in cases of refractory or recurrent hypercapnia, and those with no predisposing conditions, consideration to uncommon causes should be given (Table 1).

Amyotrophic lateral sclerosis (ALS) is a progressive neurological condition characterised by degeneration of motor neurons [5]. Although respiratory failure is the most common cause of death in patients with ALS, it is rarely the presenting symptom [6]. Loss of phrenic nerve function leads to diaphragmatic weakness causing hypoventilation. Non-invasive ventilation for patients with respiratory failure due to motor neurone disease has both survival and quality of life benefits [6, 7].

4 Other Gems

- Mean inspiratory and expiratory pressures, often abbreviated to "MIPS and MEPS", are a non-invasive measure of respiratory muscle strength performed in the lung function laboratory. The major limitation of this test is that it is entirely

Table 1 Aetiology of hypercapnic respiratory failure. (Adapted from Roussos et al. [4])

Decreased central respiratory drive	Pharmacological sedatives (opiates, benzodiazepines, antipsychotic medications, anaesthetic, some antidepressant drugs) Neurological disease (stroke, encephalitis, brainstem disease) Sleep apnoea (central and obstructive) Obesity hypoventilation Metabolic causes (severe hypothyroidism, starvation)
Decreased respiratory neuromuscular or thoracic cage function	Primary spinal cord disorders (Spinal cord trauma, transverse myelitis) Amyotrophic lateral sclerosis Myasthenia gravis Guillain-Barre syndrome Phrenic nerve injury Poliomyelitis Critical illness polymyoneuropathy Muscle abnormalities (muscular dystrophy) Toxins (organophosphate poisoning, botulism, tetanus) Tick paralysis Acute intermittent porphyria Neuralgic amyotrophy Periodic paralysis Glycogen storage and mitochondrial diseases Chest wall disease (kyphoscoliosis, thoracoplasty, flail chest, pectus excavatum, fibrothorax) Metabolic disorders (hypophosphataemia, hypomagnesaemia, hypothyroidism, hyperthyroidism)
Lung and airway disease	Obstructive airways disease (acute exacerbations of asthma, COPD, bronchiectasis) Severe interstitial lung disease Pulmonary embolism or pulmonary vascular disease (usually severe)

dependent on the participants effort, and therefore lacks specificity [8], although it is frequently used as an endpoint in motor neuron disease research [6, 7].

- Reduction in forced vital capacity (FVC) has a direct relationship to survival in motor neurone disease, with an FVC of <50% considered to be an imminent risk of respiratory failure [6].
- Calculation of the Alveolar to arterial oxygen gradient (A-a gradient) readily identifies hypoventilation as the cause of hypoxia, and thus an arterial blood gas is an essential diagnostic test in respiratory failure [9].
- To quickly determine chronicity of hypercapnia:
  - In acute respiratory acidosis, bicarbonate will increase by 1 mEq/L for every 10 mmHg in $paCO_2$.
  - In chronic respiratory acidosis, bicarbonate will increase by 4 mEq/L for every 10 mmHg in $paCO_2$ [10].

- Hypercapnic respiratory failure related to COPD occurs in people with severe obstruction, and is incredibly uncommon in non-smokers.

References

1. Davidson AC, Banham S, Elliott M, Kennedy D, Gelder C, Glossop A, et al. BTS/ICS guideline for the ventilatory management of acute hypercapnic respiratory failure in adults. Thorax. 2016;71 Suppl 2:ii1–ii35.
2. Marhong J, Fan E. Carbon dioxide in the critically ill: too much or too little of a good thing? Respir Care. 2014;59(10):1597–605.
3. Chung Y, Garden FL, Marks GB, Vedam H. Population prevalence of hypercapnic respiratory failure from any cause. Am J Respir Crit Care Med. 2022;205(8):966–7.
4. Roussos C, Koutsoukou A. Respiratory failure. Eur Respir J Suppl. 2003;47:3s–14s.
5. Niedermeyer S, Murn M, Choi PJ. Respiratory failure in amyotrophic lateral sclerosis. Chest. 2019;155(2):401–8.
6. Tateno F, Sakakibara R, Kawashima K, Kishi M, Tsuyusaki Y, Aiba Y, et al. Amyotrophic lateral sclerosis presenting respiratory failure as the sole initial manifestation. Case Rep Neurol. 2014;6(2):213–6.
7. Walsh LJ, Murphy DM. The benefit of non-invasive ventilation in motor neuron disease. Open Respir Med J. 2020;14:53–61.
8. American Thoracic Society/European Respiratory S. ATS/ERS statement on respiratory muscle testing. Am J Respir Crit Care Med. 2002;166(4):518–624.
9. Petersson J, Glenny RW. Gas exchange and ventilation-perfusion relationships in the lung. Eur Respir J. 2014;44(4):1023–41.
10. Martinu T, Menzies D, Dial S. Re-evaluation of acid-base prediction rules in patients with chronic respiratory acidosis. Can Respir J. 2003;10(6):311–5.

Wheeze in COPD

Ashleigh Witt and Alistair Miller

1 Clinical Pearl

The presence or absence of wheeze doesn't distinguish severity of a COPD exacerbation.

2 Clinical Case

A 65 year-old man presents to the emergency department after a fall and is found to be in profound hypercapnic respiratory failure. His respiratory rate is 40 breaths per minute and he remains hypoxic despite supplemental oxygen via high-flow nasal prongs and is transitioned to non-invasive ventilation. His chest is clear to auscultation. A CT pulmonary angiogram performed to exclude pulmonary emboli (PE) shows a small non-occlusive clot suspected to be chronic and significant airway wall thickening and mucous plugging. He is commenced on a 3-day course of prednisolone and intravenous antibiotics.

His medical background includes Chronic Obstructive Pulmonary Disease (COPD) with ongoing smoking, prior PE with poor adherence with therapy, and

A. Witt
Department of Respiratory and Sleep Medicine, Royal Melbourne Hospital, Melbourne, VIC, Australia

A. Miller (✉)
Department of Respiratory and Sleep Medicine, Royal Melbourne Hospital, Melbourne, VIC, Australia

Department of Internal Medicine, Peter MacCallum Cancer Centre, Melbourne, VIC, Australia

Department of Medicine—RMH, Faculty of Medicine, Dentistry and Health Services, The University of Melbourne, Melbourne, VIC, Australia

R. Junckerstorff et al. (eds.), *Beyond Evidence-Based Medicine*,
https://doi.org/10.1007/978-981-99-4440-8_63

Hepatitis C with cirrhosis. The severity of his COPD is unknown, but he has been prescribed an Inhaled Corticosteroid (ICS)/Long-Acting Beta-Agonist (LABA)/ Long-Acting Muscarinic-Antagonist (LAMA) inhaler. After 5 days in hospital, he remains hypoxic with a clear chest and no response to subsequent attempts at diuresis. Oral prednisolone is restarted along with bronchodilator therapy, with progressive improvement in oxygenation and he is able to be weaned from oxygen and discharged home.

3 Discussion

Acute exacerbations of COPD are of great significance to both disease progression for the individual and the burden on the health care system [1]. In 2015–16, more than half all expenditure on COPD was for hospital admissions ($536 m), which does not take into account the cost of exacerbations managed in the community [2]. However, while it is clearly true that exacerbations are important, defining them and grading their severity is poorly elucidated.

Wheeze is considered a cardinal examination finding in COPD; however it is neither necessary for a diagnosis nor specific to COPD. It is described as a musical sound which can occur during both inspiration and expiration, occurring as a result of airway narrowing, turbulent airflow and oscillation of the airway. The volume and frequency of the sound will depend on the location of the narrowing within the bronchial tree [3]. If the airway is not sufficiently narrowed or turbulent airflow is not adequate to lead to airway oscillation, or indeed if sputum plugging results in no airflow into inflamed segments, then wheeze will not be clinically evident. COPD describes a broad spectrum of disease, with increasing phenotypic delineation occurring in recent years [4]. A wheezy phenotype has been described [5] and absence of wheeze has been associated with late or under-diagnosis [6]. To further cloud the picture, upper airway dystonias may also cause noisy breathing and be described as wheeze by patients and clinicians alike [7].

Previous grading of COPD exacerbation severity has relied on retrospective analysis of healthcare utilisation, but a new schema has been proposed, providing both a definition of an exacerbation and factors which delineate severity [8]. The proposed definition for an exacerbation takes into account both the natural variation of symptoms and a time frame of any change that may signal an exacerbation. The proposed definition is: 'In a patient with COPD, an exacerbation is an event characterised by dyspnoea and/or cough and sputum that worsens over ≤ 14 days, which may be accompanied by tachypnoea and/or tachycardia and is often associated with increased local and systemic inflammation caused by airway infection, pollution, or other insult to airways'. The authors also propose a method of delineating severity using only commonly collected clinical and pathology results (see Table 1). While awaiting external validation, this allows for a repeatable and reliable assessment of severity without reliance on inconsistent clinical signs.

Table 1 Classification of COPD Exacerbation Severity. (Adapted from [8])

Severity	Criteria
Mild (default)	• Dyspnoea VAS <5 • RR <24 breaths/min • HR <95 bpm • Resting $SaO_2 \geq 92\%$ breathing ambient air (or patient's usual oxygen prescription) AND change ≤3% (when known) • CRP <10 mg/L (if obtained)
Moderate (meets at least 3 of 5 criteria)	• Dyspnoea VAS ≥5 • RR ≥24 breaths/min • HR ≥95 bpm • Resting $SaO_2 < 92\%$ breathing ambient air (or patient's usual oxygen prescription), AND/OR change >3% (when known) • CRP ≥10 mg/L If obtained, ABG may show hypoxemia ($PaO_2 < 60$ mmHg) and/or hypercapnia ($PaCO_2 > 45$ mmHg) but no acidosis (pH >7.35)
Severe	• ABG show hypercapnia and acidosis ($PaCO_2 \geq 45$ mmHg and pH <7.35)

VAS visual analogue scale, *CRP* C-reactive protein, *ABG* arterial blood gas, *HR* heart rate, *RR* respiratory rate, SaO_2 oxygen saturation, $PaCO_2$ partial pressure of carbon dioxide in arterial blood

4 Other Gems

- Many conditions can mimic exacerbations of chronic obstructive pulmonary disease, and in particular heart failure, pneumonia and pulmonary embolism should be considered as key differentials [8].
- Deaths from chronic obstructive pulmonary disease exceed three million per year and account for 6% of all deaths worldwide [9].
- Asthma and COPD can co-exist, in an entity called asthma-COPD overlap syndrome (ACOS) [9].
- In an exacerbation, systemic corticosteroids improve lung function and shorten recovery time and hospital length of stay [9].

References

1. Waeijen-Smit K, Jacobsen PA, Houben-Wilke S, Simons SO, Franssen FME, Spruit MA, et al. All-cause admissions following a first-ever exacerbation-related hospitalization in COPD. ERJ Open Res. 2022;9:00217–2022.
2. AIHW. Chronic obstructive pulmonary disease (COPD). 2020; updated 25 Aug 2020. https://www.aihw.gov.au/reports/chronic-respiratory-conditions/copd/contents/impact.
3. JR GH. Wheezing and asthma. Clinical methods: the history, physical, and laboratory examinations. 3rd ed. Boston, MA: Butterworths; 1990.
4. Mirza S, Benzo R. Chronic obstructive pulmonary disease phenotypes: implications for care. Mayo Clin Proc. 2017;92(7):1104–12.

5. Huang WC, Tsai YH, Wei YF, Kuo PH, Tao CW, Cheng SL, et al. Wheezing, a significant clinical phenotype of COPD: experience from the Taiwan obstructive lung disease study. Int J Chron Obstruct Pulmon Dis. 2015;10:2121–6.
6. Camargo CA, Hasegawa K. Absence of wheezing is associated with underdiagnosis of chronic obstructive pulmonary disease: analysis of the NHANES, 2007–2012. In: A49 COPD: CARE DELIVERY; 2016. p. A1703.
7. Leong P, Ruane LE, Phyland D, Koh J, MacDonald MI, Baxter M, et al. Inspiratory vocal cord closure in COPD. Eur Respir J. 2020;55(5):1901466.
8. Celli BR, Fabbri LM, Aaron SD, Agusti A, Brook R, Criner GJ, et al. An updated definition and severity classification of chronic obstructive pulmonary disease exacerbations: the rome proposal. Am J Respir Crit Care Med. 2021;204(11):1251–8.
9. GOLD. Global strategy for the diagnosis, management, and prevention of chronic obstructive pulmonary disease. Fontana, WI: Global Initiative for Chronic Obstructive Lung Disease; 2021.

Exercise Testing Can Uncover Early Respiratory Disease

Ashleigh Witt and Alistair Miller

1 Clinical Pearl

Early pulmonary vascular disease/pulmonary hypertension may be picked up with exertional desaturation in the presence of otherwise normal lung function.

2 Clinical Case

A 27-year-old female presents with pleuritic chest pain and dyspnoea and is found to have bilateral pulmonary emboli on computed tomography pulmonary angiogram (CTPA). Her medication history is significant for the combined oral contraceptive pill, and she has recently undertaken a 4-h flight from Perth to Melbourne.

Observations on presentation demonstrate an oxygen saturation of 96% on room air, a heart rate of 85 bpm, respiratory rate 18 and non-invasive blood pressure of 115/70 mmHg. Her high sensitivity troponin is elevated at 31 ng/L (normal range < 26 ng/L) and she has mild radiological right heart strain on both CTPA and transthoracic echocardiogram. She is commenced on rivaroxaban, undergoes 48 h

A. Witt
Department of Respiratory and Sleep Medicine, Royal Melbourne Hospital, Melbourne, VIC, Australia

A. Miller (✉)
Department of Respiratory and Sleep Medicine, Royal Melbourne Hospital, Melbourne, VIC, Australia

Department of Internal Medicine, Peter MacCallum Cancer Centre, Melbourne, VIC, Australia

Department of Medicine—RMH, Faculty of Medicine, Dentistry and Health Services, The University of Melbourne, Melbourne, VIC, Australia

R. Junckerstorff et al. (eds.), *Beyond Evidence-Based Medicine*,
https://doi.org/10.1007/978-981-99-4440-8_64

of monitoring for an intermediate-high risk PE and is discharged home once symptomatically improved.

Six months later she is reviewed in the general respiratory clinic and undergoes respiratory function testing which demonstrates normal spirometry and normal diffusing capacity for carbon monoxide. Repeat transthoracic echocardiogram is normal, although notably there is insufficient tricuspid regurgitation to estimate right ventricular systolic pressure (RVSP). Aside from mild dyspnoea on moderate exertion, she feels otherwise back to baseline.

A 6-min walk test is performed which demonstrates baseline oxygen saturations of 99% and baseline heart rate of 70 bpm. After 6 min, the patient has walked 560 m; oxygen saturations are 91% on room air and heart rate is 130 bpm. Based on these findings, a right heart catheterisation is organised which demonstrates a mean pulmonary artery pressure of 31 mmHg, and a diagnosis of chronic thromboembolic pulmonary hypertension is made.

3 Discussion

Six minute walk tests (6MWT) are commonly used as an objective functional assessment in respiratory disease. Although cardiopulmonary exercise testing (CPET) remains the gold standard in physiological testing under conditions of exertion, CPET requires complicated equipment and skilled technicians [1]. A 6-min walk test is a low resource alternative and consists of the patient walking as fast as possible along a corridor of defined length for a period of 6 min, with walk distance, oxygen saturations and heart rate measured [1].

When a patient with pulmonary hypertension increases their cardiac output through exercise, the pulmonary circulation is unable to dilate, increasing pulmonary arterial pressure and right ventricular (RV) afterload. While at rest the RV may be able to maintain systolic function, with the increase in afterload associated with exercise, the RV is unable to respond to increasing metabolic demands. This leads to a reduction in LV filling as the RV fails to maintain appropriate output, and mechanical compression of the LV as the RV dilates. To compensate for the reduction in stroke volume, heart rate (HR) is increased in an attempt to maintain cardiac output [2]. This is often associated with breathlessness "out-of-proportion" to radiological disease as there is significant mismatch between perfusion and ventilation, which gets worse with exercise. This is exacerbated by an early transition from aerobic to anaerobic metabolism [3].

The two salient features characteristic of pulmonary hypertension during exercise seen on a 6MWT are an abnormally rapid increase to the maximum predicted heart rate and impaired intrapulmonary gas exchange [2]. Further characteristics which are seen on formal cardiopulmonary exercise testing include reduced oxygen uptake (VO_2) with a normal ventilatory reserve, and reduced ventilatory efficiency as demonstrated by an elevation of the ventilation required to manage CO_2 levels (VE/VCO_2) [2]. Especially in the presence of normal spirometry, exertional

Table 1 Clinical classification of Pulmonary Hypertension (PH) [4]

Group	Classification	Prevalence
1	Pulmonary arterial hypertension	Rare
2	PH associated with left heart disease	Very common
3	PH associated with lung disease	Common
4	PH associated with pulmonary artery obstruction	Rare
5	PH with unclear and/or multifactorial mechanisms	Rare

desaturation and marked tachycardia on a 6MWT is suspicious for pulmonary hypertension.

Pulmonary hypertension is a disease of many aetiologies, all associated with increased mortality, and frequently associated with poor quality of life [4]. Pulmonary hypertension is classified into 5 groups as listed in Table 1 below. Delineation of the underlying cause and thus classification is essential, as it determines what treatments are both appropriate and available. As an example, pulmonary vasodilators are effective in Group 1 pulmonary hypertension, but are ineffective in those with Group 3 disease, and may worsen gas exchange. The patient described above has group 4 pulmonary hypertension associated with pulmonary artery obstruction, a condition for which surgery or vascular intervention may be appropriate, but for which medication is also available for those not suitable for surgery.

4 Other Gems

- The concept of "provoked" vs. "unprovoked" venous thromboembolic disease is a false dichotomy, and risk is better delineated according to the presence or absence of known risk factors for recurrence.

References

1. Agarwala P, Salzman SH. Six-minute walk test: clinical role, technique, coding, and reimbursement. Chest. 2020;157(3):603–11.
2. Neder JA, Ramos RP, Ota-Arakaki JS, Hirai DM, D'Arsigny CL, O'Donnell D. Exercise intolerance in pulmonary arterial hypertension. The role of cardiopulmonary exercise testing. Ann Am Thorac Soc. 2015;12(4):604–12.
3. Sun XG, Hansen JE, Oudiz RJ, Wasserman K. Exercise pathophysiology in patients with primary pulmonary hypertension. Circulation. 2001;104(4):429–35.
4. Humbert M, Kovacs G, Hoeper MM, Badagliacca R, Berger RMF, Brida M, et al. 2022 ESC/ERS guidelines for the diagnosis and treatment of pulmonary hypertension. Eur Respir J. 2022;

Vaping and Risks to Lung Health

Ashleigh Witt and Alistair Miller

1 Clinical Pearl

The use of e-cigarettes/vaping to reduce combustible cigarette use (dual-use) does not significantly reduce your cancer risk.

2 Clinical Case

A 40 year-old man is admitted to hospital with a moderate severity community acquired pneumonia. He reports that he is a smoker, with no other past medical history aside from a previous presentation with breathlessness. On revisiting the history on the consultant ward round, it is discovered that the patient reduced his combustible cigarette use after his last presentation by taking up vaping. The patient believes e-cigarettes to be a risk-free alternative to smoking cigarettes and made the change as he was concerned about developing lung cancer like his father.

A. Witt
Department of Respiratory and Sleep Medicine, Royal Melbourne Hospital, Melbourne, VIC, Australia

A. Miller (✉)
Department of Respiratory and Sleep Medicine, Royal Melbourne Hospital, Melbourne, VIC, Australia

Department of Internal Medicine, Peter MacCallum Cancer Centre, Melbourne, VIC, Australia

Department of Medicine—RMH, Faculty of Medicine, Dentistry and Health Services, The University of Melbourne, Melbourne, VIC, Australia

R. Junckerstorff et al. (eds.), *Beyond Evidence-Based Medicine*,
https://doi.org/10.1007/978-981-99-4440-8_65

3 Discussion

Electronic cigarettes (e-cigarettes, vaping devices or vapes) have rapidly increased in popularity since their initial development in 2003 as a smoking cessation product. They have now been seconded by tobacco companies, with marketing targeted at children and young adults. Vaping may have a potential benefit to adult smokers if they are used as a complete substitute for regular cigarettes and subsequent cessation of vaping, however most people continue to smoke (dual-use) [1, 2] or at best continue to vape [3]. Cutting down to quit is a valid smoking cessation method but is less effective (~5% vs. 16% abstinence at 12 months) and generally requires considerably more clinician input than complete cessation [4]. Interestingly, one study showed no improvements in self-reported health in those who switched to sole vape or dual-use, and no reduction in smoking related diseases, albeit only over a 4-year follow-up period [5].

E-cigarette and vaping fluids contain both definite and probable carcinogens [6] and while they have been widely quoted as being 95% safer than combustible cigarettes, there is no reasonable scientific rationale to this claim [7]. They are known to lead to airway inflammation [8], alter the bronchial proteome [9] and have been associated with small airway obstruction [10]. In tobacco smoking, there is a lag time from smoking commencement until diagnosis of lung cancer of approximately 20 years [6], so it will be some time until we know with any certainty regarding the absolute risk of vaping or dual-use, but we can draw some conclusions from existing data.

Whilst there is a clear linear relationship between intensity of cigarette smoking and risk of cancer, there is no established safe level. In a large cohort study, those who smoked 1–10 cigarettes per day had a higher all-cause mortality than never smokers (Hazard Ratio [HR] 1.87), and a nine fold increase in lung cancer risk [11]. In those who do not vape, there is reduction in risk of lung cancer in those who reduce their use of combustible cigarettes by >50% (HR 0.73), but it is significantly less than quitting completely (HR 0.5) [12]. However, we do not know what effect dual-use has on this reduction. Other respiratory disease has also been shown to be associated with dual-use. In a large Korean cohort study, dual users had the highest rate of COPD, even when compared to those who smoked combustible cigarettes alone [2].

At a broader level, there is significant concern that e-cigarette use in youths is associated with higher rates of combustible cigarette use [13]. Given the association between earlier onset of smoking and risk of lung cancer [14], anything that promotes uptake of smoking in children must be avoided.

4 Other Gems

- The improvements in cardiovascular outcomes associated with smoking cessation are lost or attenuated by ongoing vaping [15].

References

1. QuickStats: cigarette smoking status* among current adult e-cigarette users,(†) by age group—National health interview survey,(§) United States, 2015. MMWR Morb Mortal Wkly Rep. 2016;65(42):1177.
2. Kim T, Kang J. Association between dual use of e-cigarette and cigarette and chronic obstructive pulmonary disease: an analysis of a nationwide representative sample from 2013 to 2018. BMC Pulm Med. 2021;21(1):231.
3. Hajek P, Phillips-Waller A, Przulj D, Pesola F, Myers Smith K, Bisal N, et al. A randomized trial of E-cigarettes versus nicotine-replacement therapy. N Engl J Med. 2019;380(7):629–37.
4. Wang D, Connock M, Barton P, Fry-Smith A, Aveyard P, Moore D. 'Cut down to quit' with nicotine replacement therapies in smoking cessation: a systematic review of effectiveness and economic analysis. Health Technol Assess 2008;12(2):iii-iv, ix-xi, 1–135.
5. Flacco ME, Ferrante M, Fiore M, Marzuillo C, La Vecchia C, Gualano MR, et al. Cohort study of electronic cigarette use: safety and effectiveness after 4 years of follow-up. Eur Rev Med Pharmacol Sci. 2019;23(1):402–12.
6. Bracken-Clarke D, Kapoor D, Baird AM, Buchanan PJ, Gately K, Cuffe S, et al. Vaping and lung cancer—a review of current data and recommendations. Lung Cancer. 2021;153:11–20.
7. Gotts JE, Jordt S-E, McConnell R, Tarran R. What are the respiratory effects of e-cigarettes? BMJ. 2019;366:l5275.
8. Kim MD, Baumlin N, Guerrero-Cignarella A, Schmid A, Aguiar C, Mohiuddin M, et al. Persistence of airway inflammation in smokers who switch to electronic cigarettes. ERJ Open Res. 2022;8(2):00117.
9. Ghosh A, Coakley RC, Mascenik T, Rowell TR, Davis ES, Rogers K, et al. Chronic E-cigarette exposure alters the human bronchial epithelial proteome. Am J Respir Crit Care Med. 2018;198(1):67–76.
10. Hariri LP, Flashner BM, Kanarek DJ, O'Donnell WJ, Soskis A, Ziehr DR, et al. E-cigarette use, small airway fibrosis, and constrictive bronchiolitis. NEJM Evid. 2022;1(6):EVIDoa2100051.
11. Inoue-Choi M, Liao LM, Reyes-Guzman C, Hartge P, Caporaso N, Freedman ND. Association of long-term, low-intensity smoking with all-cause and cause-specific mortality in the national institutes of health–aarp diet and health study. JAMA Intern Med. 2017;177(1):87–95.
12. Godtfredsen NS, Prescott E, Osler M. Effect of smoking reduction on lung cancer risk. JAMA. 2005;294(12):1505–10.
13. McDonald CF, Jones S, Beckert L, Bonevski B, Buchanan T, Bozier J, et al. Electronic cigarettes: a position statement from the Thoracic Society of Australia and New Zealand. Respirology. 2020;25(10):1082.
14. Hegmann KT, Fraser AM, Keaney RP, Moser SE, Nilasena DS, Sedlars M, et al. The effect of age at smoking initiation on lung cancer risk. Epidemiology. 1993;4(5):444–8.
15. Kim C-Y, Paek Y-J, Seo HG, Cheong YS, Lee CM, Park SM, et al. Dual use of electronic and conventional cigarettes is associated with higher cardiovascular risk factors in Korean men. Sci Rep. 2020;10(1):5612.

Part IX
Infectious Diseases

Clinical Significance of Staphylococcal Bacteriuria

Denis Spelman

1 Clinical Pearl

Staphylococcus aureus is not recognised as urinary tract pathogen. However, if *S. aureus* is isolated from urine, then consideration should be given to the possibility of concurrent or recent *S. aureus* bacteraemia.

2 Clinical Case

A 45-year-old-man was a victim of an assault which resulted in pain and bruising across his left chest wall. One week later, he presented to the Emergency Department (ED) with chest pain, and 3 days of sweats, cough, and sputum. Chest Xray and computed tomography (CT) scan revealed a fractured left sided ninth rib. His C-reactive protein (CRP) was 138 mg/L. On this presentation he also had urine specimen taken for microscopy and culture. He was discharged with oxycodone for analgesia and was for follow-up with his General Practitioner. Subsequently the mid-stream urine (MSU) sample was finalised the day following his discharge: microscopy revealed 10–50 polymorphs/μL and Methicillin Susceptible *Staphylococcus aureus* (MSSA) was cultured from the urine specimen.

Four weeks later he returned to the ED, with intermittent fever and sweats. He also had developed thoracic back pain and gave a 3-day history of paraesthesia down his lower legs. On the day of this presentation, he had noticed loss of power

D. Spelman (✉)
Department of Infectious Diseases and Microbiology, Alfred Hospital, Melbourne, VIC, Australia

Monash University, Melbourne, VIC, Australia

R. Junckerstorff et al. (eds.), *Beyond Evidence-Based Medicine*,
https://doi.org/10.1007/978-981-99-4440-8_66

in both legs. An urgent spinal magnetic resonance imaging (MRI) scan revealed a T8–9 epidural abscess with cord compression. His white cell count was 12.9×10^9/L, CRP 155 mg/L and erythrocyte sedimentation rate (ESR) 107 mm/h. He underwent urgent neurosurgical decompression and drainage. *S. aureus* was isolated from the operative tissue. This was the same organism as was identified 4 weeks earlier from his urine.

3 Discussion

At the initial presentation a fractured rib was confirmed by imaging and was managed appropriately. However, there were some features which were not well explained by chest wall trauma. The sweats, sputum and elevated CRP of 138 mg/L are more in keeping with infection. An MSU was collected on the day of his ED presentation and *S. aureus* was subsequently isolated from this specimen. Importantly *S. aureus* in urine is an unusual cause of primary urinary tract infection. *S. aureus* in urine can originate from another site (e.g., endocarditis or in this case the site of this man's trauma) through concurrent *S. aureus* bacteraemia [1, 2]. In one study of 339 patients with MSSA isolated in urine, 12% had concurrent *S. aureus* bacteraemia [3]. Thus, *S. aureus* bacteriuria is an indication for blood cultures to be taken. Because of the potential significance of *S. aureus* bacteriuria, the microbiology laboratory which isolated the *S. aureus* in urine should inform the ordering doctor of this result at that time and suggest that blood cultures be taken.

In contrast, the isolation of *S. aureus* from urine taken in the presence of a urinary catheter is most likely due to catheter colonisation and therefore does not have the same clinical significance as a non-catheter specimen.

It is unfortunate with the above case that the urine culture result was not followed up at that time of positive growth. Ideally the patient should have been contacted at the time *S. aureus* was isolated, asked to return to hospital, have a clinical review and have blood cultures taken. If this had been undertaken, *S. aureus* bacteraemia, if present, would have been diagnosed and treated and the subsequent events may have been prevented. Unfortunately, only a minority of patients who have *S. aureus* bacteriuria have concomitant blood cultures taken.

Even if such a patient is followed up and the blood cultures are taken but prove negative, *S. aureus* bacteriuria should be a flag to the physician that this patient should have close clinical follow-up. If a blood culture is taken 1 to 2 weeks after the episode of *S. aureus* bacteriuria, then bacteraemia which was present at the time of the bacteriuria may be no longer present. Such a patient would be at risk of subsequently presenting with metastatic staphylococcal infection, such as staphylococcal bone, cardiac or other localised infection.

Similarly, salmonella species if isolated in urine may also indicate salmonella bacteraemia, and such a patient should also have blood cultures and close clinical follow-up.

4 Take Home Messages

- *S. aureus* bacteriuria can indicate concurrent or recent *S. aureus* bacteraemia.
- If *S. aureus* bacteriuria occurs with a urinary catheter in place this is more likely due to catheter colonisation rather *S. aureus* bacteraemia.
- All patients with *S. aureus* isolated from non-catheter urine samples should have timely clinical review and blood cultures taken.
- When a laboratory isolates *S. aureus* from a non-catheter urine, the ordering doctor should be informed at that time.

References

1. Al Mohajer M, Darouche RO. *Staphylococcus aureus* bacteriuria: source, clinical relevance, and management. Curr Infect Dis Rep. 2012;14:601–6.
2. Muder RR, Brennen C, Rihs J. Isolation of Staphylococcus aureus from the urinary tract: association of isolation with symptomatic urinary tract infection and subsequent Staphylococcal bacteremia. Clin Infect Dis. 2006;42:46–60.
3. Trevillyan J, Spelman D. Testing the golden rules of infectious diseases: Staphylococcal bacteriuria is predictive of Staphylococcal bacteremia. Med J Aust. 2012;197(3):149–50.

Fever of Unknown Origin

Denis Spelman

1 Clinical Pearl

The management of a patient presenting with prolonged fever without an obvious cause (FUO) requires a complete medical history and a skilled physical examination before embarking on rounds of investigations. In this clinical scenario there are specific parts of the history and examination that may not be a part of routine practice but may lead to the diagnosis.

2 Clinical Case

A 25-year-old man was admitted to hospital with a 6-week history of daily fevers, with shivers and sweats. He had measured his temperature with regular readings up to 38.5 °C. There were no localising clinical symptoms. He had lost 2 to 3 kg in weight during this time. He was not taking any specific medications, had no allergies, no history of intravenous drug use, animal contacts and no recent overseas travel. He worked as an automobile mechanic and lived with his long-term partner. He had attended his general practitioner during this time, took a 10-day course of amoxicillin without benefit. Prior to this illness, he had been well with no history of past significant illness or hospitalisation.

On admission, he was afebrile and did not appear acutely unwell. His pulse was 72/min and regular, blood pressure 110/60 mmHg and a respiratory rate 12/min. There was no cervical, axillary or inguinal lymphadenopathy. His throat, tonsils,

D. Spelman (✉)
Department of Infectious Diseases and Microbiology, Alfred Hospital, Melbourne, VIC, Australia

Monash University, Melbourne, VIC, Australia

R. Junckerstorff et al. (eds.), *Beyond Evidence-Based Medicine*, https://doi.org/10.1007/978-981-99-4440-8_67

palate, gums and teeth were normal. He had normal heart sounds, with no cardiac murmurs. The lung fields were clear. His abdomen was lax and non-tender without hepatosplenomegaly or any other intra-abdominal mass. There was no rash, no peripheral stigmata of endocarditis and no peripheral oedema.

On admission a chest X-ray, full blood examination, electrolytes, C-reactive protein and liver function were ordered and all returned normal results. Blood cultures were taken on admission and were repeated that evening when he developed a fever of 37.8 °C. The next morning, he was reviewed by a second physician who confirmed the clinical findings. The decision was made to await pending blood cultures results, but also to perform a blood film, serological screen (for Epstein-Barr virus (EBV), cytomegalovirus (CMV), human immunodeficiency virus (HIV) and toxoplasma), and a midstream urine for full ward test, microscopy and culture and to consider an abdominal computed tomography (CT) scan, if these extra tests were non-diagnostic.

That afternoon a trained nurse approached the medical staff with a concern. When instructing the patient on how to produce a mid-stream urine, she noticed that there was significant swelling of his left testis. He was reviewed and the nurse's finding was confirmed: a significant non-tender swelling of left testis. On further questioning, the patient reported that he had noted some swelling 2–3 weeks earlier but it was non tender and he had not worried. This clinical finding resulted in urology review, specific scans and histological diagnosis of testicular seminoma at orchiectomy.

3 Discussion

This patient presented with 6 weeks of fever without any initial localising clues on history or routine clinical examination. Swelling of the testis was missed on clinical assessment by 2 experienced clinicians. Once the testicular swelling was detected, the road to investigation, diagnosis and treatment was straightforward.

Tumours that can present with fever include lymphoma, renal cell carcinoma, hepatic tumours, atrial myxoma and metastatic liver disease. If the swollen testis had been missed for longer, the patient may have undergone further rounds of unnecessary investigations and delays in diagnosis.

In this clinical scenario of prolonged fever without any localising findings, then re-taking of the history and re-examination of the patient is recommended with emphasis on those parts of the history and the examination that may need further clarification or may not be a part of a physician's usual clinical practice.

Re-taking the history should concentrate on aspects which were not fully covered in the initial conversation such as medications, other possible exposures, possible relevant epidemiology, including occupation and hobbies and taking a collateral history from a family member.

- Questions about medications should include not only prescription medications but also over the counter or substances that a patient may not consider to be a medication. For example, with one patient, we did not discover until day 5 of his admission that he was taking tablets for leg cramps. He had not told us because he did not consider this to be a medication but rather a health supplement. It eventuated that this tablet contained quinine, which was the cause of his fever.

- Asking the patient to bring in all the medications that he is taking can sometimes produce surprises. We have seen an event of a pharmacy dispensing error in which the medication on the label of the container was different to the medication inside the container.
- Enquiries about occupation and hobbies may give rise to an important clue. Gardening with use of potting mix raises the possibility of Legionnaire's disease. The mowing of grass after the spring rains raises the possibility of aerosolisation of bird excreta resulting in psittacosis.
- A collateral history from a partner or family member of the patient may be useful. An example of this was a when a young woman presented with a FUO: at that time her partner was working at an abattoir where there were cases of Q fever. It was she who handled and laundered his work clothes each day, raising the possibility of her acquiring Q fever form his work clothes.

On re-examination of the patient with a FUO, it is important to realise there are specific parts of the clinical examination which, although not be routinely undertaken, may be relevant in this clinical setting. Table 1 summarises these sites, commencing anatomically from above and working downwards.

I have included in this list any site of recent trauma or surgical intervention now covered by a dressing or plaster. The covering should be removed and area examined for evidence of infection or other pathology, which may be the cause of fever. This is a longstanding Golden Rule of Infectious Diseases (Petersdorf's Law) [1]. "When a patient has fever post-operatively, it is usually related to the surgical procedure" [1].

In a patient with prolonged fevers, in whom no localising clue has been found after some time in hospital, a fruitful strategy may be starting the admission process again or "re-admit" the patient. The diagnosis may only be made with finding of a new symptom or sign not present on admission or when a test that was normal but then becomes abnormal.

4 Take Home Messages

- Prolonged fever is an important clinical presentation with many possible causes.
- Skilled history with general and targeted examination should be undertaken.
- History should include details on over-the-counter substances, health supplements and contacts or exposures at work or hobbies.
- Examination of anatomical sites which may not be a part of routine examination should be considered.
- Collateral history from a family member may be useful.

Table 1 Sites of clinical examination considered in a patient presenting with FUO

Clinical examination	Clinical finding	Cause of fever
Temporal arteries	Tenderness	Giant cell arteritis
Conjunctivae	Haemorrhages	Endocarditis
Palate	Palatal petechiae	Epstein Barr Virus
Fundoscopy	Roth spots Haemorrhages Retinal infarction Choroid tubercles	Endocarditis Retinitis Toxoplasma, CMV TB
Teeth and gums	Swollen inflamed gums Broken tooth Tooth sensitivity	Gingivitis Dental infection/abscess
Thyroid	Swelling Tenderness	Subacute thyroiditis
Skin sites	Evidence of intravenous drug use	Blood-borne virus infection
Back	Spinal tenderness	Vertebral osteomyelitis Still's disease
Testes	Swelling Epididymitis	Testicular cancer Tuberculosis
Rectal /vaginal examination	Mass Tenderness	Tumour, abscess, pelvic or Pouch of Douglas abscess, retrocecal appendicitis Prostatitis
Any site under a dressing or plaster	Erythema Unhealed wound	Wound infection

Reference

1. Petersdorf RG, Beeson PB. Fever of unexplained origin: report of 100 cases. Medicine. 1961;40:1–30.

Gastro-Enteritis Complicated by Mycotic Aneurysm

Denis Spelman

1 Clinical Pearl

When a patient presents with acute gastroenteritis, especially if over the age of 60 and especially if salmonella is isolated from faeces or blood, it is important to be aware of the possibility of salmonella aortitis as a complication at the time of the initial or subsequent presentation.

2 Clinical Case

A 67-year-old man presented with 3 days of acute bloody diarrhoea and fever. He gave a past history of hypertension and peripheral vascular disease, but no history of previous gastro-intestinal disease. On examination he was febrile at 38 °C, had mild dehydration with tender abdomen but no rigidity. Investigations demonstrated an elevated white cell count of 15.0×10^9/L, a raised C-reactive protein (CRP) of 155 mg/L, with normal electrolytes except for eGFR of 64 ml/min/1.73m^2. An abdominal x-ray was normal. Faeces microscopy showed white blood cells 2+ and red blood cells 2+. After 48 hours, faeces culture was reported positive with *Salmonella* species. His acute symptoms resolved, and he had almost fully recovered by the time faeces culture result was finalised. He received no antibiotic therapy and was well when discharged home.

D. Spelman (✉)
Department of Infectious Diseases and Microbiology, Alfred Hospital, Melbourne, VIC, Australia

Monash University, Melbourne, VIC, Australia

R. Junckerstorff et al. (eds.), *Beyond Evidence-Based Medicine*,
https://doi.org/10.1007/978-981-99-4440-8_68

Three weeks later he represented with severe abdominal and lumbar back pain with vomiting. On examination, he had fever of 38.5 °C, generalised lower abdominal tenderness with rigidity. CT abdominal imaging demonstrated an infrarenal aortic aneurysm with changes suggestive of aortitis. There were calcified plaques throughout the abdominal aorta and iliac vessels. The white cell count was elevated to 18.5×10^9/L with a CRP of 194 mg/L. Blood cultures were negative. He was commenced on a combination of ceftriaxone and ciprofloxacin, targeting the previously isolated salmonella. He was referred to the Vascular Surgical unit and after a course of antimicrobial treatment he underwent resection of the aneurysm and replacement with a bifurcated synthetic graft attached to both common iliac arteries. He subsequently made a complete recovery.

3 Discussion

Salmonella has a proven propensity to attach to and infect vascular endothelium, especially in the presence of atheromatous plaques. This can occur in the setting of salmonella gastroenteritis which may have concurrent short-lived bacteraemia. Infective arteritis can occur with any artery but most commonly involves the infrarenal aorta. This can be followed by weakening of the aortic wall, with the production of an aneurysm and the possibility of rupture. This sequence of events with silent seeding of the aortic wall can occur even while the initial salmonella gastroenteritis symptoms settle and then completely resolve. This was the likely sequence of events in the patient described here.

Infection of the aorta was probably made more likely by this patient's known vascular disease, which was demonstrated by CT imaging. Either infection of a pre-existing atherosclerotic aneurysm or primary infection of the aorta wall with aneurysm formation could result in the CT demonstrated infrarenal aortic aneurysm. Symptoms caused by this infected aneurysm resulted in his second presentation to hospital.

Apart from endothelium infection, salmonella can also seed and infect cardiac (usually prosthetic) valve endocardium and orthopaedic implants.

In both this patient's presentations to hospital, blood cultures were taken but no bacteraemia was documented. On both occasions only one blood culture was taken. Ideally if bacteraemia is being considered, then 3 sets of blood cultures would be optimal. Most likely the bacteraemia was short lived and occurred during the pre-admission part of the initial illness with seeding of the aorta at that stage. The symptoms on initial presentation resolved spontaneously and he did not receive any antimicrobial therapy for salmonella.

The risk of vascular infection in salmonella septicaemia is significant. In one series 3 (10%) of 30 patients with documented salmonella bacteraemia developed a *mycotic aneurysm* [1]. The risk appears to be greatest in males, over the age of 60 and in those with known or unknown vascular disease [2]. The patient described belonged to this at-risk patient group. Because of the demonstrated risk, management of salmonella gastroenteritis in this age group should include consideration for a course of anti-salmonella antibiotics at the time of his initial presentation. Also, such patients should undergo imaging of the abdominal aorta by CT, MRI or PET/CT scan and subsequent close and regular clinical follow-up. Choice of antimicrobial will be dependent on susceptibility testing e.g., ciprofloxacin 500 mg–750 mg bd with usual duration of 4 to 6 weeks but dependent on clinical and scan follow up.

4 Take Home Messages

- Salmonella infection especially in the presence of bacteraemia can result in endovascular infection.
- The presence of new abdominal pain sometime after an episode of acute gastro-enteritis raises the possibility of an infective aortic aneurysm, especially if salmonella infection is proven or suspected.
- Patients over the age of 60 and/or with a history of vascular disease and presenting with acute salmonella gastro-enteritis, should undergo screening for aortic infection e.g., CT, MRI or PET scan.
- A treatment course of antibiotics should be considered in patients over the age of 60 years with known vascular disease who present with possible or proven salmonella infection.
- Such patients should be warned of the symptoms of this complication and advised to return to hospital if any concerns.
- If the patient has a prosthetic joint or other implant, there is also a risk of salmonella infection of these devices.

References

1. Hsu RB, Lin FY. Risk factors for bacteraemia and endovascular infection due to non-typhoid salmonella: a reappraisal. QJM. 2005;98(11):821.
2. Benenson S, Raveh D, Schlesinger Y, Alberton J, Rudensky B, Hadas-Halpern I, Yinnon AM. The risk of vascular infection in adult patients with nontyphi *Salmonella bacteremia*. Am J Med. 2001;110(1):60.

A Neuropathy in Infectious Disease

Denis Spelman

1 Clinical Pearl

In patients with chronic foot infections in the presence of longstanding diabetes, the cause of the foot infection is usually diabetes. Conditions commonly seen are the common diagnoses, but this dictum is not always correct.

2 Clinical Case

A 42-year-old man was referred because of a longstanding discharging right foot ulcer in the presence of poorly controlled diabetes. The letter of referral introduced his problem as a diabetic foot infection. On history he had initially developed the plantar ulcer 3 years earlier and it had gradually worsened with intermittent episodes of purulent discharge. He had worn a supportive moonboot over the past 2 years. He was born in the Pacific Islands, had spent some years playing high level rugby and now worked as an accountant. His only other medical condition was diabetes, which was diagnosed 10 years before, when he took oral medication for 6 months, but this had no more recent active follow-up. Surprisingly he did not appear greatly concerned about the ulcer: when asked why not, his response was that there was no pain. On examination he had a 3 cm diameter discharging plantar foot ulcer with the metatarsal head on view. He had sensory loss, to touch and pinprick, of his right leg below the knee. Sensory examination of his left leg was normal. There were three 2 cm hypopigmented anaesthetic lesions on his upper thigh.

D. Spelman (✉)
Department of Infectious Diseases and Microbiology, Alfred Hospital, Melbourne, VIC, Australia

Monash University, Melbourne, VIC, Australia

R. Junckerstorff et al. (eds.), *Beyond Evidence-Based Medicine*,
https://doi.org/10.1007/978-981-99-4440-8_69

On palpation, the right common fibular nerve was thickened as it crossed the neck of the right fibula bone. He was admitted to hospital for management of the ulcer, the underlying metatarsal osteomyelitis and to optimise his diabetes control.

3 Discussion

Over recent years this man had presented on a number of occasions for medical care most often at times when there was increased discharge, often with odour, from his foot. On each occasion he was told that this was a diabetic foot infection with the ulcer secondary to diabetic peripheral neuropathy. On these occasions, he was treated with courses of antibiotics and foot rest, usually with a clinical response.

The admissions team considered that his abnormal peripheral neurological signs were not diabetic in origin. The asymmetrical loss of sensation, the painless foot ulcer, the hypopigmented anaesthetic skin lesions, and thickened peripheral nerve on palpation all supported a diagnosis of leprosy. When this diagnosis was raised with the patient, he then reported that this diagnosis had been made 3 years earlier, before he had come to Australia. He had commenced on dual medications at that time but had ceased these after 1–2 months and had not returned for follow-up care.

Leprosy is usually a clinical diagnosis, with occasionally a biopsy of a skin lesion revealing acid fast bacilli. Peripheral nerve enlargement is a feature of leprosy. Neuropathy can be variable, including a mononeuritis, such as isolated ulnar nerve involvement, or a polyneuritis and resulting in motor, sensory or autonomic dysfunction [1]. Both peripheral and cranial nerves can be involved. In the patient described here, the common fibular nerve and posterior tibial nerve involvement likely resulted anaesthesia of his foot, resulting in plantar ulcer formation and then underlying metatarsal bone osteomyelitis.

In many parts of the world where leprosy is rare, this diagnosis is a challenge for medical practitioners who may not have seen any patient with this diagnosis [2]. Also, if the diagnosis is considered then they may not be confident in their ability to clinically screen, investigate and manage this. However, the initial and most critical step is to consider this diagnosis. This is more important at that stage than a detailed knowledge of the leprosy. In the patient described here, the treating clinicians realised his neuropathy was not the pattern usually seen with diabetes, leading to a search for another cause. Clinical evaluation for possible leprosy includes examination of the skin, peripheral nerves, eyes, and nasal mucosa. Examination of the skin includes a search for hypopigmented lesions, painless wounds, and areas of anaesthesia. Peripheral nerve examination targets those superficial peripheral nerves that are open to palpation and where increased nerve thickness can be identified. These include the ulnar nerve at the elbow, median and superficial radial cutaneous nerves at the wrist, fibular nerve at the neck of the fibula, great auricular nerve in the neck, and the facial nerve as it crosses the zygoma. Later clinical features of leprosy are clawing of fourth and fifth fingers, foot drop, facial paralysis, perforated nasal septum, and loss of hair especially eyebrow and eyelashes.

Early diagnosis is vital for treatment and prevention of neuropathy, deformity, tissue loss and disability.

4 Take Home Messages

- Not all foot infections in patients with diabetes are diabetic foot infections.
- Initial clinical screening for leprosy includes a detailed history, palpation for thickened peripheral nerves, and a search for anaesthetic skin lesions.
- Leprosy is largely a clinical diagnosis and is followed by an assessment for and management of any disability.
- Early diagnosis and treatment of leprosy may prevent disability to hands and feet.
- If disability has occurred, this requires life-long care.
- Following the diagnosis, consultation with a physician experienced in leprosy is recommended.

References

1. Nascimento OJM. Leprosy neuropathy: clinical manifestations. Arq Neuropsiquiatr. 2013;71(9B):661–6. https://doi.org/10.1590/0004-282X20130146.
2. WHO Guidelines for the diagnosis, treatment and prevention of leprosy. 2018.

Management of Suspected Epidural Abscess

Denis Spelman

1 Clinical Pearl

There are multiple causes of new onset acute severe back pain. For the diagnosis of an epidural abscess, the initial critical step is to actively consider this diagnosis. If an epidural abscess is suspected, this should be considered a medical emergency, as a delay in diagnosis and treatment can result in paralysis from spinal cord compression. The suspicion of an epidural abscess is an indication for URGENT neurosurgical or orthopaedic consultation and an URGENT spinal magnetic resonance imaging (MRI).

2 Clinical Case

A 19-year-old apprentice butcher presented to the Emergency Department with lumbar back pain. He reported he had injured his back at work one week earlier, had taken one day off, then returned to work. He now presented with 2 days of severe lumbar back pain with radiation down his left leg. On examination his spinal flexion was restricted because of pain, he had mild tenderness from L1 to L3, an absent left ankle reflex with a temperature of 37.7 °C. The provisional diagnosis was a prolapsed disc with sciatica. He was admitted for analgesia. Investigations on the day of admission demonstrated normal lumbar spine Xray, white cell count of 14.0 (normal 4-11 × 10^9/L) and a C-reactive protein (CRP) of 108 mg/L. An MRI was organised for the next afternoon. However, on the next morning he had a fever of 38.5 °C, he complained of difficulty passing urine and by lunchtime he had increasing

D. Spelman (✉)
Department of Infectious Diseases and Microbiology, Alfred Hospital, Melbourne, VIC, Australia

Monash University, Melbourne, VIC, Australia

R. Junckerstorff et al. (eds.), *Beyond Evidence-Based Medicine*,
https://doi.org/10.1007/978-981-99-4440-8_70

bilateral leg weakness. On that day, he underwent an urgent MRI followed by urgent decompression of a L1 to L3 epidural abscess.

3 Discussion

It is unfortunate that this patient developed cord compression while an inpatient and awaiting a spinal MRI. He presented with acute severe back pain with the initial provisional diagnosis of a prolapsed disc. However, his fever, the elevated white cell count and high CRP may not be explained by this diagnosis and are more in keeping with infection. If the diagnosis of an epidural abscess had been suspected at that time, an urgent MRI on the day of admission would have been undertaken and the subsequent paralysis may well have been prevented.

The diagnosis of epidural abscess may not be straightforward. The classic diagnostic triad is severe back pain, fever, and abnormal neurological signs. However, this triad is only present on initial presentation in 15% of cases [1], with the neurological deficit present in only 33% of patients at the time of initial presentation [2]. Tell-tale signs of cord compression include new bladder or bowel symptoms, reduced anal tone, diminished perineal sensation and loss of leg power. However, the clinical aim is to make the diagnosis of epidural abscess prior to the onset of abnormal neurology, in which case surgical drainage would then prevent the occurrence of such neurological deficits.

Unfortunately, diagnosis may be missed early in the clinical course, especially in the absence of neurological symptoms or signs. In such a patient with acute back pain there are certain RED FLAGS that support the diagnosis of an epidural abscess [1, 2]:

- Severity and type (lancinating, sharp) of pain with distal radiation.
- Unexplained fever and signs of sepsis.
- Recent spinal instrumentation.
- Spinal tenderness.
- Repeated presentations to medical care.
- Elevated inflammatory markers: white cell count >12.5 (normal 4-11 × 10^9/L), CRP > 115 mg/L and erythrocyte sedimentation rate (ESR) >95 mm/h.
- The presence of recognised risk factors: intravenous drug use, urosepsis, recent back trauma, diabetes.

The symptoms and signs may be absent or subtle and require active questioning and careful physical examination. The patient should have frequent clinical reviews searching for neurological signs whilst awaiting MRI or surgical review.

The patient described here had severe back pain with RED FLAGS supportive of the diagnosis of epidural abscess: fever, recent back trauma, and elevated inflammatory markers. Unfortunately, this diagnosis was not considered on the day of presentation, and he was not managed with the urgency that suspicion of this diagnosis warranted. An MRI was only organised for the following day. The absence of abnormal neurology should not delay the urgency of the MRI if this diagnosis is suspected. If the MRI had been performed on the day of admission, surgical decompression would have occurred and subsequent paralysis in all likelihood would have been prevented.

This case supports the recommendation that any suspicion of an epidural abscess should be regarded as a medical emergency requiring urgent discussion with neurosurgery or orthopaedics, and an urgent MRI should be performed regardless of the time of day or night. An urgent MRI often needs conversation between treating physician, neurosurgeon/orthopaedics, and the radiologist. Generally, a total spinal MRI is recommended because about 5 to 10% of epidural abscesses have skip lesions.

4 Take Home Messages

- An epidural abscess should be included in the differential diagnosis of acute back pain especially if any of the RED FLAGS are present.
- If an epidural abscess is suspected, an URGENT whole spine MRI is indicated.
- The absence of abnormal neurology should not delay an MRI, as neurology may be prevented by early diagnosis.
- Frequent clinical examination should be undertaken until this diagnosis is made or excluded.
- Optimal investigation and management need discussion between treating physician, neurosurgeon/orthopaedics and MRI radiologist.

References

1. Sendi P, Bregenzer T, Zimmerli W. Spinal epidural abscess in clinical practice. QJM. 2008;101(1):1–12. https://doi.org/10.1093/qjmed/hcm100; Epub 2007 Nov 3.
2. Reihsaus E, Waldbaur H, Seeling W. Spinal epidural abscess: a meta-analysis of 915 patients. Neurosurg Rev. 2000;23(4):175–204. https://doi.org/10.1007/pl0001195; discussion 205.

Hypervirulent *Klebsiella pneumoniae* with Hepatic Abscess and Endophthalmitis

Denis Spelman

1 Clinical Pearl

There are multiple microbiological causes of a liver abscess, including mixed enteric bacteria, hydatid, and amoebic disease. Over recent years a newly described hypervirulent strain of *Klebsiella pneumoniae* has been added to this list. This entity has significant differences in epidemiology, clinical manifestations, and optimal management approach.

2 Clinical Case

A 52-year-old gentleman was admitted to hospital with a 3-day history of fever, rigors, right sided upper quadrant abdominal pain and diarrhoea. He was born in Taiwan and emigrated to Australia 10 years earlier. On admission, he was unwell with fever of 38 °C and systolic blood pressure of 100 mm Hg. Initial blood investigations revealed a white cell count of 13.6×10^9/L with a neutrophilia, toxic granulations and left shift, a C-reactive protein (CRP) of 259 mg/L and mild derangement of liver function. An ultrasound (US) followed by abdominal computed tomography (CT) scan revealed a 8 × 7 × 4 cm abscess in the right hepatic lobe. He had blood cultures taken on arrival which flagged positive at 24 h with a Gram negative bacillus. On the following day he underwent a US-guided aspiration of the liver lesion. Gram stain revealed neutrophils (3+) and Gram negative bacilli. Both Gram negative bacilli from blood cultures and the liver aspirate were identified as *Klebsiella pneumoniae*, the colonies had a mucoid phenotype on culture with a 5 cm positive

D. Spelman (✉)
Department of Infectious Diseases and Microbiology, Alfred Hospital, Melbourne, VIC, Australia

Monash University, Melbourne, VIC, Australia

R. Junckerstorff et al. (eds.), *Beyond Evidence-Based Medicine*,
https://doi.org/10.1007/978-981-99-4440-8_71

string test. He was screened for other possible sites of metastatic infection including fundoscopy, all of which were negative. The patient was treated initially with ceftriaxone for 10 days, with good clinical response and then completed a 4-week antimicrobial course with oral ciprofloxacin.

3 Discussion

A liver abscess in a middle-aged patient can be due to any of a spectrum of organisms. Classically hydatid (*Echinococcus granulosis*) infection is well described, as well as amoebic disease in immigrants from, and travellers to, highly endemic countries. Pyogenic abscesses also occur most often in older patients, with a history of abdominal surgery or intra-abdominal pathology such as diverticulitis.

Confirming the presence of an abscess is usually performed initially by imaging, although at times there may be still some uncertainty concerning the possibility of alternate diagnoses such as primary hepatic malignancy or metastatic disease. Needle aspiration or insertion of a pigtail catheter with the production of abscess material is usually diagnostic.

A diagnosis of hydatid disease is usually based on the patient's epidemiology, serology, and microscopy of aspirated fluid (scolices, hooklets). For amoebic disease, useful diagnostic tools include epidemiology, amoebic serology, macroscopic appearance ("anchovy source") of an aspirate, with microscopy (amoebae trophozoites may be seen but not always) and/or molecular identification (e.g. polymerase chain reaction of amoebae on aspirated fluid). With both hydatid and amoebic infection, the diagnosis may be accepted on the basis of positive serology together with appropriate epidemiology, although drainage may be still indicated as a part of treatment. For pyogenic liver abscess, there is often polymicrobial infection with a mixture of enteric organisms such as Gram negative bacilli, streptococci and/or anaerobes. Polymorphs and the causative organisms are often identified by microscopy and culture of the fluid aspirate or from blood culture ideally taken before antimicrobial therapy is commenced.

Over that last 2 decades a new clinical syndrome has been described: a monomicrobial bacterial hepatic abscess with other sites of metastatic infection due to a new hypervirulent strain of *K. pneumoniae* [1]. This often has different epidemiological, clinical and microbiological features that separates it from other enteric flora. This entity is mostly described in patients living in or from for Taiwan or East Asia [2]. Unlike the classical pyogenic abscess, there is usually an absence of predisposing hepatobiliary or intra-abdominal disease with this syndrome. Most importantly there is a significant risk of concurrent metastatic pyogenic disease at extra-hepatic sites, especially of the eye resulting in a pyogenic endophthalmitis [3]. This may result in the loss of vision or even loss of an eye secondary to this infection. Other sites of metastatic spread have been brain, lung, skin and soft tissue, meninges, and vertebrae. Many other klebsiella strains are healthcare-associated but this new strain is most often community acquired infection.

These strains of *K. pneumoniae* have been labelled "hypervirulent" because of the clinical features above and because of distinctive laboratory features. On blood agar culture plates, the organism has very mucoid phenotype and very often has a positive string test (Figs. 1 and 2) which is a measure of this organism's capsular viscosity. This mucoid capsule may be a virulence factor for this organism. It usually belongs to a K1 or K2 capsular types. The presence of specific genes e.g. rmpA gene may be predictors of likelihood of metastasis.

The reasons why these strains of *K. pneumoniae* have appeared over recent years is uncertain. The geographical localisation raises the possibility of a genetic predisposition. Others have suggested antimicrobial use within the community, or the acquisition of new virulence factors may have played a role.

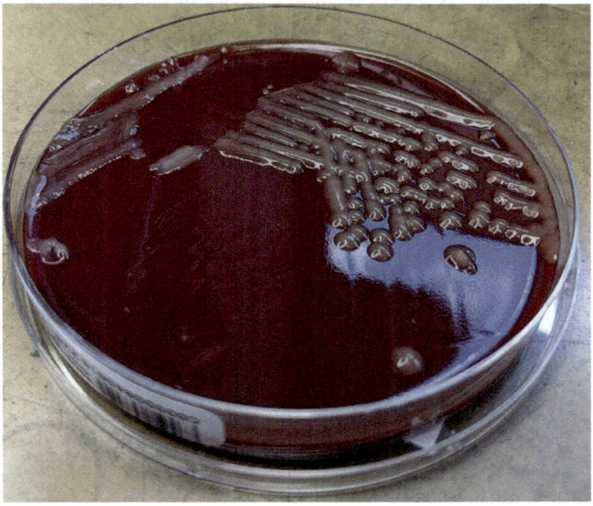

Fig. 1 Mucoid colonies of *K. pneumoniae* on horse blood agar. (Photo source: Dr. Sadid Khan, Microbiology, Alfred Hospital)

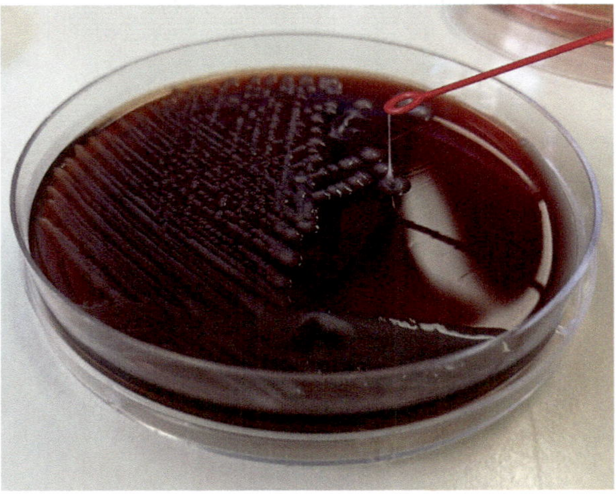

Fig. 2 Demonstration of positive string test with a loop on one of the colonies. (Photo source: Dr. Sadid Khan, Microbiology, Alfred Hospital)

The importance of this entity for the clinician is that if this diagnosis is considered, then there needs to be awareness of the possible presence of metastatic infection and the need to screen the likely sites. Initial and repeated fundoscopy with review by an ophthalmologist may be eye or vision saving if ophthalmitis identified and treated early. Education of the patient to urgently report any visual or eye symptoms is important. If careful clinical assessment suggests another possible metastatic site, this warrants timely investigation and management.

4 Take Home Messages

- A broad spectrum of infective organisms (bacterial, protozoal, and metazoal) can cause a liver abscess.
- The recently described invasive or hypervirulent strain of *K. pneumoniae* can cause liver abscess and, unlike other bacterial causes of pyogenic liver abscess, has a high incidence of metastatic disease.
- Suspicion or proof of the organism should result in careful screening of potential metastatic sites, especially the eye, orbit and meninges.
- Review by an ophthalmologist is indicated.

References

1. Zou Q, Li Y. Hypervirulent *Klebsiella pneumoniae*. N Engl J Med. 2021;385(9):833.
2. Wang JH, Liu YC, Lee SS, Yen MY, Chen YS, Wang JH, Wann SR, Lin HH. Primary liver abscess due to *Klebsiella pneumoniae* in Taiwan. Clin Infect Dis. 1998;26(6):143.
3. Fung CP, Chang FY, Lee SC, Hu BS, Kuo BI, Liu CY, Ho M, Siu LK. A global emerging disease of *Klebsiella pneumoniae* liver abscess: is serotype K1 an important factor for complicated endophthalmitis? Gut. 2002;50(3):420.

Protean Clinical Manifestations of *Strongyloides stercoralis*

Denis Spelman

1 Clinical Pearl

Investigation of a patient with repeated episodes of Gram negative bacteraemia usually includes a search for a localised site of untreated infection or other localised gastrointestinal pathology. However, in a patient with appropriate epidemiology, investigation should include the search for *Strongyloides stercoralis*. This roundworm can result in both Gram negative bacteraemia and other clinical manifestations such as adult onset asthma and recurrent skin urticaria.

2 Clinical Case

A 75-year-old man presented to Emergency Department with new onset asthma and responded to a 2-week course of prednisolone at a starting dose of 50 mg daily. Two weeks later he re-presented with fevers up to 39 °C and rigors. Blood cultures, taken on arrival, isolated *Klebsiella pneumoniae*. Treatment included intravenous ceftriaxone followed by oral ciprofloxacin with complete resolution of symptoms. A peripheral eosinophilia of 3.52×10^9/L (Normal 0.0–0.5%) was noted during this admission. Ten months later he again developed fevers and rigors, and *K. pneumoniae* was again isolated from blood cultures. He again fully recovered with antimicrobial therapy. On this second admission he reported that he was a World War 2 veteran with over 2 years' service in the Middle East. He had subsequently emigrated from Russia. Both this epidemiology and the eosinophilia documented in the previous admission, resulted in the consideration of a parasitic infection.

D. Spelman (✉)
Department of Infectious Diseases and Microbiology, Alfred Hospital, Melbourne, VIC, Australia

Monash University, Melbourne, VIC, Australia

R. Junckerstorff et al. (eds.), *Beyond Evidence-Based Medicine*, https://doi.org/10.1007/978-981-99-4440-8_72

Strongyloides stercoralis was identified in faeces and by positive serology. He received a course of Ivermectin. He has had no further episode of Gram negative bacteraemia or asthma during a four year follow-up period.

3 Discussion

Strongyloides is a roundworm (nematode), with a unique life cycle that includes larval migration from skin, through the lungs and the gastrointestinal tract and can cause disease at each of these 3 sites. Infection is often associated with poor living conditions. This patient most likely acquired infection decades before his initial presentation, most likely during World War 2. This parasite can live for many years in the human host through a process of autoinoculation whereby after excretion through the rectum it can re-inoculate its human host by piercing and re-infecting through the perianal skin. This cycle often results in lifelong infection.

Many infected patients remain asymptomatic for long time periods. Some do have low grade nonspecific symptoms such as intermittent pruritus, urticarial rash, diarrhoea, or weight loss.

Suggestive epidemiology for strongyloidiasis is immigration from or travellers from an endemic country such as in Asia, Africa, or the Middle East [1]. This parasite is also endemic in some rural communities in northern Australia.

The life cycle explains the clinical manifestations in this case. After infective larvae penetrate skin, the nematode enters the venous circulation and travels to the lungs, where infection can result in asthma. From the lungs it then ascends the bronchus, is swallowed to the reach bowel. At this site there is development into filariform larvae, which can penetrate bowel mucosa and perianal skin leading to autoinfection. During this bowel penetration the parasite can carry bowel Gram negative bacilli resulting in Gram negative septicaemia [2].

Because of this life cycle, treatment of an episode of Gram negative sepsis will not necessarily prevent future episodes. Ongoing and repeated cycles of larval migration can result in repeated episodes of Gram negative bacteraemia if the parasite is not considered, diagnosed and treated.

This parasite was the likely cause of this patient's onset of asthma even at the age of 75 years. The diagnosis of new onset asthma in a patient with such appropriate epidemiology should result in investigation for strongyloides. The elevated eosinophil count documented on the first admission is consistent with parasitic infection, but no further action was taken at that time.

Steroids as used to treat asthma in this case can precipitate increased strongyloides migration resulting in life-threatening disseminated strongyloidiasis or the hyperendemic syndrome [3]. Ideally screening for strongyloides should occur before commencement of immunosuppressive therapy. Screening usually consists of an eosinophil count, faeces for ova, cysts and parasites and serology. It should be remembered that the use of corticosteroids can cause a decrease in the eosinophil count. One faecal sample is positive in <50% cases because of intermittent larval excretion, and 3 specimens are often recommended. Faecal polymerase chain reaction (PCR) testing for strongyloides may have greater sensitivity and greater specificity than stool examination, but this testing is not widely available [4]. The sensitivity of serology does vary between patient cohorts (68–98%). A positive serology test does not distinguish between past and present infection, although antibody levels may decrease over 2 years following treatment.

Treatment usually consists of ivermectin or albendazole which are generally safe medications. On occasion, a patient with strong epidemiology and about to commence immunosuppressive therapy may undergo strongyloides treatment without a confirmative diagnosis. Treatment failures can occur. Normalisation of eosinophil count, negative faeces sample and improvement in the serological titre may indicate treatment success.

4 Take Home Messages

- Adult-onset asthma and Gram negative sepsis can both be caused by underlying strongyloides infection.
- Long term asymptomatic infection can convert to severe clinical disease especially if the patient receives corticosteroids or other immunosuppressive agents.
- Screening for strongyloides is recommended for: persons with suggestive symptoms and appropriate epidemiology, immigrants and return travellers from high endemic countries, and those from endemic countries who are taking or about to commence immunosuppressive therapy (e.g. pre-transplantation).
- Screening methods include faeces for the detection of ova, cysts and parasites, strongyloides serology and peripheral blood eosinophil count.

References

1. Einsiedel L, Spelman D. *Strongyloides stercoralis*: risks posed to immigrant patients in an Australian tertiary referral centre. Intern Med J. 2006;36:632–7.
2. Ghosal UC, Ghosal U, Jain M, et al. *Strongyloides stercoralis* infestation associated with septicaemia due to intestinal transmural migration of bacteria. J Gastroenterol Hepatol. 2002;17(12):1331.
3. Lim L, Biggs BA. Fatal disseminated strongyloidiasis in a previously treated patient. MJA. 2001;174:355–6.
4. Robertson GJ, Koehler AV, Bradbury RS. Application of PCR-based tools to explore strongyloides Infection in people in parts of Northern territory. Trop Med Infect Dis. 2017;2(4):62. https://doi.org/10.3390/tropicalmed2040062.

Vibrio Necrotising Fasciitis (“Bubblewrap” Disease)

Denis Spelman

1 Clinical Pearl

A diagnostic challenge is to separate cellulitis from deeper necrotising soft tissue infections (NSTI) such as necrotising fasciitis and myonecrosis. These entities can be caused by a spectrum of invasive bacteria. Timely diagnosis with identification of the causative organism and instigation of early treatment may be limb or lifesaving.

2 Clinical Case

A 55-year-old man developed an area of tenderness and redness on the front of his left lower leg. There had been no preceding injury. Two days earlier he had visited a coastal region where he had spent time with his legs in sea water. Over the next 24 h he developed fever, and the pain increased such that he was unable to walk. The next day his General Practitioner noted the redness and tenderness with the severity of his pain appearing out of proportion compared to the clinical signs. A diagnosis of cellulitis was made, and he started a course of cephalexin. The following day, he complained of more severe pain, increased leg swelling, with ongoing fever, sweats, and rigors. His wife noticed and felt small skin “bubbles” in the area of redness which she described as looking like “bubblewrap”.

Because of this deterioration he was taken by ambulance to the Emergency Department at a local hospital. On arrival, he was febrile at 38.5 °C, sweating, mildly confused with tachycardia (100/min) and a blood pressure of 95/70 mmHg.

D. Spelman (✉)
Department of Infectious Diseases and Microbiology,
Alfred Hospital, Melbourne, VIC, Australia

Monash University, Melbourne, VIC, Australia

R. Junckerstorff et al. (eds.), *Beyond Evidence-Based Medicine*,
https://doi.org/10.1007/978-981-99-4440-8_73

There was marked swelling of his left lower leg with a large area of erythema and 2 areas of black skin of the dorsum of his foot. Subcutaneous crepitus was palpable.

Initial investigations revealed leucocytosis (18.2×10^9/L) with a left shift and toxic granulations, and C-reactive protein (CRP) of 305 mg/L. Necrotising fasciitis or myonecrosis was suspected. Broad spectrum antibiotics were commenced. He was taken to the operating theatre and underwent an open exploration revealing necrotising fasciitis involving the anterior, posterior, and lateral compartments of his lower leg. Debridement of non-viable tissue, including skin, fat, fascia, and muscle of his lower leg was undertaken. An exploratory lateral thigh incision was made to reveal healthy tissues. Gram staining of the resected tissue revealed Gram negative bacilli. He was subsequently transferred to the intensive care unit of a large metropolitan hospital.

Both the blood cultures taken at his initial presentation and the resected tissue isolated *Vibrio vulnificus*. The initial broad spectrum antibiotic regime was expanded to insure coverage of this organism. He subsequently underwent 4 further surgical debridements and a course of hyperbaric therapy. Unfortunately, he had lost significant muscle from the lower leg, which could not be salvaged, and an above knee amputation was necessary. After a long inpatient stay, he was finally discharged to undertake rehabilitation.

3 Discussion

The challenge in this scenario is to separate uncomplicated cellulitis from deeper, more severe infection such as necrotising fasciitis or myonecrosis. NSTI is a medical emergency requiring urgent surgical intervention. There were red flags of more severe clinical infection early in the course of his illness, especially the description of pain out of proportion to the clinical signs. Other suggestive features were the rapidity of onset and the progression of the illness despite the initial antibiotic therapy. Later signs of this diagnosis were the development of crepitus and areas of skin necrosis.

V. vulnificus is a Gram negative bacillus which is found in coastal sea waters [1] most often in the warmer months, this case occurring during the Australian summer. This vibrio can also cause primary septicaemia, wound infections and gastroenteritis. A history of sea water contact or less frequently with raw seafood [2] may alert the physician to infection with this organism. It is a well described cause of necrotising fasciitis, often resulting in fulminant clinical disease as in the case described here.

Other organisms that can cause the same clinical syndrome are *Clostridium perfringens, Clostridium septicum* and Group A streptococcus (*Streptococcus pyogenes*). *C. perfringens* necrotising fasciitis most often occurs in the setting of an infected traumatic or surgical wound. *C. septicum* is notorious for causing spontaneous myonecrosis and is usually a harbinger of co-existent, often clinically silent, colonic carcinoma. *S. pyogenes* causes necrotising fasciitis in a number of clinical settings including intravenous drug use. Each of these has a similar aggressive clinical course with a high incidence of morbidity, such as limb amputation as in this case, and mortality. In each of these scenarios the organism is usually identified in blood culture or operative tissue or both. Prior to the identification of the causative organism, empiric antibiotics need to cover anaerobic (clostridium), Gram positive(streptococci) and Gram negative(vibrio) bacteria.

The mainstays of treatment of necrotising fasciitis are surgical debridement [3], antimicrobials, and often intensive care. In many cases with severe disease, hyperbaric oxygen therapy, if available, is included in management. The benefit of hyperbaric oxygen therapy may be the salvage of some tissue which would otherwise become non-viable.

Early diagnosis and intervention may be limb-saving or lifesaving. In the present case if the diagnosis was made earlier, then this would have resulted in earlier surgical debridement, earlier antimicrobial therapy, and possibly successful treatment without amputation. When the diagnosis is not clear cut, early and frequent review of the patient is warranted. Radiological imaging (computed tomography scan, magnetic resonance imaging or ultrasound) may be useful in the demonstration of tissue oedema and the presence of gas in tissue.

The usefulness of a collateral history from a family member is demonstrated in this case. The patient's wife gave a superb description of the tissue crepitus, which she described as "bubblewrap". This is included as the title of this topic.

4 Take Home Messages

- Necrotising fasciitis is a medical emergency requiring urgent surgical debridement and empiric broad spectrum antimicrobial treatment.
- Recent water exposure suggests *V vulnificus* as the causative organism.
- When the diagnosis is suspected but not proven, early and frequent clinical review is strongly recommended.
- Beware when the severity of a patient's pain is out of proportion to the clinical signs.
- The presence of tissue crepitus, haemorrhagic bullae and skin necrosis heralds a poor outcome and demands urgent surgical debridement.
- Early intervention may be limb or lifesaving.

References

1. Tsai Y-H, Huang T-Y, Chen J-L, Hsiao C-T, Kuo L-T, Huang K-C. Bacteriology and mortality of necrotizing fasciitis in a tertiary coastal hospital with comparing risk indicators of methicillin-resistant Staphylococcus aureus and Vibrio vulnificus infections: a prospective study. BMC Infect Dis. 2021;21(1):771. https://doi.org/10.1186/s12879-021-06518-5.
2. Hau V, Ho CO. Necrotising fasciitis caused by Vibrio vulnificus in the lower limb following exposure to seafood on the hand. Hong Kong Med J. 2011;17(4):335.
3. Chao WN, Tsai CF, Chang HR, Chan KS, Su CH, Lee YT, Ueng KC, Chen CC, Chen SC, Lee MC. Impact of timing of surgery on outcome of Vibrio vulnificus-related necrotizing fasciitis. Am J Surg. 2013;206(1):32–9; Epub 2013 Feb 12.

Why Did This Patient Develop Invasive *Streptococcus pneumoniae* Infection?

Denis Spelman

1 Clinical Pearl

When *Streptococcus pneumoniae* presents as invasive infection, it is often associated with significant morbidity and mortality. Such a presentation should generate the questions as to what is the underlying predisposition for severe sepsis in this patient, what investigations should be undertaken to detect that predisposition and what can be done to prevent future episodes of such sepsis?

2 Clinical Case

A 45-year-old female presented to the Emergency Department (ED) with 2 days of cough, runny nose, fevers, and diarrhoea. She gave a history of long-term inflammatory bowel disease, had required immunosuppressive therapy in the past, but minimal treatment in the past 2 years. She underwent basic investigations including chest Xray, full blood examination, electrolytes, and liver function. She also had a COVID-19 PCR test which was negative. She was not considered to be very unwell and was discharged home with symptomatic treatment, to be followed up by her general practitioner. However, 2 days later the blood culture taken on that ED visit was reported as growing a Gram positive cocci, which was identified as *Streptococcus pneumoniae*. The patient was recalled and admitted to hospital. At the time of admission, she was unwell with high fever, tachycardia, and hypotension. She spent 5 days in hospital, treated with intravenous penicillin and fully recovered. At the end

D. Spelman (✉)
Department of Infectious Diseases and Microbiology,
Alfred Hospital, Melbourne, VIC, Australia

Monash University, Melbourne, VIC, Australia

R. Junckerstorff et al. (eds.), *Beyond Evidence-Based Medicine*,
https://doi.org/10.1007/978-981-99-4440-8_74

of that admission the presence of Howell-Jolly Bodies (HJB), indicating hyposplenia or asplenia was noted on a blood film. It was also then discovered that HJBs had been reported on previous blood films dating back 5 years. This patient did not know she had hyposplenia/asplenia and had not previously had pneumococcal vaccination.

3 Discussion

This patient initially presented with fever and respiratory symptoms, was not considered to be very unwell and was discharged home. However, she was then recalled and admitted when *S pneumoniae* grew from her blood cultures. She received antimicrobial therapy and subsequently made a complete recovery. At that time neither the patient nor the medical staff knew of her hyposplenia/asplenia. It was only towards the end of this admission that HJBs were noted on her blood film report. Such patients without a functioning spleen are at increased risk of overwhelming sepsis, with capsulated organisms especially *S pneumoniae*, *Neisseria meningitidis* and *Haemophilus influenzae* type b, which have significant morbidity and mortality. The previous blood films in this patient which also reported HJBs were missed opportunities to manage her hypo/asplenia, and such interventions in all likelihood would have prevented this and any future episodes of overwhelming sepsis with these organisms.

Any patient presenting with invasive *S pneumoniae* infection should undergo screening for a number of conditions which predispose to this infection. Asplenia or hyposplenia has many causes. The commonest cause is splenectomy most often for trauma or malignancy and such causes would be apparent from the medical history. However, there are a number of medical conditions that can cause hyposplenia/asplenia. These include haemoglobinopathies, coeliac disease, lupus, splenic irradiation and inflammatory bowel disease. There are also reports of congenital or familial asplenia in which case the patient may be unaware of the medical condition. In the case presented here, the hyposplenia or asplenia was most likely caused by inflammatory bowel disease.

Screening for hyposplenia/asplenia is usually through a blood film looking for Howell Jolly Bodies, which is a measure of the filtering function of the spleen. IgM memory B cells is also a test for spleen immune function but less commonly performed. Ultrasound and computed tomography (CT) scan can give a useful measurement of spleen size, but this may not reflect spleen function.

With this patient following the diagnosis of hyposplenia/asplenia, she was registered with Spleen Australia [1], received an education kit and person to person introduction to following preventive strategies [2] to prevent recurrence of invasive sepsis (see Fig. 1):

It has been demonstrated that for patients with hyposplenia/asplenia, registration with Spleen Australia has been associated with a 69% decrease in the incidence of overwhelming sepsis [3].

*Education of her and her family about the risks and strategies to minimise that risk.

*Carriage of medical alert: wallet card, medallion or bracelet

*Her Vaccine plan was prepared and included:

- -13 valent Pneumococcal Conjugate Vaccine (13vPCV)
- -23 valent Polysaccharide Pneumococcal Vaccine (23vPPV)
- -Meningococcal conjugate quadrivalent ACWY vaccine: 2 doses
- -Meningococcal B recombinant vaccine (MenB): 2 doses
- -Haemophilus influenzae type b vaccine

*She had the 1st dose of COVD-19 vaccine and annual influenza vaccine

*She commenced on daily amoxicillin 250mg prophylaxis for at least 3 years

*She also now has an emergency supply of antibiotics (amoxicillin 500mg x 4) and instructions to take this if she develops acute significant symptoms and to attend her local medical officer or hospital emergency department as soon as possible

*Because of the increased risk of malaria in people without a functioning spleen, she should seek specialist travel medicine advice if future travel plans include malaria endemic regions.

*She was warned of the potential risks from animal bites and scratches, which may cause acute sepsis with organisms from animal's oropharyngeal flora such as *Capnocytophagia canimorsus*

For more information, see Spleen Australia (www.spleen.org.au)

Fig. 1 Preventive strategies for a patient without a functioning spleen (Asplenia/hyposplenia)

Apart from hyposplenia/asplenia there are other medical conditions that predispose to invasive *S pneumoniae* infection. These include HIV, congenital immunodeficiencies, myeloma, diabetes, chronic liver disease, transplantation, and complement deficiency. Screening for these conditions should also be considered. If the invasive infection is meningitis, then an anatomical skull base deficit, such as a cribriform plate defect or fracture, may be the predisposition, which would only be detected by cranial imaging [4].

4 Take Home Messages

- With invasive pneumococcal infection, an underlying predisposing condition should be sought.
- Screening should include FBE, blood film with a request for HJBs, Immunoglobulin quantitation, IgG subclasses determination, CD4, HIV serology, and HbA1c.
- Other tests for spleen function less commonly performed are IgM memory B cells and ultrasound or CT scanning of the splenic bed to estimate spleen size.
- If the invasive pneumococcal infection is meningitis, consider cranial imaging to determine anatomical bone defects or fracture.
- Be aware that some medical conditions can result in a poorly functioning spleen e.g. inflammatory bowel disease, coeliac disease, haemoglobinopathies. Screening for spleen function in these conditions should be considered.
- If hyposplenia/asplenia is documented, then the outlined infection preventive strategies should be introduced.

References

1. www.spleen.org.au.
2. Kanhutu K, Jones P, Cheng A, Grannell G, Best E, Spelman D. Spleen Australia guidelines for the prevention of sepsis in patients with asplenia and hyposplenism in Australia and New Zealand. Intern Med J. 2017;47:848–55.
3. Arnott A, Jones P, Franklin L, Spelman D, Leder K, Cheng A. A registry for patients with Asplenia/Hyposplenism reduces the risk of infections with encapsulated organisms. Clin Infect Dis. 2018;67(4):557–61.
4. Verma Nm Sayy LE, Lund V, et al. An important diagnosis to consider in recurrent meningitis. JRSM Short Rep. 2013;4:1–6.

Part X
Gastroenterology

Acute Diarrhoea is Likely Infectious

Adam Peterson and Ray Boyapati

1 Clinical Pearl

Acute diarrhoea is likely infectious.

2 Clinical Case

A 36-year-old lady presents to the emergency department with 5 days of loose, watery diarrhoea, anorexia and cramping abdominal pain. A CT abdomen and pelvis is performed and is reported as 'thickening of the transverse and descending colon'. Initial laboratory tests reveal an elevated white cell count (14) and C-reactive protein (230).

3 Discussion

Acute diarrhoea without alarm features should be diagnosed and managed as acute infectious diarrhoea. For uncomplicated presentations, further investigations are not indicated and management should prioritise rehydration and prevention of dehydration [1].

A. Peterson · R. Boyapati (✉)
Monash Health, Melbourne, VIC, Australia

Faculty of Medicine Nursing and Health Sciences, Monash University, Melbourne, VIC, Australia

R. Junckerstorff et al. (eds.), *Beyond Evidence-Based Medicine*,
https://doi.org/10.1007/978-981-99-4440-8_75

Clinical characteristics such as fever and dysentery, as well as epidemiological factors such as employment in food services should guide the decision of whether to perform stool culture or multiplex PCR [1, 2].

Whilst computed tomography imaging in patients with abdominal pain without trauma is established, it is not recommended in the evaluation of diarrhoea with abdominal pain and has not been shown to change management [3]. Colonic thickening seen on imaging is consistent with infectious colitis and does not necessarily suggest an alternate cause of diarrhoea such as inflammatory bowel disease.

The most useful discriminating factor between infectious and non-infectious aetiologies of diarrhoea is a thorough clinical history to determine the chronicity of symptoms.

4 Other Gems

- Other red flags for alternate causes of diarrhoea include significant weight loss, hypoalbuminaemia, iron and B12 deficiency.
- Any hospitalised patient who develops diarrhoea, and those at high risk in the community (e.g., immunosuppressed, post antibiotic use) should be evaluated for *Clostridioides difficile.*

References

1. Riddle MS, DuPont HL, Connor BA. ACG Clinical Guideline: diagnosis, treatment, and prevention of acute diarrheal infections in adults. Am J Gastroenterol. 2016;111(5):602–22.
2. DuPont HL. Acute infectious diarrhea in immunocompetent adults. N Engl J Med. 2014;370(16):1532–40.
3. Aisenberg GM, Grimes RM. Computed tomography in patients with abdominal pain and diarrhoea: does the benefit outweigh the drawbacks? Intern Med J. 2013;43(10):1141–4.

Always Ask About Medicines and Supplements When Faced with Elevated Liver Enzymes

Adam Peterson and Ray Boyapati

1 Clinical Pearl

Elevated liver enzymes? Ask about prescription, over the counter, supplements, internet, naturopathic, homeopathic and Chinese herbal medications. Then ask again!

2 Clinical Case

A 29-year-old man is referred to the gastroenterology outpatient clinic with elevated alanine transaminase (ALT) of 708 U/L and aspartate transaminase (AST) of 687 U/L. His medical history is unremarkable, he reports no regular medications and does not drink alcohol. Abdominal ultrasound is normal and hepatitis B and C serology show no evidence of infection. Anti-nuclear antibody and anti-smooth muscle antibodies are negative. After a detailed medication history, he reveals he has been prescribed a Chinese herbal tea by a Chinese medicine practitioner for the management of gastro-oesophageal reflux disease.

A. Peterson · R. Boyapati (✉)
Monash Health, Melbourne, VIC, Australia

Faculty of Medicine Nursing and Health Sciences, Monash University, Melbourne, VIC, Australia

R. Junckerstorff et al. (eds.), *Beyond Evidence-Based Medicine*,
https://doi.org/10.1007/978-981-99-4440-8_76

3 Discussion

The use of herbal and dietary supplements is increasing. They are commonly considered safe by patients and may not be volunteered when taking a medication history. Patients often take multiple products, and these often contain more than one ingredient. Furthermore, the ingredient lists may not be accurate as these products are less regulated than prescription medications and are often sourced from other countries. Patients using these products are commonly from culturally and linguistically diverse backgrounds. Herbal and dietary supplements are often used in traditional medicine in the developing world and migrants may transport these practices to their new homes in developed countries [1].

Drug induced liver injury (DILI) is the most common cause of acute liver failure in developed nations [2]. DILI from herbal and dietary supplements is increasing both in Australia [3] and abroad [4]. Concerningly, DILI arising from herbal and dietary products can be severe and is associated with poorer outcomes than that of paracetamol toxicity. DILI remains a clinical diagnosis of exclusion with judicious use of pathologic and radiologic testing to exclude alternate differential diagnoses [5].

A thorough clinical history should be conducted with a particular focus on:

- Complete list of medications and herbal and dietary supplements (particularly over the preceding 6 months)
- Indication for use, and exposure time to product
- History of alcohol use and other liver disorders
- History of other drug reactions

4 Other Gems

- Antibiotics are the most common non-paracetamol cause of DILI and are commonly missed.
- The pattern of liver injury may provide insight to the causative agent [2].
- 'LiverTox' [6] is an online resource that provides information on the diagnosis, cause, frequency, and clinical patterns of liver injury attributable to medications and selected herbal and dietary supplements.

References

1. Ekor M. The growing use of herbal medicines: issues relating to adverse reactions and challenges in monitoring safety. Front Pharmacol. 2014;4:177.
2. Hoofnagle JH, Björnsson ES. Drug-induced liver injury — types and phenotypes. N Engl J Med. 2019;381(3):264–73.

3. Nash E, et al. Drug-induced liver injury in Australia, 2009-2020: the increasing proportion of non-paracetamol cases linked with herbal and dietary supplements. Med J Aust. 2021;215(6):261–8.
4. Navarro VJ, et al. Liver injury from herbals and dietary supplements in the U.S. Drug-Induced Liver Injury Network. Hepatology. 2014;60(4):1399–408.
5. Chalasani NP, et al. ACG clinical guideline: diagnosis and management of idiosyncratic drug-induced liver injury. Am J Gastroenterol. 2021;116(5):878–98.
6. LiverTox: clinical and research information on drug-induced liver injury. 2012. Available from https://www.ncbi.nlm.nih.gov/books/NBK547852/.

Never Miss the Digital Rectal Examination

Adam Peterson and Ray Boyapati

1 Clinical Pearl

Never miss the digital rectal examination.

2 Clinical Case

A 67-year-old man is referred with altered bowel habit and bright rectal bleeding following a prostate biopsy for the monitoring of known low grade prostate cancer. A perianal examination is unremarkable, but on digital rectal examination (DRE) a hard mass is felt anteriorly in a hemi-circumferential distribution. Colonoscopy confirms a malignant appearing 5 cm partially obstructing rectal mass.

A. Peterson · R. Boyapati (✉)
Monash Health, Melbourne, VIC, Australia

Faculty of Medicine Nursing and Health Sciences, Monash University, Melbourne, VIC, Australia

R. Junckerstorff et al. (eds.), *Beyond Evidence-Based Medicine*, https://doi.org/10.1007/978-981-99-4440-8_77

3 Discussion

Despite no longer being indicated in routine screening for prostate cancer, the platitudinous adage of “if you don’t put your finger in it, you’ll put your foot in it” continues to hold truth in evaluation of rectal diseases. To perform a rectal examination, the patient should be positioned in the left lateral position. Careful inspection of the perianal area is followed by using the gloved index finger to assess for intramural and extramural findings. Finally, the glove should be examined for evidence of blood, mucous or melaena [1, 2]. DRE is a key aspect of the physical examination for patients presenting with symptoms of rectal disease including rectal bleeding, abdominal pain, constipation, tenesmus, and anaemia. A positive finding will affect the triage of further investigations including colonoscopy [3]. Failure to perform DRE for further evaluation of concerning gastrointestinal symptoms may lead to a delay in diagnosis of rectal cancer [4]. It has previously been demonstrated to have sensitivity of 76.2% and specificity of 91.7% in detecting rectal cancer in primary care. Importantly, this study demonstrated a high negative predictive value of 98.8% [5].

4 Other Gems

- Rectal examination should be performed for patients who present with suspected gastrointestinal bleeding and has been shown to alter subsequent diagnostic tests and management [6].
- A commonly cited reason for not performing the DRE is a lack of confidence, but this can be overcome with supervised practice and training [7].

References

1. Williams N, Bulstrode C, O’Connell PR. Bailey & Love’s short practice of surgery. 25th ed. Boca Raton: CRC Press; 2018.
2. Talley NJ. How to do and interpret a rectal examination in gastroenterology. Am J Gastroenterol. 2008;103(4):820–2.
3. Emery J, Freeman V, Brown G, Macrae F, Bell C; Cancer Council Australia Colorectal Cancer Guidelines Working Party. Clinical question: symptoms predictive of colorectal cancer. In: Clinical practice guidelines for the prevention, early detection and management of colorectal cancer. Available from: https://wiki.cancer.org.au/australia/Guidelines:Colorectal_cancer.
4. Young CJ, Sweeney JL, Hunter A. Implications of delayed diagnosis in colorectal cancer. Aust N Z J Surg. 2000;70(9):635–8.
5. Ang CW, et al. The diagnostic value of digital rectal examination in primary care for palpable rectal tumour. Color Dis. 2008;10(8):789–92.
6. Shrestha MP, Borgstrom M, Trowers E. Digital rectal examination reduces hospital admissions, endoscopies, and medical therapy in patients with acute gastrointestinal bleeding. Am J Med. 2017;130(7):819–25.
7. Patel MI, Kakala B, Beattie K. Teaching medical students digital rectal examination: a randomized study of simulated model vs rectal examination volunteers. BJU Int. 2019;124(1):14–8.

Proton Pump Inhibitors Should be Dosed 30 Minutes Prior to Meals

Adam Peterson and Ray Boyapati

1 Clinical Pearl

Proton pump inhibitors should be dosed 30 minutes prior to meals.

2 Clinical Case

A 50-year-old lady presents to the outpatient clinic with a recurrent rising, burning epigastric and retrosternal pain that is worse after eating. She has no past medical history although she has gained 10 kg over the past 2 years. She is diagnosed with gastro-oesophageal reflux disease (GORD) and prescribed pantoprazole 40 mg daily. Unfortunately, she returns the following week as her symptoms have not improved despite taking the medicine with meals.

3 Discussion

GORD is a commonly encountered clinical presentation in the Western world and thought to be associated with the increasing prevalence of metabolic diseases including obesity [1]. Fortunately, proton pump inhibitors (PPIs) have transformed the management of GORD and most patients can achieve excellent symptomatic

A. Peterson · R. Boyapati (✉)
Monash Health, Melbourne, VIC, Australia

Faculty of Medicine Nursing and Health Sciences, Monash University, Melbourne, VIC, Australia

R. Junckerstorff et al. (eds.), *Beyond Evidence-Based Medicine*,
https://doi.org/10.1007/978-981-99-4440-8_78

relief. In a patient with GORD symptoms and no identifiable red flags, a therapeutic trial of PPI should be prescribed before further evaluation [2]. However, careful attention should be taken to adherence and timing of doses for these medications to yield their full effect. A careful clinical history should establish a pattern of symptoms and the medicine should be timed to have a maximum effect. Importantly, PPIs should be administered 30 minutes prior to meals, rather than with the meal itself, to permit maximum effect of gastric acid secretion. Patients with persistent symptoms despite appropriate adherence to PPI therapy should be referred for specialist review and endoscopic evaluation.

4 Other Gems

- There is a lack of evidence to support any specific dietary modification for GORD, however identifying patient specific precipitants can be helpful in allaying symptoms.
- Obesity is associated with GORD, and weight gain may be the precipitant to symptoms onset [3]. Conversely, weight loss may help alleviate symptoms [4].
- Functional dyspepsia often coincides with irritable bowel syndrome and can be managed with the same armamentarium of low-FODMAP diet, neuro-modulatory medication, and cognitive behavioural therapy.
- A diagnosis of gastroparesis should be considered when patients with risk factors such as diabetes mellitus present with severe reflux symptoms.
- Red flags indicating a need for further evaluation include: recurrent vomiting, dysphagia/odynophagia, weight loss, gastrointestinal bleeding, age of onset >50, epigastric mass and duration of symptoms >5 years or <6 months [5].

References

1. Dent J, et al. Epidemiology of gastro-oesophageal reflux disease: a systematic review. Gut. 2005;54(5):710–7.
2. Katz PO, Gerson LB, Vela MF. Guidelines for the diagnosis and management of gastroesophageal reflux disease. Am J Gastroenterol. 2013;108(3):308–28; quiz 329.
3. Locke GR, et al. Risk factors associated with symptoms of gastroesophageal reflux. Am J Med. 1999;106(6):642–9.
4. Singh M, et al. Weight loss can lead to resolution of gastroesophageal reflux disease symptoms: a prospective intervention trial. Obesity. 2013;21(2):284–90.
5. Keung C, Hebbard G. The management of gastro-oesophageal reflux disease. Aust Prescr. 2016;39(1):6–10.

Hypovolaemia is a Common Precipitant of Hepatic Encephalopathy

Adam Peterson and Ray Boyapati

1 Clinical Pearl

Hypovolaemia is a common precipitant of hepatic encephalopathy.

2 Clinical Case

A 52-year-old gentleman with known alcoholic associated cirrhosis is brought to the emergency department by his partner having developed confusion. On examination he is disorientated and exhibits asterixis. A non-contrast CT brain is unremarkable, and a blood alcohol level is negligible. He is diagnosed with hepatic encephalopathy (HE) and commenced on hourly lactulose therapy. Further investigation to identify a cause of his decompensation including abdominal ultrasound and infective screen are unrevealing. An astute junior doctor returns to re-examine the patient and notes decreased tissue turgor and dry mucous membranes.

A. Peterson · R. Boyapati (✉)
Monash Health, Melbourne, VIC, Australia

Faculty of Medicine Nursing and Health Sciences, Monash University, Melbourne, VIC, Australia

R. Junckerstorff et al. (eds.), *Beyond Evidence-Based Medicine*,
https://doi.org/10.1007/978-981-99-4440-8_79

3 Discussion

HE is a brain dysfunction caused by liver insufficiency and commonly portosystemic shunting. Its incidence and prevalence are proportional to the severity of an individual's underlying liver disease, and the diagnosis of overt HE defines decompensated liver disease [1].

The diagnosis and management of HE should involve excluding alternate diagnoses, addressing the underlying cause of liver disease, and commencing empirical treatment. However, a commonly missed aspect of HE evaluation is the identification of a precipitating event. This includes infection, gastrointestinal bleeding, constipation, electrolyte disorders and over diuresis or dehydration.

Patients with cirrhosis are commonly prescribed diuretics for the management of ascites and empirical treatment of HE involves the administration of nonabsorbable disaccharides such as lactulose, which have a laxative effect, increasing the risk that this group may develop dehydration. Correction of precipitating events can resolve HE, and careful fluid resuscitation when appropriate is an important aspect of care for a cirrhotic patient.

4 Other Gems

- Low grade encephalopathy may present with more subtle clinical features including an altered sleep wake cycle.
- A normal plasma ammonia level calls into question the diagnosis of HE, but as there are many causes of elevated plasma ammonia, a high result is not diagnostic of HE.
- Patients who present with unprovoked HE, should be considered for secondary prophylaxis.
- A high protein diet is not a cause of HE. An early referral to a dietician to aid in the identification and management of malnutrition should be made.

Reference

1. Vilstrup H, et al. Hepatic encephalopathy in chronic liver disease: 2014 practice guideline by the American Association for the Study Of Liver Diseases and the European Association for the Study of the Liver. Hepatology. 2014;60(2):715–35.

Part XI
Haematology

Describing Lower Limb Deep Vein Thrombosis: Needs More Than Just the Knee

Harry Gibbs and David Buxton

1 Clinical Pearl

Proximal deep vein thrombosis (DVT) may occur below the knee.

2 Clinical Case

A 36-year-old woman developed pain and swelling of the left calf 6 days after a long distance flight. She had previously been healthy and her only medication was the combined oral contraceptive pill containing ethinylestradiol and drospirenone. She was currently menstruating. A duplex ultrasound was performed and reported, "Thrombus is present in one of the gastrocnemius veins, extending into the popliteal vein to a point 4 cm below the knee crease. Conclusion: Below knee DVT". The patient was reviewed and advised that the treatment options were serial ultrasound examination or anticoagulation. The treating clinician felt that anticoagulant therapy may increase the amount of menstrual bleeding and advised her to have a repeat ultrasound examination in 4 days. She developed breathless and chest pain 2 days later and was found to have pulmonary embolism (PE) on computed tomography (CT) scanning. She was admitted to hospital and anticoagulant therapy was commenced.

H. Gibbs (✉)
Department of General Medicine, Alfred Health, Melbourne, VIC, Australia

Monash University, Melbourne, VIC, Australia

D. Buxton
Department of General Medicine, Alfred Health, Melbourne, VIC, Australia

R. Junckerstorff et al. (eds.), *Beyond Evidence-Based Medicine*,
https://doi.org/10.1007/978-981-99-4440-8_80

3 Discussion

The anatomical extent of DVT has a significant impact on the risk of both the development of acute pulmonary embolism and of recurrent venous thromboembolism (VTE) and is a major determinant of treatment decision making. If thrombus is confined to veins distal to the popliteal vein, it is termed "distal" and if it involves the popliteal or any more proximal vein (including the femoral, external iliac or common iliac veins or the inferior vena cava) it is termed "proximal". The popliteal vein commences at the confluence of the tibial and fibular veins which is below the knee crease. Proximal DVT can, therefore, be confined to the calf. Treatment decisions are made according to whether the DVT is proximal or distal and not according to whether it is above or below the knee crease (Fig. 1).

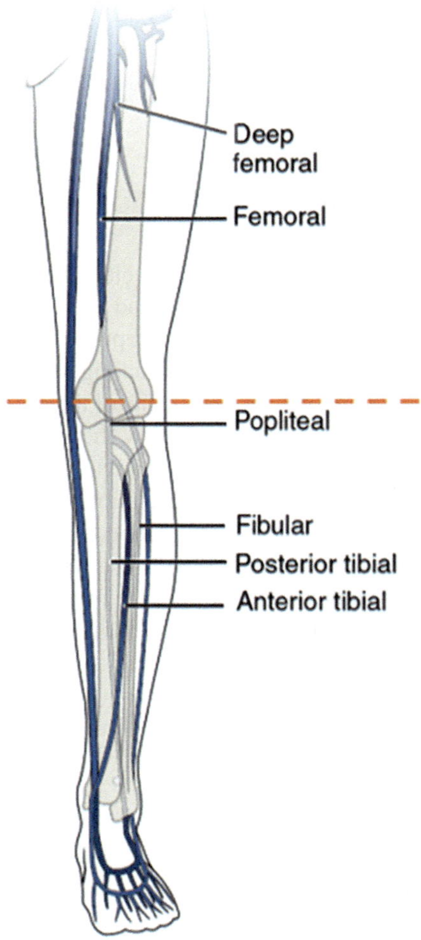

Fig. 1 Schematic of deep venous system of the leg. The Popliteal vein commences at the confluence of the tibial and fibular (peroneal) veins below the dotted orange line which corresponds to the 'knee crease'. Thus a popliteal thrombus is considered a high risk 'proximal' DVT, could also erroneously be considered 'below knee'. The Adapted from OpenStax College—http://cnx.org/content/col11496/1.6/ CC BY 3.0

If anticoagulant therapy is not administered in patients with acute DVT, the risk of developing PE is at least 35% if the DVT is proximal and only about 5% if it is distal [1]. For this reason, anticoagulant therapy is indicated for proximal DVT but serial ultrasound examination or anticoagulant therapy may be used for distal DVT [2]. Serial ultrasound examination is usually recommended if the risk of bleeding is increased [1]. If clot propagation from distal to proximal is demonstrated on serial ultrasound, treatment should change to anticoagulant therapy [1].

Following a course of anticoagulation for 3–6 months, recurrent VTE occurs infrequently if the original DVT was distal and extended duration anticoagulation is rarely indicated [2]. However, the recurrence rate following a course of anticoagulation for proximal DVT is significant and extended duration anticoagulation is frequently recommended [2].

4 Take Home Messages

- The terms "above knee DVT" and "below knee DVT" should not be used as they may lead to inappropriate and potentially dangerous treatment decisions; refer to DVT as proximal or distal depending on the involved veins.
- When deciding between serial monitoring and anti-coagulant therapy in distal DVT a tailored approach should be instigated, taking into account individualised risk of proximal thrombus propagation against bleeding risk secondary to treatment.

References

1. Tran HA, Gibbs H, Merriman E, Curnow JL, Young L, Bennett A, Tan CW, Chunilal SD, Ward CM, Baker R, Nandurkar H. New guidelines from the Thrombosis and Haemostasis Society of Australia and New Zealand for the diagnosis and management of venous thromboembolism. Med J Aust. 2019;210(5):227–35. https://doi.org/10.5694/mja2.50004. Epub 2019 Feb 10. Erratum in: Med J Aust. 2019 Jul;211(2):94. Erratum in: Med J Aust. 2020 Feb;212(3):108. PMID: 30739331.
2. Stevens SM, Woller SC, Kreuziger LB, Bounameaux H, Doerschug K, Geersing GJ, Huisman MV, Kearon C, King CS, Knighton AJ, Lake E, Murin S, Vintch JRE, Wells PS, Moores LK. Antithrombotic therapy for VTE disease: second update of the CHEST guideline and expert panel report. Chest. 2021;160(6):e545–608. https://doi.org/10.1016/j.chest.2021.07.055. Epub 2021 Aug 2. Erratum in: Chest. 2022 Jul;162(1):269. PMID: 34352278.

Fishing for Cancer After VTE: A Costly Expedition with Little Benefit

Harry Gibbs and David Buxton

1 Clinical Pearl

Extensive screening for occult malignancy is not warranted in patients presenting with the first episode of unprovoked venous thromboembolism.

2 Clinical Case

A 56-year-old man presented with 3 days of pain and swelling of the right calf and breathlessness on exertion. He had a past history of gout but had otherwise been well. He had no recent history of surgery, hospitalisation, or long-distance travel. On physical examination there was tenderness and swelling of the right calf and a tachycardia at rest. The remainder of the physical examination was normal and, in particular, there were no masses or lymphadenopathy present. Ultrasound examination of the right leg demonstrated thrombus in the posterior tibial vein, popliteal vein and the femoral vein extending to the mid-thigh. Computed tomography (CT) scanning of the chest showed pulmonary embolism (PE) in segmental pulmonary arteries bilaterally. The diagnosis of unprovoked venous thromboembolism (VTE) was made, and anticoagulant therapy was commenced. Screening for occult

H. Gibbs (✉)
Department of General Medicine, Alfred Health, Melbourne, VIC, Australia

Monash University, Melbourne, VIC, Australia

D. Buxton
Department of General Medicine, Alfred Health, Melbourne, VIC, Australia

R. Junckerstorff et al. (eds.), *Beyond Evidence-Based Medicine*,
https://doi.org/10.1007/978-981-99-4440-8_81

malignancy was performed and included CT scanning of the abdomen and pelvis, CT colonoscopy, ultrasound of prostate, positron emission scanning and tumour marker assays. These were all normal, which reassured the referring clinician but the patient, however, was unhappy that he missed work and accrued significant medical costs.

3 Discussion

Cancer is an important and potent cause of VTE. About 10% of patients with cancer will develop VTE during their illness and about 20% of all cases of VTE occur in patients with active cancer [1]. Most cases of cancer associated thrombosis (CAT) develop after the diagnosis of cancer has been established but VTE may precede this diagnosis. Approximately 5–10% of individuals who present with unprovoked VTE will be found to have cancer during the following 6 months [1, 2].

The value of screening for occult malignancy in this cohort of patients has been studied in two prospective randomised controlled trials. In these trials, patients with unprovoked VTE were randomised to extensive screening for malignancy or routine care. Cancer was detected earlier in patients undergoing extensive screening but there was no mortality benefit demonstrated in either trial with extensive screening [3, 4]. Similar conclusions were found in a systematic review of the literature [2].

It is recommended that all patients with VTE have the recommended cancer screening appropriate for their age and sex, and relevant past medical history [1]. Examples of age, sex and risk-stratified screening activities include skin checks for individuals at high risk of melanoma, pap-smears for cervical cancer, mammography for breast cancer, faecal occult blood testing or colonoscopy for colorectal cancer [5]. Cancers for which routine screening is not currently recommended in Australia include: lung, prostate, testicular, and ovarian cancer [5]. Additional investigations should be performed if appropriate for any concerning symptoms or if abnormalities on physical examination are detected [1, 5]. Routine extensive screening for malignancy should not be performed in patients with unprovoked VTE [1–3].

4 Take Home Messages

- Whilst cancer is a common precipitating aetiology of VTE, evidence suggests that extensive investigations for occult malignancy does not change long term outcomes
- The presence of an unprovoked VTE should prompt the astute clinician to ensure age-appropriate cancer screening has been implemented

References

1. Tran HA, Gibbs H, Merriman E, Curnow JL, Young L, Bennett A, Tan CW, Chunilal SD, Ward CM, Baker R, Nandurkar H. New guidelines from the Thrombosis and Haemostasis Society of Australia and New Zealand for the diagnosis and management of venous thromboembolism. Med J Aust. 2019;210(5):227–35. https://doi.org/10.5694/mja2.50004. Epub 2019 Feb 10. Erratum in: Med J Aust. 2019 Jul;211(2):94. Erratum in: Med J Aust. 2020 Feb;212(3):108. vPMID: 30739331.
2. Robertson L, Broderick C, Yeoh SE, Stansby G. Effect of testing for cancer on cancer- or venous thromboembolism (VTE)-related mortality and morbidity in people with unprovoked VTE. Cochrane Database Syst Rev. 2021;10(10):CD010837. https://doi.org/10.1002/14651858.CD010837.pub5. PMID: 34597414; PMCID: PMC8486018.
3. Carrier M, Lazo-Langner A, Shivakumar S, Tagalakis V, Zarychanski R, Solymoss S, Routhier N, Douketis J, Danovitch K, Lee AY, Le Gal G, Wells PS, Corsi DJ, Ramsay T, Coyle D, Chagnon I, Kassam Z, Tao H, Rodger MA, SOME Investigators. Screening for occult cancer in unprovoked venous thromboembolism. N Engl J Med. 2015;373(8):697–704. https://doi.org/10.1056/NEJMoa1506623. Epub 2015 Jun 22. PMID: 26095467.
4. Piccioli A, Lensing AW, Prins MH, Falanga A, Scannapieco GL, Ieran M, Cigolini M, Ambrosio GB, Monreal M, Girolami A, Prandoni P, SOMIT Investigators Group. Extensive screening for occult malignant disease in idiopathic venous thromboembolism: a prospective randomized clinical trial. J Thromb Haemost. 2004;2(6):884–9. https://doi.org/10.1111/j.1538-7836.2004.00720.x. PMID: 15140122.
5. The Royal Australian College of General Practitioners. Guidelines for preventive activities in general practice. 9th ed. Melbourne: RACGP; 2016.

Not All Laboratory Abnormalities Are In Vivo Problems

Krystal Bergin

1 Clinical Pearl

Always consider the possibility of EDTA-associated pseudo-thrombocytopenia in a patient with thrombocytopenia without any bleeding history.

2 Clinical Case

A clinically well 31-year-old woman with no bleeding history is noted on routine full blood examination (FBE) to have a moderate thrombocytopenia (platelets 95 × 10^9/L; normal range 150–450 × 10^9/L). She was known to have a normal platelet count 1 year prior. Her past medical history is significant only for Graves' disease, for which she underwent radioactive iodine ablation therapy and now on thyroxine replacement. She is on no other medications and has no allergies. Repeat FBE confirms a further drop in platelet count to 75 × 10^9/L. She is otherwise well with no prior personal history or family history of bleeding, thrombosis, or other haematological condition. She does not recall any recent viral infections. She is referred to a haematologist for investigation of thrombocytopenia. Her malignancy symptom screen and laboratory thrombocytopenia screen (including FBE, blood film examination, urea and electrolytes, liver function tests, coagulation screen, antinuclear antibody, extractable nuclear antigen, C-reactive protein, serum protein electrophoresis, free light chains, thyroid function tests and geographically appropriate viral screening) are all normal. Given the lack of concerning features for true

K. Bergin (✉)
Alfred Health, Melbourne, VIC, Australia

Monash University, Melbourne, VIC, Australia

R. Junckerstorff et al. (eds.), *Beyond Evidence-Based Medicine*,
https://doi.org/10.1007/978-981-99-4440-8_82

thrombocytopenia, a diagnosis of ethylenediaminetetraacetic acid (EDTA) pseudo-thrombocytopenia was considered and a repeat FBE was collected in both a heparin and sodium citrate tube. The platelet count returned a result of 155×10^9/L in the heparin tube and 180×10^9/L in the sodium citrate tube. A diagnosis of EDTA pseudo-thrombocytopenia was made. As this is an in vitro only phenomenon, the woman was given reassurance and discharged from the haematology clinic.

3 Discussion

EDTA-associated pseudo-thrombocytopenia is due to a naturally occurring IgG or IgM antibody directed against a cryptic glycoprotein platelet antigen (GPIIbIIIa, fibrinogen receptor) that is only exposed by EDTA [1]. Generally, platelet clumps result which are not recognised as platelets by the automated blood analyser but can be seen on morphological examination. Platelet counts in citrate-anticoagulated blood are often, but not always, normal as alteration of the GPIIbIIIa molecule is prevented by calcium chelation by citrate. Alternatively, pseudo-thrombocytopenia occasionally occurs secondary to leukocyte platelet satellitism. EDTA-associated pseudo-thrombocytopenia can be seen in the normal population but has been reported to be associated with autoimmune conditions, liver disease, cardiac disease, malignancy and cold-agglutin disease [2]. It occurs in 0.1% of the normal population and is transient in some patients but the responsible antibody can persist indefinitely in others [3]. No haemostatic or thrombotic abnormalities have been attributed to this antibody. If undiagnosed these antibodies have led to unnecessary platelet transfusion, investigations (bone marrow biopsies), interventions (steroids, intravenous immune globulin or even splenectomy) as well as appropriate therapies being withheld such as anticoagulants and delayed surgery.

If suspected (in a well patient with no bleeding issues), ask your laboratory to have a closer look at the blood film for any evidence of platelet clumping and repeat FBE in a different anticoagulant as well as consider FBE re-assessment in a warmed sample (37 °C).

4 Other Gems

- Haemoglobin and haematocrit are not, strictly speaking, measures of total red cell volume and are influenced if plasma volume is altered disproportionately. For example, if a patient is very dehydrated, the haemoglobin and haematocrit will be artificially elevated, with the converse occurring in a fluid-overloaded patient.
- Haemoglobin is expressed in g/L, therefore if a patient loses whole blood rapidly (massive bleeding), their haemoglobin level may seem normal if the FBE has been taken soon after the blood loss, as there has not been enough time for the body to attempt to improve circulating blood levels or for fluid resuscitation to

occur. Never be reassured by a "normal" haemoglobin level in a patient with acute blood loss.
- Mean corpuscular volume (MCV) should not vary significantly over a short space of time (for example, within a few days). If there is a significant change to the MCV, make sure to consider it being the wrong patient's blood in the tube!
- When interpreting the FBE, asking for a blood film examination can be helpful to identify potential causes for a specific abnormality.

References

1. Lardinois B, Favresse J, Chatelain B, Lippi G, Mullier F. Pseudothrombocytopenia-a review on causes, occurrence and clinical implications. J Clin Med. 2021;10(4):594.
2. Sahin C, Kırlı I, Sozen H, Canbek TD. EDTA-induced pseudothrombocytopenia in association with bladder cancer. BMJ Case Rep. 2014;2014:205130.
3. Shabnam I, Chuphal DS, Joshi BC. Ethylenediaminetetraacetic acid (EDTA) - dependent pseudothrombocytopenia: a case report. J Clin Diagn Res. 2014;8(10):103–4.

Low von Willebrand Levels, von Willebrand Disease Does not Make

Krystal Bergin

1 Clinical Pearl

Easy bruising and being 'a bleeder' are common presentations in general practice. Von Willebrand disease is common, but the diagnosis is not always straightforward and requires a comprehensive clinical history, repeat testing and often referral to a specialist centre.

2 Clinical Case

An 18-year-old woman presents with dysmenorrhoea and menorrhagia. She describes heavy, painful periods, lasting 6–7 days with 2–3 heavier days requiring tampon or sanitary pad change 5–6 times in 24 h but does not bleed through onto clothes or sheets. After review with her gynaecologist, she was found to have abnormal von Willebrand factor (VWF) testing. She also reports prolonged bleeding post tooth extraction in the past. Haemostasis was achieved with local pressure application with packing by her dental practitioner without need for presentation to hospital. She had a tonsillectomy as a child without any bleeding complications and has never required medical attention due to uncontrolled bleeding. She has infrequent epistaxis with no cutaneous bleeding but has occasional mild bleeding after brushing her teeth, without significant bleeding after a minor wound. She has never been pregnant.

Her testing revealed a VWF antigen level of 33% (normal range 50–200%), Factor VIII level 44% (normal range 50–200%) and von Willebrand Activity of 33% (normal range 50–200%) with an APTT of 44 (normal range 23–38 s). Her blood

K. Bergin (✉)
Alfred Health, Melbourne, VIC, Australia

Monash University, Melbourne, VIC, Australia

R. Junckerstorff et al. (eds.), *Beyond Evidence-Based Medicine*,
https://doi.org/10.1007/978-981-99-4440-8_83

group is O positive. Her full blood evaluation was normal (haemoglobin 142 g/L, platelets 250 × 10^9), with normal thyroid, renal and liver function.

Repeat von Willebrand screen three months later returned normal levels of both VWF antigen (54%), von Willebrand Activity (55%) and Factor VIII levels (54%).

3 Discussion

Von Willebrand disease (VWD) is the most common inherited bleeding disease (1% of the population) and affects males and females equally [1]. VWF is encoded on chromosome 12 and produced predominantly in the vascular endothelial cells and less so by megakaryocytes. Importantly approximately 13% of the N-linked glycans on VWF molecules terminate in an ABO blood group antigen [2]. There is a well described approximately 25% decrease in VWF levels in patients with blood group O compared to non-O patients. VWD level variations in individual patients have been reported with menstruation cycle changes as well as use of the oral contraceptive pill. Despite potential changes in VWF due to these factors, current expert consensus guidelines do not recommend blood group-specific reference ranges or the use of timed samples for menstrual cycles [3, 4]. Increased plasma VWF due to increased synthesis occurs physiologically as part of the acute phase response and can be seen in pregnancy, intercurrent illness, inflammation, hyperthyroidism, and other conditions [2].

Traditionally three major types of VWD have been recognised—type 1 (partial VWF deficiency), type 2 (qualitative defects in VWF (abnormal functioning VWF)) and Type 3 (almost total absence of VWF).

Type 1 VWD is most common and in recent years international clinical guidelines have suggested patients with partial quantitative VWF deficiency should be considered in two separate categories. Patients with consistently markedly decreased VWF levels (<30 IU/dL or 30%) should be labelled "type 1 VWD". This group often exhibit an autosomal-dominant inheritance pattern, and are more likely to have a known VWF gene mutation. In contrast, patients with consistently intermediate VWF levels (30–50 IU/dL or 30–50%) are now labelled "low VWF levels" [2, 3]. Patients labelled as "low VWF" often do not have known VWF genetic variants and present with variable bleeding phenotypes [5].

4 Other Gems

- The inheritance of VWD is often more complex than the classical autosomal dominant pattern.
  - Penetrance can be weak or variable
- Never forget a good family history particularly regarding maternal menstrual or obstetric history and circumcision.

- Always repeat von Willebrand testing on two separate occasions at least 3 months apart.
- Always consider referral to a specialised bleeding centre for assessment.
- Always use a standardised bleeding assessment tool (BAT) [6]:
  - The most commonly used questionnaires are the condensed molecular and clinical markers for the diagnosis and management of type 1 (MCMDM-1) VWD score and the International Society of Thrombosis and Hemostasis (ISTH) BAT score
  - Remember that younger patients often have undergone fewer previous haemostatic challenges and therefore may have misleadingly low (or even negative BAT scores)
  - BAT scores may not always accurately predict future surgical bleeding risk
- Remember laboratory reference ranges are specific to individual laboratories and are based on a specified range (usually 95%) of results from "healthy" individuals, therefore 2.5% of "healthy" patients would be expected to have VWF levels below the normal range.

References

1. Lillicrap D. von Willebrand disease: advances in pathogenetic understanding, diagnosis and therapy. Blood. 2013;122(23):3735–40.
2. Laffan MA, Pasi KJ. Inherited bleeding disorders. In: Hoffbrand AV, Catovsky D, Tuddenham EGD, Green AR, editors. Postgraduate haematology. 6th ed. West Sussex: Blackwell Publishing; 2011. p. 804–12.
3. Nichols WL, Hultin MB, James AH, Manco-Johnson MJ, Montgomery RR, Ortel TL, Rick ME, Sadler JE, Weinstein M, Yawn BP. von Willebrand disease (VWD): evidence-based diagnosis and management guidelines, the National Heart, Lung, and Blood Institute (NHLBI) Expert Panel report (USA) 1. Haemophilia. 2008;14(2):171–232.
4. Laffan MA, Lester W, O'Donnell JS, Will A, Tait RC, Goodeve A, Millar CM, Keeling DM. The diagnosis and management of von Willebrand disease: a United Kingdom Haemophilia Centre Doctors Organization guideline approved by the British Committee for Standards in Haematology. Br J Haematol. 2014;167(4):453.
5. Lavin M, O'Donnell JS. How I treat low von Willebrand factor levels. Blood. 2019;133(8):795–804. https://doi.org/10.1182/blood-2018-10-844936.
6. Bowman ML, James PD. Bleeding scores for the diagnosis of von Willebrand disease. Semin Thromb Hemost. 2017;43(5):530–9.

Thrombophilia: To Test or Not to Test, That Is the Question

Krystal Bergin

1 Clinical Pearl

Thrombophilia testing is very rarely of clinical benefit to an individual patient and should not be used to decide acute venous thrombosis management or duration of anticoagulation.

2 Clinical Case

A 47-year-old woman presents with shortness of breath in the setting of newly diagnosed atrial fibrillation and commencement of the combined oral contraceptive pill for management of peri-menopausal hot flushes. She has no other significant past medical history or family history. Of note she has no personal or family history of thrombosis, a normal body mass index (BMI), no known active cancer, and has previously had multiple long-haul flights and two uncomplicated pregnancies without any thrombotic complications.

On assessment in the emergency department, imaging confirms a bilateral pulmonary embolism. She is commenced on apixaban 10 mg orally twice daily for 7 days followed by 5 mg orally twice daily and blood for a thrombophilia screen was taken prior to her first dose.

On review a week later with her GP, she was found to be a compound heterozygote for factor V Leiden (FVL) mutation and prothrombin gene mutation (PTG) mutation. She continued her apixaban for a total of 6 months and was referred to a haematologist for assessment of the need for ongoing anticoagulation.

K. Bergin (✉)
Alfred Health, Melbourne, VIC, Australia

Monash University, Melbourne, VIC, Australia

R. Junckerstorff et al. (eds.), *Beyond Evidence-Based Medicine*,
https://doi.org/10.1007/978-981-99-4440-8_84

3 Discussion

Thrombophilia testing is now easy to perform and widely available, requiring only a simple blood test. The benefit of this testing in most patients is dubious with little to no evidence base of improved outcomes or change in management, but the financial cost is significant. Factors positively associated with the presence of inherited thrombophilia include venous thromboembolism (VTE) at a young age (less than 50 years of age), strong family history (first-degree relative with VTE at less than 50 years of age), VTE in unusual sites (e.g., cerebral veins, splanchnic veins) and recurrent VTE.

Basic thrombophilia screening tests include factor V Leiden and prothrombin gene mutational analysis, protein S, protein C, anti-thrombin levels and anti-phospholipid antibodies. There is no role for thrombophilia testing in patients with first episode of VTE provoked by strong risk factors (such as major surgery, trauma or immobility). Duration of anticoagulation should be guided by whether a VTE is provoked or unprovoked and if it is a first episode or recurrent VTE. Proximal DVT/PE associated with a transient non-surgical risk factor should be treated with anticoagulant therapy for 3–6 months [1]. The risk of VTE recurrence in patients with VTE provoked by nonsurgical triggers is low if the provoking factor is removed and is similar in patients with and without thrombophilia. In the context of reversible provoking factors, even patients who are homozygous or compound heterozygote for FVL and PTG mutations do not require lifelong anticoagulation [2, 3]. Women with confirmed inherited thrombophilia presenting with an oestrogen-associated provoked VTE do not need lifelong anticoagulation if the exogenous oestrogens are ceased [3].

4 Other Gems

- Positive inherited thrombophilia testing has no bearing on acute VTE management—all patients with acute VTE require therapeutic dose anticoagulant therapy regardless of the cause of the VTE.
- Protein C, S and anti-thrombin levels as well as anti-phospholipid antibodies testing can be affected by acute thrombosis, pregnancy and anticoagulants. Testing for these should be delayed until the patient has ceased anticoagulation.
- If the risk of recurrent VTE from ceasing anticoagulation to perform these tests is considered too high, the testing result is essentially irrelevant as the decision to continue anticoagulation long-term has already been made.
- A negative inherited thrombophilia screen in a patient with a strong family history of VTE does not equate to low risk for VTE.
- Inherited thrombophilia screening is not appropriate as routine work-up for patients with myocardial infarction, stroke or peripheral arterial thrombosis [4].

References

1. Tran HA, Gibbs H, Merriman E, Curnow JL, Young L, Bennett A, et al. New guidelines from the Thrombosis and Haemostasis Society of Australia and New Zealand for the diagnosis and management of venous thromboembolism. Med J Aust. 2019;210(5):227–35.
2. Lijfering WM, Middeldorp S, Veeger NJ, Hamulyák K, Prins MH, Büller HR, et al. Risk of recurrent venous thrombosis in homozygous carriers and double heterozygous carriers of factor V Leiden and prothrombin G20210A. Circulation. 2010;121(15):1706–12.
3. Connors JM. Thrombophilia testing and venous thrombosis. N Engl J Med. 2017;377(12):1177–87.
4. Boekholdt SM, Kramer MH. Arterial thrombosis and the role of thrombophilia. Semin Thromb Hemost. 2007;33(6):588–96.

Myeloma: Hiding in Plain Sight

Krystal Bergin

1 Clinical Pearl

> The presentation of multiple myeloma can be varied, and symptoms or abnormal laboratory findings can easily be attributed to other common conditions leading to delayed diagnosis and suboptimal patient outcomes.

2 Clinical Case

A 70-year-old man presents with body aches, worst in his left hip and thigh. His past history is significant for hypertension, type-2 diabetes and osteoarthritis. Left hip x-ray confirms features consistent with osteoarthritis and blood tests show mild-moderate renal impairment (eGFR 43 mL/min/m^2, normal range >90 ml/min/m^2), which is attributed to diabetic or hypertensive nephropathy. He is managed with regular paracetamol and oxycodone as required for break-through pain with reasonable pain control. Six months later he presents to the emergency department with a right humeral fracture after minimal trauma, with a large lytic lesion seen on CT scan. He is subsequently found to have an IgA paraprotein of 8 g/L with serum free lambda light chains of 500 mg/L. A low dose whole body CT scan demonstrates widespread lytic lesions (as well as osteoarthritic changes in the left hip). His renal function further deteriorates with an eGFR of 28 mL/min/m^2, and he develops anaemia (haemoglobin 99 g/L, normal range 130–180 g/L). Bone marrow biopsy confirms a diagnosis of multiple myeloma with 30–40% bone marrow plasma cells and he is commenced on induction myeloma therapy.

K. Bergin (✉)
Alfred Health, Melbourne, VIC, Australia

Monash University, Melbourne, VIC, Australia

R. Junckerstorff et al. (eds.), *Beyond Evidence-Based Medicine*,
https://doi.org/10.1007/978-981-99-4440-8_85

3 Discussion

Multiple myeloma is the second most common haematological malignancy and is characterised by the proliferation of malignant plasma cells [1]. Clinical features include hyperCalcaemia, Renal dysfunction, Anaemia and Bone lesions (the so-called CRAB criteria) [2]. A report from the Australian and New Zealand Myeloma and Related Diseases Registry analysing 2405 newly diagnosed multiple myeloma patients found 59% presented with bone lesions, 25% with renal impairment, 8% with anaemia and 7% with hypercalcaemia [3]. Up to 60% of patients will develop a fracture during their disease course. Myeloma-related bone disease can be asymptomatic and is often associated with non-healing fractures despite effective anti-myeloma therapy. It is associated with increased morbidity and mortality, shorter survival, inferior quality of life, and increased healthcare utilisation and treatment cost.

Delayed diagnosis of myeloma can be associated with inferior outcomes due to morbidity and mortality related to the disease, but also reduced therapeutic options are available for patients presenting later in their disease course with greater co-morbidity and/or poorer performance status. For example, this patient who may have worsened performance status due to his fracture and impaired renal function, may be considered too frail for an autologous stem cell transplant, a standard of care therapy with proven survival advantage, and therefore be offered less intensive therapy.

4 Other Gems

- Traditional bone scans (bone scintigraphy) are not useful to detect myeloma-related bone disease. Bone scintigraphy is useful in detecting osteoblastic lesions such as bony metastasis from solid organ tumours but has no role in myeloma detection as these bone lesions are typically caused by increased osteoclastic bone destruction with suppressed osteoblastic activity [4].
- IgA myeloma behaves differently to IgG myeloma subtypes with adverse events more common at lower paraprotein levels. This may be partly due to inherent worse prognosis but is compounded by unreliable IgA monoclonal protein quantification on serum protein electrophoresis due to co-migration, leading to under-estimation of tumour burden. Quantitative IgA is the recommended monitoring method [5].
- Autologous stem cell transplantation should be considered in patients up to the age of 70–75 years in otherwise well patients. Referral to an experienced transplant centre should be strongly considered for all patients up to 70 years of age and for fit patients up to 75 years of age [6].

References

1. Australian Institute of Health and Welfare. Cancer in Australia: an overview in 2014. CAN 88. Canberra: Australian Institute of Health and Welfare; 2014. Available https://www.aihw.gov.au/reports/cancer/cancer-data-in-australia/contents/cancer-rankings-data-visualisation. Accessed May 2023.
2. Kyle RA, Rajkumar SV. Criteria for diagnosis, staging, risk stratification and response assessment of multiple myeloma. Leukemia. 2009;23:3–9.
3. Bergin K, Wellard C, Moore E, McQuilten Z, Blacklock H, Harrison SJ, Ho PJ, King T, Quach H, Mollee P, Walker P, Wood E. Spencer A; Australian and New Zealand Myeloma and Related Diseases Registry. The myeloma landscape in Australia and New Zealand: the first 8 years of the myeloma and related diseases registry (MRDR). Clin Lymphoma Myeloma Leuk. 2021;21(6):e510–20. https://doi.org/10.1016/j.clml.2021.01.016. Epub 2021 Jan 30. PMID: 33785297.
4. Creeper K, Augustson B, Kusel K, Fulham MJ, Ho J, Quach H, Mollee P, Weber N, Talaulikar D, Johnston A, Murphy N, Joshua D, Ward C, Ling S, Gibson J, Szer J, Harrison S, Zannettino A, Jaksic W, Lee C, Spencer A, Kalff A, Szabo F, Romeril K, Chan H, Gibbs S, Horvath N, Prince HM. Imaging of patients with multiple myeloma and associated plasma cell disorders: consensus practice statement by the Medical Scientific Advisory Group to Myeloma Australia. Intern Med J. 2021;51:1707–12. https://doi.org/10.1111/imj.15457.
5. Kumar S, Paiva B, Anderson KC, Durie B, Landgren O, Moreau P, et al. International Myeloma Working Group consensus criteria for response and minimal residual disease assessment in multiple myeloma. Lancet Oncol. 2016;17:e328–e46.
6. Quach H, Joshua D, Ho J, Szer J, Spencer A, Harrison SJ, et al. Treatment of patients with multiple myeloma who are eligible for stem cell transplantation: position statement of the Myeloma Foundation of Australia Medical and Scientific Advisory Group. Intern Med J. 2015;45:94–105.

Part XII
Oncology

The Complications of Prostate Cancer Treatment

Peter Briggs

1 Clinical Pearl

Patients with prostate cancer on Androgen Deprivation Therapy (ADH) are at risk of developing ischaemic heart disease, osteoporosis, venous thromboembolism and neurocognitive decline.

2 Clinical Case

A 72-year old man attends his General Practitioner (GP) complaining of recent back pain. He is accompanied by his wife who says that the patient has not been well for at least 6 months with lethargy, inactivity, forgetfulness and low mood. His previous health had been good until 18 months earlier when the patient was found incidentally to have prostate cancer in curettings obtained at transurethral resection of prostate (TURP) for symptoms of prostatism. Investigations at that time had shown an elevated prostate specific antigen (PSA) of 130 mcg/L (reference range 0.0–4.0) and a number of asymptomatic bone lesions were seen on bone scan. Treatment commenced with the gonadotropin releasing hormone agonist, goserelin. The patient's urologist reported over following months that the PSA had returned to normal and the patient had no further prostatic symptoms.

To investigate the back pain, the GP organises X-rays and blood tests. X-rays of the spine reveal diffuse osteopenia with a superior end plate compression fracture of L2. Several areas of sclerosis are noted in the pelvis. Blood tests show a mild normocytic anaemia with a Haemoglobin of 109 g/L (reference range 125–175g/L) but normal haematological parameters otherwise. Renal function is moderately impaired

P. Briggs (✉)
Monash Health, Melbourne, VIC, Australia

R. Junckerstorff et al. (eds.), *Beyond Evidence-Based Medicine*,
https://doi.org/10.1007/978-981-99-4440-8_86

with an estimated glomerular filtration rate (eGFR) of 55 mL/min (normal >90 mL/min) but electrolytes including calcium are normal. The patient has normal thyroid function but a fasting blood glucose is elevated at 8.5 mM/L (reference range 3.0–7.7 mM/L) and total cholesterol is 6.9 mM/L (reference range 0–5.5 mM/L). The PSA is 0.2 mcg/L (reference range 0–4.0 mcg/L).

The patient is instructed to take regular paracetamol and is given a 2 week course of tramadol. At subsequent review he reports his pain has improved but states that he is experiencing hot flushes two or three times daily. Although he had expected these from his androgen deprivation therapy (ADT) the symptom is getting more bothersome. Prompted by his wife the patient admits that life is no longer enjoyable. He also complains that he has no libido and feels he has lost his masculinity. A bone mineral density scan is ordered and shows osteoporosis with a T score of −2.5. Subsequent management includes commencement of the anti-bone resorptive agent denosumab with calcium and vitamin D supplementation. After further discussion with the patient's urological oncologist the patient commences venlafaxine at 37.5 mg daily for his hot flushes and is referred to an exercise physiologist.

3 Discussion

Many men with advanced prostate cancer are managed with long term androgen deprivation therapy with Luteinizing Hormone Releasing Hormone (LHRH) agonists with or without anti-androgen drugs. Many years of disease control can be obtained during a phase of 'castrate sensitivity'. The impact of androgen deprivation is well understood in terms of sexual function and vasomotor instability however other short and long term effects of androgen deprivation therapy are under appreciated. Acceleration of bone mineral loss with the complications of osteoporosis, progressive vascular disease manifesting as cerebrovascular, renal or ischaemic heart disease, venous thromboembolism, diabetes and development of neurocognitive decline are all well described associations. All men on long term therapy for prostate cancer should be monitored for these toxicities [1].

Treatment strategies involve multidisciplinary management. Often a comprehensive geriatric assessment will be useful to identify the major risks for an individual and facilitate allied health involvement. At the oncological level, use of an intermittent ADT treatment strategy is often considered. There is evidence that single agent anti-androgen therapy produces less toxicity than LHRH therapy. The treatment of hot flushes overlaps with that for women on anti-oestrogen therapy. Antidepressants can be useful and the treatment of depression per se may be necessary. The metabolic changes including diabetes and hyperlipidaemia need specific treatment as the mortality from complications of vascular disease are significantly increased in men on ADT [1].

The management of osteoporosis is intensive and requires long term monitoring. At a symptom level it may be challenging to distinguish between the impact of osteoporosis and prostate cancer metastases. The use of Prostate-Specific Membrane

Antigen Positron Emission Tomography (PSMA PET) scans may be helpful in this context. Management of the side effects of androgen deprivation therapy in older men is challenging and ideally should be multidisciplinary. This is a patient population known to typically under report their symptoms but appropriate and holistic management can have a major impact on patients' overall health and quality of life.

4 Other Gems

- Vasomotor instability causing unpleasant hot flushes occur in more than half of men receiving ADT. Symptoms increase over the first few months of treatment and are persistent with significant impact on quality of life [2]. Both hormonal agents such as medroxyprogesterone 200 mg daily and non-hormonal agents including the alpha-adrenergic agent clonidine and selective serotonin reuptake inhibitors (SSRI) are effective [3].
- Treating hot flushes requires balancing potential toxicities with benefit. SSRIs for example may be effective at doses lower than used to treat depression and doses should be titrated slowly.
- Bisphosphonates and denosumab are effective in preventing bone mineral density loss in men treated with ADT and should be considered. Exercise is insufficient in isolation but should be encouraged to mitigate sarcopenia and as an adjunct to holistic care [4].

References

1. Nguyen C, Lairson DR, Swartz MD, Du XL. Risks of major long-term side effects associated with androgen-deprivation therapy in men with prostate cancer. Pharmacotherapy. 2018;38(10):999–1009.
2. Mohile SG, Mustian K, Bylow K, Hall W, Dale W. Management of complications of androgen deprivation therapy in the older man. Crit Rev Oncol Hematol. 2009;70(3):235–55.
3. Irani J, Salomon L, Oba R, Bouchard P, Mottet N. Efficacy of venlafaxine, medroxyprogesterone acetate, and cyproterone acetate for the treatment of vasomotor hot flushes in men taking gonadotropin releasing hormone analogues for prostate cancer: a double blind randomised trial. Lancet Oncol. 2010;11(2):147–54.
4. Joseph JS, Lam V, Patel MI. Preventing osteoporosis in men taking androgen deprivation therapy for prostate cancer: a systematic review and meta-analysis. Eur Urol Oncol. 2019;2(5):551–61.

Dyspnoea in Lung Cancer

Peter Briggs

1 Clinical Pearl

Increasing dyspnoea in a lung cancer patient responding to chemo-immunotherapy—consider immune related pneumonitis.

2 Clinical Case

A 62-year old woman presents to the Emergency Department (ED) with increasing dyspnoea over the preceding 24 hours. She is receiving 4 weekly infusions of durvalumab, an immune checkpoint inhibitor (ICI), as maintenance treatment for adenocarcinoma of the lung treated definitively 6 months earlier with chemoradiotherapy. The patient has a past history of smoking related Chronic Obstructive Pulmonary Disease (COPD) having quit smoking at the diagnosis of her lung cancer. Routine medications include inhaled steroid and beta agonist therapy and rivaroxaban since an episode of pulmonary embolism (PE) during her radiation treatment.

At presentation the patient has laboured breathing with a respiratory rate (RR) of 24 breaths/min, a heart rate (HR) of 110 beats/min, her temperature is 37.8 °C and O_2 saturation is 84% improving to 92% with O_2 therapy at 3 L/min via nasal prongs. Notable findings on physical examination include a soft wheeze throughout both phases of respiration and scattered coarse crackles. Blood tests are essentially unremarkable although the white cell count (WCC) is mildly increased to 12×10^9/L

P. Briggs (✉)
Monash Health, Melbourne, VIC, Australia

R. Junckerstorff et al. (eds.), *Beyond Evidence-Based Medicine*,
https://doi.org/10.1007/978-981-99-4440-8_87

(reference range 4–11) and CRP to 45 mg/L (reference range 0–5). A computed tomography pulmonary angiogram (CTPA) is performed which shows no evidence of pulmonary embolus. Significant emphysematous changes are noted particularly through the upper zones and there is dense fibrotic change extending from the left hilum to the left upper lobe (LUL) but no definable lung mass or lymphadenopathy is noted. Patchy interstitial opacities are present bilaterally. The LUL changes correspond to the previous radiotherapy field.

A working diagnosis of infective exacerbation of COPD is made and the patient is admitted to hospital and commenced on intravenous (IV) antibiotics, oral prednisolone 20 mg daily and oxygen therapy as required. A sputum sample could not be obtained and a blood culture is sterile. No further fever is noted but the patient's clinical condition does not improve. The possibility of radiation pneumonitis or immune related pneumonitis is raised and IV methylprednisolone is commenced at 2 mg/kg. The patient's condition improves significantly over the next 24 hours and a repeat CT chest on day 5 shows significant clearing of the interstitial opacities.

3 Discussion

Most patients with metastatic or locally advanced non-small cell lung cancer are currently treated with regimens including ICIs. The potential for immune related adverse events due to auto-inflammatory reactions is increasingly recognised. Less well appreciated is the potential for rapid and potentially fatal toxicity emerging within a couple of weeks or many months after initiation of treatment. Such toxicities typically respond well to corticosteroids but awareness of the possibility of immune related pneumonitis is important in patients with acute deterioration of dyspnoea in the context of lung cancer therapy.

Clinical management is compounded by the fact that the differential diagnosis is often broad and includes infection, progressive cancer, radiation pneumonitis or fibrosis and cardiac failure. Classical radiological changes of symmetrical perihilar opacities are often not present in immune related pneumonitis especially in patients with underlying emphysema and scarring related to previous radiotherapy. The diagnosis is often one of exclusion. High dose corticosteroids may be necessary during the diagnostic process in view of the possibility of rapid progression if untreated.

In the above case, radiation pneumonitis remained a differential diagnosis because idiosyncratic or sporadic radiation pneumonitis (as opposed to classical in-field radiation pneumonitis) can occur outside the irradiated field from about 6 weeks to 6 months following radiation therapy. This condition is presumed to have an immunological basis to explain inflammation outside the treatment field and is steroid responsive. Typically, the onset is earlier than 6 months. As in this case, 6 months following radiotherapy, the radiation lung injury in the treatment field often evolves into fibrosis. Radiation fibrosis can continue to evolve over the longer term [1]. Therefore, it is very likely that in the above clinical case that the ICI is the cause of the pneumonitis. Prior lung irradiation and pre-existing chronic obstructive pulmonary disease are documented risk factors for ICI induced pneumonitis [2].

Severe pneumonitis (grade 3 or 4 with greater than 50% of lung parenchyma involved) requiring inpatient management and oxygen therapy is an indication to permanently cease the ICI. Steroid treatment should be commenced at 1–2 mg/kg daily. In the presence of severe symptoms requiring non-invasive respiratory support or even intubation, high doses of intravenous methylprednisolone should be given over several days. Steroid doses are weaned slowly and as symptoms allow over a period of 4–12 weeks. The half-life of ICIs is long (durvalumab half-life approximately 18 days) and a flare in symptoms is possible.

A recent analysis of pneumonitis in a real-world population of patients treated with durvalumab following chemo-radiotherapy for lung cancer found 17.9% experienced some degree of pneumonitis. Almost 10% of the population discontinued treatment due to pneumonitis but mortality from this adverse event was relatively rare (0.1%) [3]. Immune related pneumonitis can be a fulminant condition and early recognition and treatment is essential.

4 Other Gems

- Immune related pneumonitis can occur within a couple of weeks or after many months of ICI therapy [2]
- Specific tyrosine kinase inhibitors are standard treatments for Epidermal Growth Factor Receptor (EGFR) mutated lung cancer and can also rarely induce pneumonitis. This risk may be potentiated by exposure to ICI therapy.

References

1. Hanania AN, Mainwaring W, Ghebre YT, Hanania NA, Ludwig M. Radiation-induced lung injury: assessment and management. Chest. 2019;156(1):150–62.
2. Suresh K, Voong KR, Shankar B, Forde PM, Ettinger DS, Marrone KA, Kelly RJ, Hann CL, Levy B, Feliciano JL, Brahmer JR, Feller-Kopman D, Lerner AD, Lee H, Yarmus L, D'Alessio F, Hales RK, Lin CT, Psoter KJ, Danoff SK, Naidoo J. Pneumonitis in non-small cell lung cancer patients receiving immune checkpoint immunotherapy: incidence and risk factors. J Thorac Oncol. 2018;13(12):1930–9.
3. Girard N, Bar J, Garrido P, Garassino MC, McDonald F, Mornex F, Filippi AR, Smit HJM, Peters S, Field JK, Christoph DC, Sibille A, Fietkau R, Haakensen VD, Chouaid C, Markman B, Hiltermann TJN, Taus A, Sawyer W, Allen A, Chander P, Licour M, Solomon B. Treatment characteristics and real-world progression-free survival in patients with unresectable stage III NSCLC who received durvalumab after chemoradiotherapy: findings from the PACIFIC-R study. J Thorac Oncol. 2023;18(2):181–93.

Diarrhoea in the Setting of Immune Checkpoint Inhibitor Therapy

Peter Briggs

1 Clinical Pearl

If a cancer patient on an immune checkpoint inhibitor develops diarrhoea, consider immune related enterocolitis and manage with aggressive fluid support and immunosuppression.

2 Clinical Case

A 64-year old man recently commenced treatment for metastatic squamous cell lung cancer. He has a 40 pack/year smoking history and a chronic dry cough but was otherwise previously well. Baseline haematological and biochemical blood tests are normal. There is no history of autoimmune disease. The patient received chemotherapy with carboplatin/paclitaxel in addition to combination immune checkpoint inhibitors (ICI) ipilimumab and nivolumab. He presented to his GP with a 2 day history of diarrhoea and colicky abdominal pain. He denied fever, nausea or vomiting and maintained fluid and food intake. No other household members had symptoms. Initial treatment was with loperamide and increased oral fluids, however the diarrhoea persisted with 4–6 loose stools per day.

The patient feels increasingly unwell and presents to the Emergency Department (ED). Examination reveals a soft non-tender abdomen, clear chest but a tachycardia of 100 beats per minute (bpm) and a blood pressure (BP) of 90/60 mmHg. His weight is 77 kg relative to his baseline of 80 kg. The patient is given a litre of intravenous normal saline and after 4 hours feels better with a BP of 110/75 mmHg and heart rate (HR) of 80 bpm. Blood tests show normal haematological and biochemical parameters however the patients CRP is elevated at 90 mg/L (reference range

P. Briggs (✉)
Monash Health, Melbourne, VIC, Australia

R. Junckerstorff et al. (eds.), *Beyond Evidence-Based Medicine*,
https://doi.org/10.1007/978-981-99-4440-8_88

0–5 mg/L). A stool sample is collected for viral PCR and *Clostridium difficile* testing.

The patient is discharged but is brought back to ED by ambulance the following day with a systolic BP of 60 mmHg, HR of 130 bpm and intractable diarrhoea of at least 10 loose stools in the last 24 hours. Blood tests reveal an acute kidney injury with an eGFR of 38 mL/min (reference range >90 mL/min), sodium of 132 mM/L (135–145 mM/L) and potassium of 2.9 mM/L (3.5–5.2 mM/L). A full blood examination (FBE) is normal. An abdominal computed tomography (CT) scan demonstrates a thickened colonic wall with no evidence of intestinal perforation. The differential diagnosis includes infective gastroenteritis, chemotherapy induced and immune related entero-colitis. Subsequently, PCR testing of the patient's faecal sample shows no evidence of infection and a faecal calprotectin level is found to be moderately elevated.

A diagnosis of immune related (IR) enterocolitis is made. The patient is treated with intensive intravenous (IV) fluid and electrolyte replacement and intravenous methylprednisolone at a dose of 2 mg/kg daily. Within 24 h the HR and BP have returned to normal and by day 3 the diarrhoea has improved to 2–3 poorly formed stools per 24 hours. Steroid therapy is converted to oral prednisolone 100 mg daily with a plan to wean off over the following 2–4 weeks. Further checkpoint inhibitor therapy is postponed. The patient is discharged home on day 5 taking prednisolone 50 mg daily with the instruction to reduce by 10 mg every 3 days pending clinic review.

Unfortunately, the patient deteriorates 5 days following discharge with a major flare in his symptoms and haemodynamic compromise. IV methyl prednisolone is recommenced at 200 mg daily and a dose of IV infliximab is given at 5 mg/kg. A repeat dose is required 2 weeks later and corticosteroids are tapered more slowly over a planned 2 month period as symptoms settle. Checkpoint inhibitor therapy is permanently discontinued but the patient resumes his chemotherapy on recovery from IR colitis and a follow up CT scan at week 6 shows a partial cancer response.

3 Discussion

Immune related entero-colitis must be considered in all patients receiving immune checkpoint inhibitors who develop diarrhoea especially if severe or persistent. The incidence varies according to the type of checkpoint inhibition with all grade colitis occurring in 1–2% of patients receiving Programmed Death 1 receptor (PD-1) or Programmed Death Ligand 1 (PD-L1) inhibitors and approximately 10% of patients receiving Cytotoxic T-lymphocyte associated Antigen 4 (CTLA-4) inhibitors such as ipilimumab [1]. Symptoms typically develop several months after commencement of ICIs but can occur within days particularly in patients on combination ICIs.

Grade 1 diarrhoea (up to 3 stools above baseline) is usually managed with anti-diarrhoea medication (if no evidence of infective cause) and increased fluid intake. Grade 2 diarrhoea (4–6 stools above baseline) may be accompanied by abdominal pain, passage of blood and mucus. In addition to supportive care, treatment with corticosteroids (prednisolone 1 mg/kg or equivalent) should be considered if symptoms exceed 3 days. Further ICI should be withheld pending recovery.

Grade 3 diarrhoea (≥7 stools above baseline) is often associated with fever and severe abdominal pain and hypovolaemic shock. Patients should be managed in hospital with intensive fluid resuscitation and IV methyl prednisolone (at least 2 mg/kg). Anti-diarrhoeals are discouraged. Failure to respond may require additional therapy such as the anti-Tumour Necrosis Factor (TNF) agent, infliximab. Further ICI therapy should be permanently discontinued although patients on dual ICI therapy who recover promptly may be offered ongoing treatment with the PD-L1 or PD-1 inhibitor and cessation of the CTLA-4 inhibitor. Grade 4 toxicity is life threatening and may include perforation, gut ischaemia, bleeding and toxic megacolon. ICI should be permanently ceased [2].

A diagnosis of IR enterocolitis should be considered in the appropriate clinical context with exclusion of alternative causes such as infection and underlying inflammatory bowel disease. The earliest CT findings include bowel wall thickening/oedema and mucosal hyper-enhancement but the negative predictive value of CT is low (50–75% sensitivity and 75–80% specificity). Endoscopic findings of inflammation and ulceration are usual but not well correlated with symptoms. More severe features tend to be associated with resistance to steroid therapy [3]. Stool calprotectin levels are not discriminatory and reflect bowel inflammation [2].

Key to successful management of IR enterocolitis is early recognition of the cause, appropriate fluid resuscitation and electrolyte replacement, and early immunosuppressive therapy with corticosteroids.

Symptom severity can escalate rapidly and it is important to recognise that symptom onset can occur at any point during therapy with ICIs and even post treatment. It is not uncommon for symptoms to recur during steroid weaning as the half-life of PD-1 inhibitors nivolumab and pembrolimumab is approximately 4 weeks and the half-life of the CTLA-4 inhibitor ipilimumab is 15 days. Steroid weaning is necessarily slow extending over a period of 4–12 weeks. Therefore, the risk of steroid toxicity is high and most patients will require prophylaxis for atypical infection and gastric ulceration. Patients should be instructed to report symptoms promptly and ongoing careful clinical monitoring during the weaning process is required.

4 Other Gems

- Immune related gut toxicity most commonly affects the colon but all levels of the gut can be involved in a diffuse or patchy distribution
- Clinical monitoring on treatment should include careful evaluation of volume status, electrolyte management, and stool frequency to evaluate disease severity and response to treatment
- Maintenance of nutrition can be challenging and requires multidisciplinary management

- Most patients respond to steroids but initial resistance occurs in at least a third of patients with grade 3 or 4 IR enterocolitis and a biological agent should be considered. The anti-TNF agent infliximab is most commonly used. Vedolizumab, an anti-T cell agent with some specificity for gut epithelium, may also be considered [3].

References

1. Wang DY, Ye F, Zhao S, Johnson DB. Incidence of immune checkpoint inhibitor-related colitis in solid tumor patients: a systematic review and meta-analysis. OncoImmunology. 2017;6(10):e1344805.
2. Som A, Mandaliya R, Alsaadi D, Farshidpour M, Charabaty A, Malhotra N, Mattar MC. Immune checkpoint inhibitor-induced colitis: a comprehensive review. World J Clin Cases. 2019;7(4):405–18.
3. Tang L, Wang J, Lin N, Zhou Y, He W, Liu J, Ma X. Immune checkpoint inhibitor-associated colitis: from mechanism to management. Front Immunol. 2021;12:800879.

Beware Back Pain in a Patient with Cancer

Peter Briggs

1 Clinical Pearl

Back and radicular pain in a patient with cancer is due to incipient cord compression unless proven otherwise.

2 Clinical Case

A 60-year old woman with metastatic hormone receptor positive breast cancer presents with acute on chronic mid thoracic back pain radiating anteriorly around her left thorax. She has required frequent use of her oxycodone for breakthrough pain despite taking regular slow release oxycodone 12 hourly. The patient has had stable metastatic bone disease on long term aromatase inhibitor therapy and received radiotherapy to a painful pelvic lesion a year earlier. The patient denies any weakness or neurological symptoms and her neurological examination is normal. A CT of the thorax shows widespread mixed sclerotic and lytic bone lesions throughout the vertebral column but there is no vertebral compression nor structural changes in the left sided ribs. The extent of disease is considered equivalent to a bone scan done 2 months earlier.

The patient is admitted for pain management. With an increased dose of oxycodone and the addition of naproxen her pain improves although she still complains of sharp left chest pain. The following morning, the patient requires nursing assistance to walk to the bathroom because of leg weakness. Neurological examination demonstrates upper motor neurone signs in the lower limbs with grade 3/5 muscle weakness bilaterally. An urgent MRI scan confirms widespread bony metastatic disease

P. Briggs (✉)
Monash Health, Melbourne, VIC, Australia

R. Junckerstorff et al. (eds.), *Beyond Evidence-Based Medicine*,
https://doi.org/10.1007/978-981-99-4440-8_89

with extensive destruction of T6 with posterior extension of soft tissue into the left nerve root foramen and spinal canal compressing the spinal cord. Dexamethasone is commenced intravenously and urgent neurosurgical decompression is scheduled.

The patient makes a good post-operative recovery and receives a course of radiotherapy to the mid-thoracic spine 2 weeks later. Her weakness slowly improves during an 8 week stay in a rehabilitation hospital. She is able to walk with the support a of walking frame at the time of discharge.

3 Discussion

The development of paraparesis due to progressive vertebral or epidural metastatic cancer is typically acute, often catastrophic and complete recovery, even when diagnosed early, is unusual. The extent of recovery is directly correlated with the degree of weakness at the time of decompression. Retrospectively, patients presenting with spinal cord compression usually give a history of progressive back pain and often lower limb weakness is preceded by pain with a radicular distribution at the level of incipient cord compression [1]. All patients with known metastatic cancer especially with bone disease should be questioned closely regarding back and neck pain in addition to sensory and motor neurological symptoms. The presence of radicular pain should prompt an urgent MRI scan with a view to neurosurgical review prior to the development of neurological signs.

Acute management includes high dose corticosteroids equivalent to 16 mg dexamethasone daily [2]. Patients with any motor weakness or sphincter disturbance that corresponds to a site of cord or corda equina compression require consideration of urgent surgical decompression [3]. Radiotherapy following surgical recovery is typically required. Patients considered to be of poor operative risk or who have multi-level sites of neural compression are candidates for urgent radiotherapy [2].

Cancer is increasingly prevalent, and the development of malignant paraplegia continues to be a major risk for our patients. In retrospect virtually all patients give a history which provides clues to the potential development of spinal cord compression. Clinicians assessing patients with cancer pain have opportunities to detect patients at high risk and diagnose incipient cord compression and initiate treatment prior to the development of paraparesis. The development of radicular pain may be an indicator of extraosseous tumour extension which also threatens the cord. A high index of clinical suspicion for cord compression in the appropriate clinical context remains the key to diagnosis.

4 Other Gems

- Using different imaging modalities to look for change over time is inaccurate and MRI scanning of the vertebral column remains the gold standard investigation for spinal cord compression.
- In patients at risk of spinal cord compression frequent clinical examination is critical because deterioration can be acute. Beware of attributing reduced mobility to pain alone.
- Urgent, including after hours scanning and intervention is required to optimise outcome of documented cord compression.

References

1. Mohme M, Mende KC, Krätzig T, Plaetke R, Beseoglu K, Hagedorn J, Steiger HJ, Floeth FW, Eicker SO. Impact of spinal cord compression from intradural and epidural spinal tumors on perioperative symptoms-implications for surgical decision making. Neurosurg Rev. 2017;40(3):377–87.
2. George R, Jeba J, Ramkumar G, et al. Interventions for the treatment of metastatic extradural spinal cord compression in adults. Cochrane Database Syst Rev. 2015;9:CD006716.
3. Patchell RA, Tibbs PA, Regine WF, Payne R, Saris S, Kryscio RJ, et al. Direct decompressive surgical resection in the treatment of spinal cord compression caused by metastatic cancer: a randomised trial. Lancet. 2005;366(9486):643–8.

Facial Swelling in a Cancer Patient

Peter Briggs

1 Clinical Pearl

Always think of Superior Vena Cava (SVC) syndrome when assessing patients with known malignant disease involving the chest.

2 Clinical Case

A 70 year-old man is referred to the oncology clinic with an exacerbation of cough and shortness of breath which has not responded to a recent course of antibiotics. The patient is a smoker of 45 pack years with a chronic productive cough but has been otherwise well. A chest x-ray (CXR) shows a right hilar mass and lung cancer is suspected. A computed tomography (CT) of the chest is requested with a view to define an appropriate biopsy technique. Over the next week, the patient's dyspnoea increases rapidly and on review the patient reports periorbital oedema. An allergic reaction to an antibiotic is suspected but the patient does not describe any benefit from several days of antihistamine therapy.

On examination, diffuse facial swelling is observed and commented upon by the patient's partner. Neck veins are prominent and careful inspection reveals a bluish discoloration over the upper chest with fine superficial telangiectatic vessels. With elevation of the arms above the head the patient becomes noticeably plethoric and distressed with dyspnoea after 30 seconds (Pemberton's sign). The CT chest demonstrates a proximal right upper lobe lung mass contiguous with enlarged hilar and right paratracheal nodes with significant compression of the superior vena cava (SVC) at the level of the azygos vein.

P. Briggs (✉)
Monash Health, Melbourne, VIC, Australia

R. Junckerstorff et al. (eds.), *Beyond Evidence-Based Medicine*,
https://doi.org/10.1007/978-981-99-4440-8_90

The patient almost certainly has malignant superior vena caval obstruction (SVCO) likely due to lung cancer. This patient requires urgent cytoreductive treatment with radiotherapy or potentially chemotherapy if small cell lung cancer is proven on biopsy. Whilst the priority is to obtain an urgent biopsy, the patient is considered high risk for bronchoscopy due to his inability to lie flat and his need for oxygen therapy. Dexamethasone is initiated at 16 mg daily and the patient is admitted for urgent stenting of his SVC. Several days later the patient's symptoms are considerably improved and a bronchoscopy is successfully performed. The cytology of needle aspirates obtained confirms small cell lung cancer.

Following 24 hours of pre-hydration and allopurinol premedication to reduce the risk of tumour lysis syndrome, chemotherapy is commenced. A positron emission tomography (PET) scan finds no disease beyond the thorax and a multidisciplinary team recommends definitive (curative) concurrent chemo-radiotherapy.

3 Discussion

SVC obstruction is an under-recognised but potentially fatal syndrome which can cause severe symptoms. The signs are characteristic if noted and it can be a classic 'end of the bed' diagnosis. However, SVCO is typically subacute in its presentation and subtle symptoms of periorbital/facial swelling are often attributed to allergic reactions. Symptoms may include diffuse swelling of the head, neck and arms with cyanotic or plethoric discolouration, dyspnoea, difficulty lying flat and even drowsiness and hoarse voice from cerebral and laryngeal oedema. Clinical signs include fixed distension of the neck and arm veins and evidence of a collateral circulation with prominent veins over the upper chest. Collateral vessels can develop over a period of days and the rate of development determines the degree of compensation of the SVCO.

Approximately 70% of cases of SVCO are due to malignancy. Lung cancer is the most common cause although lymphoma accounts for around 10% of cases [1]. Other primary mediastinal malignancies such as germ cell cancer and thymoma should be considered in addition to metastatic causes. Thrombosis can complicate SVCO and can also occur in the setting of central venous catheters and other benign causes to produce the signs of SVCO. Doppler ultrasound is most useful to assess thrombosis in the subclavian and more distal vessels. Venography remains the gold standard to assess patency of the SVC but contrast enhanced CT is usually sufficient to evaluate cases of malignant compression.

Management is determined by the underlying cause but radiation therapy is typically required for malignant SVCO. Highly chemo-responsive conditions such as small cell lung cancer and high grade lymphomas may respond more promptly to cytotoxic therapy. Interventional radiological techniques such as stenting are increasingly available and offer a rapid relief from symptoms. High dose corticosteroids equivalent to 16 mg dexamethasone daily should be commenced at diagnosis and are useful pending more definitive treatment.

Whilst SVCO has long been recognised, methodical studies of management are few. Newer treatment modalities including endovascular procedures and thrombolysis for thrombotic complications are now available. SVCO can be successfully managed in most patients, including those with obstructing cancers and is one of those medical diagnoses that is readily made if actively considered.

4 Other Gems

- SVCO below the azygos vein results in redirection of venous return via the azygos and hemi-azygos venous systems in a retrograde manner to the inferior vena cava. Obstruction at the level of the azygos vein forces the development of other chest wall collaterals such as the superior epigastric and internal mammary veins and symptoms are typically more severe [1].
- SVCO results in an elevated venous pressure from 20 to 40 mmHg proximal to the obstruction. The risk of secondary thrombosis is high and prophylactic anticoagulation should be strongly considered.

Reference

1. Azizi A, Shafi I, Shah N, et al. Superior vena cava syndrome. J Am Coll Cardiol Intv. 2020;13(24):2896–910.

Part XIII
Neurology

Autoimmune Encephalitis: A Diagnostic Challenge

Udaya Seneviratne

1 Clinical Pearl

NMDAR encephalitis should be suspected when a young female presents with rapid onset of neurological symptoms accompanied by psychiatric manifestations and/or cognitive dysfunction.

2 Clinical Case

A female in her early twenties, with no preceding medical problems, was admitted with a history of speech disturbances for 1 week. She experienced difficulties in reading and understanding the newspaper. Her mother noticed that the speech was slow and hard to understand. The examination on admission revealed both receptive and expressive dysphasia accompanied by semantic and phonemic errors as well as alexia and agraphia. Her Magnetic Resonance Imaging (MRI) brain scan was normal. The electroencephalogram (EEG) demonstrated diffuse slowing and an electrographic seizure of left temporal onset was captured. However, there were no clinical seizures witnessed. The cerebrospinal fluid (CSF) examination revealed 50 lymphocytes and normal protein and glucose. She was commenced on acyclovir for the presumed diagnosis of herpes simplex encephalitis and lacosamide for seizure prevention.

Despite antiviral therapy, she continued to deteriorate with confusion, agitation, and visual as well as auditory hallucinations. She also developed stereotypic

U. Seneviratne (✉)
Monash Medical Centre, Melbourne, VIC, Australia

R. Junckerstorff et al. (eds.), *Beyond Evidence-Based Medicine*,
https://doi.org/10.1007/978-981-99-4440-8_91

movements characterised by orofacial dyskinesia. The polymerase chain reaction test for multiplex herpes viruses in the CSF returned a negative result. The possibility of autoimmune encephalitis was considered, and she was commenced on intravenous immunoglobulins (IVIG) and methylprednisolone. The anti-N-methyl D-aspartate receptor (NMDAR) antibodies in the serum and CSF were found to be positive, confirming the diagnosis of anti-NMDAR encephalitis. Further investigations including pelvic ultrasound, computed tomography (CT), and positron emission tomography scans did not reveal any underlying tumours or malignancy including ovarian teratomas. As the response to IVIG and steroids was suboptimal, she was eventually treated with rituximab. Despite a prolonged stay in the hospital, she made a complete recovery and returned to full-time employment.

3 Discussion

Anti-NMDAR encephalitis was first described as a paraneoplastic syndrome in 2007 in twelve young women, aged 14–44 years, with teratomas (11-ovarian, 1-mediastinal) [1]. Non-paraneoplastic anti-NMDAR encephalitis has been reported subsequently. Tumours are less common in patients older than 45 years, and when tumours do occur in this group, they are more likely to be carcinomas than teratomas [2]. This condition predominantly involves young patients (95% of cases <45 years of age) with 80% female preponderance [3]. Overall, 38% of patients have an underlying tumour, and among those with neoplasia, 94–98% constitute ovarian teratomas [2, 3]. Rare cases of imaging negative, microscopic ovarian teratomas confirmed on oophorectomy have been reported [4].

The clinical presentation is commonly characterised by a prodrome of headache, low-grade fever, nausea, and upper respiratory tract symptoms followed by the typical psychiatric and neurological manifestations within two weeks. These features are summarised in Table 1. Demonstration of antibodies to NMDA receptors in both serum and CSF is recommended to confirm the diagnosis [5]. The MRI brain scans are abnormal in 33% whilst extreme delta brush pattern is the EEG hallmark of the

Table 1 Typical spectrum of symptoms in anti-NMDAR encephalitis

Psychiatric/behavioural	Delusions, hallucinations, mania, agitation, catatonia, anxiety, fear, paranoia, insomnia, aggression, hypersexuality
Movement disorder	Oro-lingual-facial dyskinesia, dystonia, choreoathetosis, opisthotonic posture, rigidity, oculogyric crisis, ballismus
Altered conscious state	Seizures, status epilepticus, coma, dissociative state, fluctuating level of consciousness
Autonomic dysfunction	Hyperthermia, tachycardia, bradycardia, hypertension, hypotension, incontinence, hypoventilation, hypersalivation
Language dysfunction	Dysphasia, echolalia, mutism
Cognitive dysfunction	Delayed verbal memory, impaired executive functioning, attention/concentration deficits, impaired visual motor functions

condition [3, 5]. The CSF demonstrates lymphocytic pleocytosis in 90% whereas oligoclonal bands are positive in 25% [6]. Confirmation of the diagnosis should be followed by screening for an underlying neoplasm.

Early and aggressive immunotherapy is the key to achieving good outcomes [7]. Intravenous methylprednisolone combined with intravenous immunoglobulins or plasma exchange is the first-line treatment [8]. If there is no improvement, rituximab is recommended as the second-line treatment [8]. Furthermore, management of the underlying neoplasm, when present, is essential. Favourable outcomes have been reported in 80% of cases [3]. Relapsing disease course is encountered in 25% of cases [2].

4 Other Gems

- Aetiologies of anti-NMDAR encephalitis are (1) idiopathic, (2) paraneoplastic, (3) postinfectious (following herpes simplex encephalitis), and (4) iatrogenic (due to immune check point inhibitors).
- Over 50% of patients present with psychiatric symptoms.
- Seizures are very common at presentation involving 60–80% of cases.
- Limbic encephalitis is a common presentation of this condition.
- NMDAR antibodies can be detected in the serum of around 1–3% of healthy individuals. Hence, a positive serum antibody test should be carefully interpreted in the clinical context.
- CSF antibody test is significantly more sensitive than serum testing (100% vs 85%). Hence, CSF testing is mandatory.
- Relapses are associated with antibody titre rise in CSF more than serum.

References

1. Dalmau J, Tüzün E, Wu H-y, et al. Paraneoplastic anti-N-methyl-D-aspartate receptor encephalitis associated with ovarian teratoma. Ann Neurol. 2007;61:25–36.
2. Dalmau J, Lancaster E, Martinez-Hernandez E, Rosenfeld MR, Balice-Gordon R. Clinical experience and laboratory investigations in patients with anti-NMDAR encephalitis. Lancet Neurol. 2011;10:63–74.
3. Titulaer MJ, McCracken L, Gabilondo I, et al. Treatment and prognostic factors for long-term outcome in patients with anti-NMDA receptor encephalitis: an observational cohort study. Lancet Neurol. 2013;12:157–65.
4. Boeck AL, Logemann F, Krauß T, et al. Ovarectomy despite negative imaging in anti-NMDA receptor encephalitis: effective even late. Case Rep Neurol Med. 2013;2013:843192.
5. Graus F, Titulaer MJ, Balu R, et al. A clinical approach to diagnosis of autoimmune encephalitis. Lancet Neurol. 2016;15:391–404.
6. Wandinger KP, Saschenbrecker S, Stoecker W, Dalmau J. Anti-NMDA-receptor encephalitis: a severe, multistage, treatable disorder presenting with psychosis. J Neuroimmunol. 2011;231:86–91.

7. Broadley J, Seneviratne U, Beech P, et al. Prognosticating autoimmune encephalitis: a systematic review. J Autoimmun. 2019;96:24–34.
8. Abboud H, Probasco JC, Irani S, et al. Autoimmune encephalitis: proposed best practice recommendations for diagnosis and acute management. J Neurol Neurosurg Psychiatry. 2021;92:757–68.

Myasthenia Gravis and Myositis Following Immune Checkpoint Inhibitor Therapy

Subramanian Muthusamy and Udaya Seneviratne

1 Clinical Pearl

Patients on immune checkpoint inhibitors may develop immune-related adverse events involving the nervous system. Prompt recognition of the clinical presentation, cessation of the offending medication and treatment with appropriate immunotherapy may prevent further neurologic deterioration and potentially reverse the disease process. The decision to reinstitute checkpoint inhibitor therapy in this group of patients requires careful multidisciplinary consideration.

2 Clinical Case

A person in their 70s was diagnosed with renal cell carcinoma and underwent a nephrectomy. Disease recurrence in the nephrectomy bed and metastatic deposits in the lung were discovered a few months later. Six weeks before presenting to the hospital, they were commenced on the immune checkpoint inhibitors-ipilimumab and nivolumab. They presented to the hospital with several days of binocular diplopia that was present in multiple directions of gaze. They also reported 'sore' thigh muscles, difficulty climbing up the stairs and orthopnoea. The patient's spouse observed 'drooping of the eyelids' and 'slurring of speech' towards the end of the day. Neurologic examination was notable for restricted gaze in the lateral and vertical directions of movement, bilateral ptosis with fatiguability, and proximal lower limb weakness.

S. Muthusamy · U. Seneviratne (✉)
Monash Medical Centre, Melbourne, VIC, Australia

R. Junckerstorff et al. (eds.), *Beyond Evidence-Based Medicine*,
https://doi.org/10.1007/978-981-99-4440-8_92

Creatinine kinase was elevated at 1453 Units per Litre (range: 30–150). Autoimmune myositis blood tests, myasthenia antibodies (antibodies against acetylcholine receptor(AChR) and muscle-specific tyrosine kinase (MuSK)), ganglioside antibodies, high sensitivity troponin and transthoracic echocardiogram were unremarkable. Brain and whole spine magnetic resonance imaging (MRI) with contrast was unremarkable. However, proximal lower limb MRI was notable for increased T2 signal in the bilateral psoas, right gluteus minimus and right adductor magnus suggestive of myositis. Single fibre electromyography of the frontalis muscle demonstrated features consistent with a disorder of the neuromuscular junction. The patient was diagnosed with immune checkpoint inhibitor related myasthenia gravis and myositis. They were treated with immunoglobulins and high-dose intravenous steroids acutely. They required ongoing treatment with immunoglobulins, pyridostigmine, prednisolone and mycophenolate mofetil and had slow but incomplete recovery. Due to the severity of the adverse event, ipilimumab and nivolumab were not restarted.

3 Discussion

Immune checkpoint inhibitors (ICIs) are a relatively novel class of immunologic therapies that have revolutionised the treatment of a range of different cancers such as melanoma, small-cell lung carcinoma and renal cell carcinoma. Cancer cells may avoid the immune system by activating 'checkpoints' that are in place to prevent the immune system from targeting normal cells in the body. Examples of these checkpoints include cytotoxic T lymphocyte-associated antigen (CTLA-4) and programmed cell death protein 1 (PD-1). Activation of these immune checkpoints results in downregulation of the T-cell response whereas inhibition of these immune checkpoints restores immune-mediated anti-tumour activity. Immune-related adverse events (irAEs) are a recognised complication of this class of therapies. Although the gastrointestinal tract, liver and endocrine system are most commonly affected by irAEs, neurologic involvement is reported to occur in up to 15% of patients treated with the ICIs [1]. Neurologic adverse events from ICIs are protean. Common (but potentially less serious) manifestations include headaches, peripheral neuropathy, dysgeusia and dizziness. On the other hand, rare (but potentially more serious) manifestations include Guillain-Barre syndrome, cranial neuropathies, seizures, myelitis, autoimmune encephalitis and myasthenia gravis [2, 3].

Immune-related myasthenia gravis (ir-MG) is a serious neurologic adverse event with a reported frequency of up to 0.5%. This condition is seen in an older cohort of patients (unlike classical MG). Patients may present with ocular, limb, bulbar or respiratory symptoms. Respiratory muscle involvement is almost twice as common in ir-MG compared with classical MG. Involvement of other organ systems is common with myositis with myocarditis being the most frequently reported. Symptoms manifest usually after one month and typically between the second and third cycle of immunotherapy. Fewer patients with ir-MG test positive for antibodies against AChR or MuSK compared with classical MG. Additionally, neurophysiologic testing may be negative more frequently in ir-MG compared with classical MG. Early recognition and treatment are critical as ir-MG has a mortality rate of approximately 30% (compared with 6% for classical myasthenia). Respiratory paralysis is the major cause of mortality in ir-MG [1, 4–7].

A wide range of therapeutic strategies have been used in the treatment of ir-MG. These include acetylcholinesterase inhibitors, steroids, immunoglobulins, plasma exchange and rituximab. Ongoing or maintenance therapy may be needed, especially if there are plans to re-challenge with ICIs. In one large series, more than 95% of patients with ir-MG required hospitalisation and 45% of patients required invasive or non-invasive ventilatory support. Prognosis was variable with only 20% of patients in this particular series demonstrating complete resolution of symptoms. Clinical improvement was observed in 55% and clinical worsening in 26% of patients [8].

4 Other Gems

- Concurrent presentation of ir-MG and ir-myositis increases the risk of myasthenic crisis that may prompt the need for invasive or non-invasive ventilatory support.
- Although, thymomas are seen in up to 15% of patients with classical MG, it is not implicated in the pathogenesis of ir-MG.
- Ir-MG is associated with the highest mortality rate of all neurologic adverse events associated with ICIs.
- Acute or chronic neuropathy occurs in as many as 3% of patients treated with ICIs although it is less frequent compared with patients who receive chemotherapy. Taxanes and platinum based chemotherapeutic agents are most commonly implicated in peripheral neuropathy.
- The frequency of Guillain-Barre syndrome in patients treated with ICIs is reported to range between 0.1–0.2%.
- Ir-Encephalitis generally has an overall favourable prognosis with appropriate treatment, except in cases where a previously undetected paraneoplastic encephalitic syndrome is triggered by ICIs.

References

1. Farooq MZ, Aqeel SB, Lingamaneni P, Pichardo RC, Jawed A, Khalid S, et al. Association of immune checkpoint inhibitors with neurologic adverse events: a systematic review and meta-analysis. JAMA Netw Open. 2022;5(4):e227722.
2. Ramos-Casals M, Brahmer JR, Callahan MK, Flores-Chávez A, Keegan N, Khamashta MA, et al. Immune-related adverse events of checkpoint inhibitors. Nat Rev Dis Primers. 2020;6(1):38.

3. Velasco R, Villagrán M, Jové M, Simó M, Vilariño N, Alemany M, et al. Encephalitis induced by immune checkpoint inhibitors: a systematic review. JAMA Neurol. 2021;78(7):864–73.
4. Huang YT, Chen YP, Lin WC, Su WC, Sun YT. Immune checkpoint inhibitor-induced myasthenia gravis. Front Neurol. 2020;11:634.
5. Lindstrom JM, Seybold ME, Lennon VA, Whittingham S, Duane DD. Antibody to acetylcholine receptor in myasthenia gravis. Prevalence, clinical correlates, and diagnostic value. Neurology. 1976;26(11):1054–9.
6. Meriggioli MN, Sanders DB. Muscle autoantibodies in myasthenia gravis: beyond diagnosis? Expert Rev Clin Immunol. 2012;8(5):427–38.
7. Oh SJ, Kim DE, Kuruoglu R, Bradley RJ, Dwyer D. Diagnostic sensitivity of the laboratory tests in myasthenia gravis. Muscle Nerve. 1992;15(6):720–4.
8. Safa H, Johnson DH, Trinh VA, Rodgers TE, Lin H, Suarez-Almazor ME, et al. Immune checkpoint inhibitor related myasthenia gravis: single center experience and systematic review of the literature. J Immunother Cancer. 2019;7(1):319.

Convulsive Syncope: A Common Seizure Mimicker

Subramanian Muthusamy and Udaya Seneviratne

1 Clinical Pearl

Brief muscle jerks, twitching, or convulsive movements are commonly observed in patients following syncope. These episodes can be mistaken for seizures. Careful history taking can help clinicians differentiate between these two entities and ensure that patients with these different conditions are managed in an appropriate fashion.

2 Clinical Case

A person in their thirties was referred to the seizure clinic following recurrent episodes of transient loss of consciousness associated with 'convulsions'. They had no chronic medical issues, family history of epilepsy or cardiac conditions, and denied excessive alcohol intake or recreational drug use. They reported chest discomfort and light-headedness prior to losing awareness. Their spouse observed that they were pale, clammy and slumped to the ground before they began to 'fit'. When asked to elaborate, the spouse described that their 'eyes rolled upwards' and there was irregular 'twitching' of the limbs for 30 s. There was no tongue bite or incontinence. They regained consciousness fairly quickly, felt nauseous, and vomited afterwards. An emotional trigger frequently preceded these spells. Neurologic and cardiac examination was unremarkable. Their 12-lead electrocardiogram (ECG) demonstrated sinus rhythm and routine electroencephalogram (EEG) was unremarkable. A 7-day ambulatory video EEG and ECG monitoring captured four typical events reported by the patient. One event was characterised by marked bradycardia with a heart rate of 26 beats per minute, while three others correlated with a sinus arrest lasting 21 s, 11 s and 6 s respectively (Fig. 1). There were three

S. Muthusamy · U. Seneviratne (✉)
Monash Medical Centre, Melbourne, VIC, Australia

R. Junckerstorff et al. (eds.), *Beyond Evidence-Based Medicine*,
https://doi.org/10.1007/978-981-99-4440-8_93

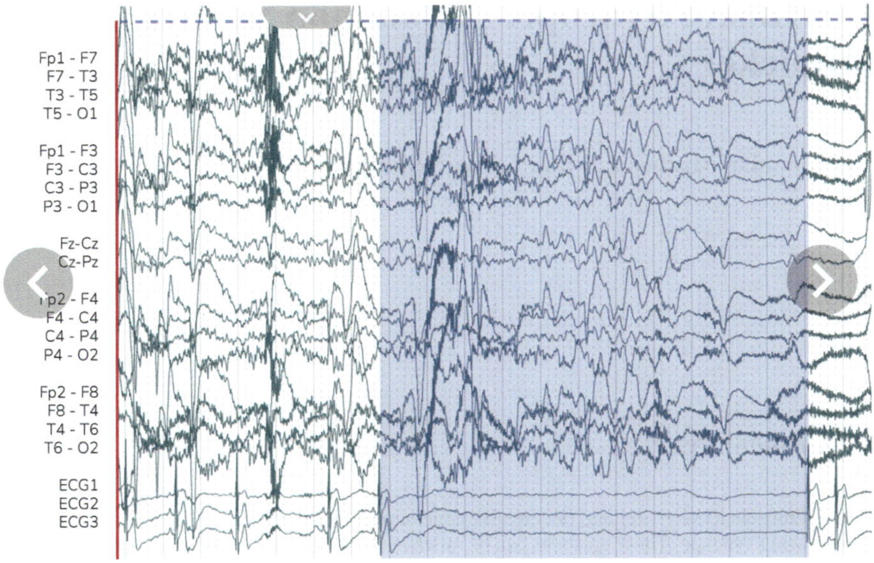

Fig. 1 Example of EEG and ECG tracing during one of patient's typical events. Time window is 20 s. Note that the ECG channels show a sinus arrest of 11 s (shaded segment). The EEG is characterised by generalised slowing followed by generalised flattening of the waveforms

nocturnal unreported events. One was characterised by sinus bradycardia with a heart rate of 20 beats per minute and the other two were characterised by sinus arrest lasting 7 s and 18 s respectively. The EEG background was notable for slowing during these episodes and there were no epileptiform abnormalities. The patient was diagnosed with neurally-mediated syncope and was initially managed with conservative measures. Due to ongoing events and failure of conservative treatment measures, a permanent pacemaker was eventually implanted resulting in complete resolution of symptoms.

3 Discussion

Seizures and syncope are the main differential diagnoses when someone presents with episodes of transient loss of consciousness. Clinicians are often required to differentiate between these conditions. Seizures are defined as 'a transient occurrence of signs and/or symptoms due to abnormal excessive or synchronous neuronal activity in the brain' [1]. Syncope is defined as abrupt and transient loss of consciousness due to cerebral hypoperfusion [2]. The lifetime prevalence of syncope in individuals under the age of 60 is reported to be between 20% and 40% [3, 4]. Abnormal motor activity such as myoclonus has been reported in up to 90% of patients during a syncope [5, 6]. This can lead to misdiagnosis, inappropriate investigations, and management. Table 1 provides a summary of the key differences in clinical phenomena between seizures and syncope.

Table 1 Summary of key differences in clinical phenomena typically observed in syncope versus seizures

	Syncope	Seizure
Position	Prolonged standing, sudden change in position	Can occur in any position
Context	Emotional distress, fear, pain, specific situations (coughing, defecation, urination)	Can occur in any context
Prodrome / Aura	Blurred vision, dizziness, light-headedness, nausea	Varies depending on region of brain involved
Duration	Usually brief (seconds)	Usually longer than syncope (seconds to minutes)
Motor phenomena	Brief multifocal arrhythmic jerks involving proximal and distal muscles Typically brief lasting seconds Onset follows loss of consciousness Lateralised head turn or increased tone with mild extensor posturing may be seen	Usually bilateral synchronous tonic-clonic or myoclonic activity Unilateral in focal seizures
Eye movements	Eyes open Brief upward deviation	Eyes open Sustained upward or lateral deviation
Vocalisation	Low pitched moan	Guttural noise
Heart rate	Usually reduced alongside blood pressure during vasovagal syncope Both bradyarrhythmias and tachyarrhythmias can be associated with syncope	Usually associated with an increase in heart rate Ictal bradycardia or asystole are rare Blood pressure usually increased
Incontinence	May occur	May occur
Tongue biting	Rare (usually tip of the tongue)	Lateral tongue bite
Associated features	Diaphoresis, pallor	Automatisms in complex partial seizures
Postictal confusion	Quick recovery of mental function	Prolonged confusion, but can be brief in some seizures

Although global cerebral hypoperfusion is the defining feature in all syncope, the underlying aetiologies vary, and the clinician needs to differentiate between benign versus serious causes. Syncope can be broadly classified into the following groups: (1) reflex (neurally-mediated) syncope, (2) syncope due to orthostatic hypotension and (3) cardiac syncope. Reflex syncope encompasses vasovagal syncope, situational syncope (e.g. micturition, cough and defecation syncope), carotid-sinus syndrome and non-classical forms (atypical cases that occur in the absence of prodrome or apparent trigger). Syncope due to orthostatic hypotension encompasses drug-induced orthostatic hypotension, volume depletion and autonomic failure. Cardiac syncope encompasses arrhythmias, structural cardiac disease and diseases of the cardiopulmonary and great vessels (e.g. pulmonary hypertension). Careful history taking and physical examination will provide clues towards a particular cause. Investigations such as ECG monitoring, transthoracic echocardiogram or head-up tilt test may be required in some cases [7–9].

4 Other Gems

- Obtain a 12-lead ECG for patients presenting with a transient loss of consciousness
- If syncope is identified as the likely cause for the patient's presentation, it is important to ascertain if there are any 'red flags' requiring emergent cardiology review. These include: [10]

  Syncope during exertion or when supine
  Associated new onset chest pain, shortness of breath, abdominal pain, or headaches
  Palpitations immediately preceding syncope
  No warning symptoms or short (<10 s) prodrome
  Abnormal cardiac examination or evidence of structural cardiac disease
  Persistent bradycardia (<40 beats per minute)
  Family history of sudden cardiac death
  ECG findings suggesting ischaemia or arrhythmic syncope

- Myoclonic activity in syncope is thought to arise from the subcortical structures, whereas it arises from the cortex in seizures

References

1. Fisher RS, Acevedo C, Arzimanoglou A, Bogacz A, Cross JH, Elger CE, et al. ILAE official report: a practical clinical definition of epilepsy. Epilepsia. 2014;55(4):475–82.
2. Goldberger ZD, Petek BJ, Brignole M, Shen WK, Sheldon RS, Solbiati M, et al. ACC/AHA/HRS versus ESC guidelines for the diagnosis and management of syncope: JACC guideline comparison. J Am Coll Cardiol. 2019;74(19):2410–23.
3. Ganzeboom KS, Mairuhu G, Reitsma JB, Linzer M, Wieling W, van Dijk N. Lifetime cumulative incidence of syncope in the general population: a study of 549 Dutch subjects aged 35-60 years. J Cardiovasc Electrophysiol. 2006;17(11):1172–6.
4. Chen LY, Shen WK, Mahoney DW, Jacobsen SJ, Rodeheffer RJ. Prevalence of syncope in a population aged more than 45 years. Am J Med. 2006;119(12):1088.e1–7.
5. Lempert T, Bauer M, Schmidt D. Syncope: a videometric analysis of 56 episodes of transient cerebral hypoxia. Ann Neurol. 1994;36(2):233–7.
6. Lin JT, Ziegler DK, Lai CW, Bayer W. Convulsive syncope in blood donors. Ann Neurol. 1982;11(5):525–8.
7. Brignole M, Moya A, de Lange FJ, Deharo JC, Elliott PM, Fanciulli A, et al. 2018 ESC Guidelines for the diagnosis and management of syncope. Eur Heart J. 2018;39(21):1883–948.
8. Runser LA, Gauer RL, Houser A. Syncope: evaluation and differential diagnosis. Am Fam Physician. 2017;95(5):303–12.
9. Cheshire WP, Jr. Syncope. Continuum (Minneap Minn). 2017;23(2, Selected Topics in Outpatient Neurology):335–58.
10. Sutton R, Ricci F, Fedorowski A. Risk stratification of syncope: current syncope guidelines and beyond. Auton Neurosci. 2022;238:102929.

Headache with Red Flags

Udaya Seneviratne

1 Clinical Pearl

New onset of headache in an immunocompromised person should raise the suspicion of an infection in the central nervous system.

2 Clinical Case

A man in his thirties was admitted with a history of headache for 2 weeks and right facial asymmetry for 5 days. He reported gradual onset persistent headache, characterised by constant pressure sensation worse over the occipital region, associated with tinnitus. The headache was worse in the morning and in the recumbent position. There was no nausea, vomiting, diplopia, or photophobia. His regular medications included mycophenolate mofetil and prednisolone for membranous nephropathy.

He was afebrile on admission and there was no neck stiffness. Fundoscopy revealed bilateral papilloedema. The neurological examination was significant for right-sided, forehead-sparing facial weakness and mild weakness of right upper and lower limbs.

The Magnetic Resonance Imaging (MRI) brain scan revealed multiple foci of restricted diffusion in both hemispheres, leptomeningeal enhancement, and an enhancing lesion in the left basal ganglia. A lumbar puncture was performed, and the opening pressure was 30 mm of water. The cerebrospinal fluid (CSF) analysis revealed an abnormally elevated cell count (lymphocytes 92×10^6/L, polymorphs 88×10^6/L), low glucose (2.3 mmol/L: normal 2.5–5.0), and slightly raised protein

U. Seneviratne (✉)
Monash Medical Centre, Melbourne, VIC, Australia

R. Junckerstorff et al. (eds.), *Beyond Evidence-Based Medicine*,
https://doi.org/10.1007/978-981-99-4440-8_94

(0.53 g/L: normal 0.15–0.45). Cryptococcal antigen was positive in both the serum and CSF. The transthoracic echocardiogram and CT scan of the chest, abdomen, and pelvis were normal.

A diagnosis of cryptococcal meningitis with an associated intracerebral cryptococcoma and multiple cerebral lacunar infarcts was made. He was treated with amphotericin B and flucytosine followed by fluconazole for the cryptococcal infection. The raised intracranial pressure was managed with repeated lumbar punctures. He made a full recovery following a prolonged hospital stay.

3 Discussion

Cryptococci are yeast-like fungi infecting both humans and animals. Inhalation is the most frequent route of infection. Infection usually occurs in immunocompromised hosts however can occur in individuals with no apparent immune deficiency. As in our case, cryptococcal meningitis usually presents in a subacute form, but acute and chronic presentations are well recognised [1, 2]. Headache is the most frequent symptom of cryptococcal meningitis and raised intracranial pressure is common. Approximately 20% of patients develop lacunar brain infarcts, which is thought to be caused by infective vasculopathy [3]. Brain imaging may reveal cerebral cryptococcoma [2]. The CSF typically shows lymphocytic pleocytosis, raised protein, and low glucose. The diagnosis can be confirmed by India Ink staining of CSF, cryptococcal antigen test, and culture. The treatment regime consists of induction therapy with amphotericin B and flucytosine followed by consolidation and maintenance phases with fluconazole [4]. All patients with cryptococcal meningitis should be tested for underlying Human Immunodeficiency Virus (HIV) infection.

Headache in clinical practice can be broadly divided into two groups; primary and secondary. In the latter, headache occurs as a symptom of another condition or disease. Examples of secondary headaches include intracranial infection, disorders of pressure or a vascular cause such as bleeding or thrombosis and disorders of the cranium and related structures. Primary headaches are more prevalent in routine practice and include migraine, tension headache, and trigeminal autonomic cephalgias. A major challenge is to identify potentially serious secondary headaches early for appropriate investigations and treatment. To achieve this goal, 'red flags' are described in the literature to guide clinicians [5, 6]. Listed below are some of those useful red flags.

4 Other Gems

4.1 Red Flags and Potential Associations

- Immunocompromised patient: opportunistic infections
- History of neoplasia: brain tumour, metastasis
- Fever: neuroinfections

- Neurological deficits (including decreased conscious state): intracranial lesion
- Thunderclap headache: subarachnoid haemorrhage
- Papilloedema: raised intracranial pressure
- Orthostatic headache: low intracranial pressure
- Headache worse on lying flat: raised intracranial pressure
- Headache precipitation by coughing, sneezing, exercise: Chiari malformation, posterior fossa lesions, mass lesions
- Headache in pregnancy and puerperium: preeclampsia, cerebral venous sinus thrombosis
- New-onset headache in old age (>65 years): temporal arteritis, neoplasms
- A recent change in the pattern of headache
- Progressive headache

References

1. Day JN. Cryptococcal meningitis. Pract Neurol. 2004;4(5):274–85. https://doi.org/10.1111/j.1474-7766.2004.00254.x.
2. Williamson PR, Jarvis JN, Panackal AA, et al. Cryptococcal meningitis: epidemiology, immunology, diagnosis and therapy. Nat Rev Neurol. 2017;13(1):13–24. https://doi.org/10.1038/nrneurol.2016.167. [published Online First: 2016/11/26].
3. Mishra AK, Arvind VH, Muliyil D, et al. Cerebrovascular injury in cryptococcal meningitis. Int J Stroke. 2018;13(1):57–65. https://doi.org/10.1177/1747493017706240. [published Online First: 2017/04/20].
4. Saag MS, Graybill RJ, Larsen RA, et al. Practice guidelines for the management of cryptococcal disease. Infectious Diseases Society of America. Clin Infect Dis. 2000;30(4):710–8. https://doi.org/10.1086/313757. [published Online First: 2000/04/19].
5. Do TP, Remmers A, Schytz HW, et al. Red and orange flags for secondary headaches in clinical practice: SNNOOP10 list. Neurology. 2019;92(3):134–44. https://doi.org/10.1212/WNL.0000000000006697. [published Online First: 2018/12/26].
6. Hainer BL, Matheson EM. Approach to acute headache in adults. Am Fam Physician. 2013;87(10):682–7. [published Online First: 2013/08/14].

Paradoxical Seizure Exacerbation with Antiseizure Medications

Udaya Seneviratne

1 Clinical Pearl

Some antiseizure medications may paradoxically exacerbate seizures. A good example is worsening of absence and myoclonic seizures even progressing to status epilepticus by carbamazepine. Hence certain antiseizure drugs such as carbamazepine and phenytoin should be avoided in genetic generalised epilepsies with absence and myoclonic seizures.

2 Clinical Case

A man in his forties was brought in by ambulance to the emergency department. He had complained of feeling unwell the day before and did not sleep well that night. He was found to be confused by his wife the next day. He was disorientated and had a slurred speech. His wife also noticed episodes of repetitive eye blinking.

His past history revealed evidence of epilepsy. His first seizure occurred at the age of 16 years, and it was a generalised tonic-clonic seizure. The Electroencephalogram (EEG) demonstrated generalised epileptiform discharges and he was commenced on carbamazepine. He used to experience occasional generalised tonic-clonic seizures due to sleep deprivation and noncompliance with carbamazepine. Subsequently, he experienced intermittent episodes of blanking out and staring into space for seconds suggestive of absence seizures. Levetiracetam was added to carbamazepine when he was admitted to the emergency department following another breakthrough tonic-clonic seizure approximately 1 year ago.

U. Seneviratne (✉)
Monash Medical Centre, Melbourne, VIC, Australia

R. Junckerstorff et al. (eds.), *Beyond Evidence-Based Medicine*,
https://doi.org/10.1007/978-981-99-4440-8_95

On examination, he was disorientated to person, place, and time. He had drooling and the speech was slurred with a vacant look on his face. Intermittently, episodes of repetitive blinking were witnessed. An urgent EEG was arranged, which demonstrated continuous generalised spike-wave discharges. He was diagnosed with absence status epilepticus and was treated with intravenous sodium valproate. Carbamazepine was ceased. He returned to his usual baseline in 48 hours and his EEG also normalised. He was discharged on sodium valproate and levetiracetam combination therapy. He remained well and seizure-free on follow-up in the outpatient clinic.

3 Discussion

Genetic generalised epilepsy (GGE) accounts for approximately 20% of all epilepsies. Onset in childhood and adolescence, positive family history, and morning preponderance for seizure occurrence are classical features of GGE. Generalised tonic-clonic, absence, and myoclonic seizures are typical seizure types in this condition [1]. The EEG is characterised by the presence of generalised epileptiform discharges (spike-wave, polyspike-wave, and polyspikes) [2]. Several syndromes are identified under the umbrella of GGE and include childhood absence epilepsy, juvenile absence epilepsy, juvenile myoclonic epilepsy, and generalised epilepsy with tonic-clonic seizures alone. The case reported here has several characteristics consistent with the diagnosis of GGE.

The most important factors in selecting the appropriate antiseizure medication in epilepsy are the seizure types and the syndrome. Sodium valproate, lamotrigine, and levetiracetam are the most frequently used drugs in GGE. Sodium valproate and ethosuximide were found to be better than lamotrigine in controlling absence seizures in a randomised controlled trial involving children [3]. However, sodium valproate is best avoided in women of child-bearing age due to the high risk of teratogenicity and cognitive problems in the offspring [4]. Sodium valproate is also quite effective in controlling myoclonic seizures whereas levetiracetam and clonazepam are less effective alternatives.

Less well-known is the fact that antiseizure drugs can paradoxically exacerbate seizures. Although it is used in the treatment of juvenile myoclonic epilepsy, lamotrigine can occasionally worsen myoclonic seizures [5]. In GGE, certain antiseizure medications such as carbamazepine, oxcarbazepine, phenytoin, gabapentin, and vigabatrin have the potential to aggravate myoclonic and absence seizures which may even progress to status epilepticus [6]. Our case is a good example of absence status epilepticus triggered by carbamazepine. Hence these drugs should be avoided in GGE patients with absence and myoclonic seizures.

4 Other Gems

- Anatomical and neurodevelopmental teratogenicity associated with sodium valproate therapy is dose dependent. Higher doses are more teratogenic.
- Anatomical teratogenicity is due to antiseizure drug exposure during the first trimester of the pregnancy, but neurodevelopmental teratogenicity extends beyond the first trimester.
- Among antiseizure medications, levetiracetam and lamotrigine are two of the safest options during pregnancy.
- The combination of sodium valproate and lamotrigine is very effective due to its synergistic effect. However, the patient should be carefully monitored for side effects such as tremors.
- Stevens-Johnson syndrome and toxic epidermal necrolysis due to carbamazepine therapy have a significant association with the Human Leukocyte Antigen (HLA)-B* 1502 allele. This allele is highly prevalent among Asians, particularly Han Chinese. Hence, the FDA recommends HLA testing for Asians before commencing carbamazepine.
- Antiseizure drugs with sodium channel modulation as the mode of action (e.g. carbamazepine, phenytoin) appear to be more effective in treating seizures in the setting of autoimmune encephalitis. However, immunotherapy is the key to controlling seizures in these patients.

References

1. Vorderwülbecke BJ, Wandschneider B, Weber Y, Holtkamp M. Genetic generalized epilepsies in adults—challenging assumptions and dogmas. Nat Rev Neurol. 2022;18(2):71–83.
2. Seneviratne U, Cook M, D'Souza W. The electroencephalogram of idiopathic generalized epilepsy. Epilepsia. 2012;53(2):234–48.
3. Glauser TA, Cnaan A, Shinnar S, Hirtz DG, Dlugos D, Masur D, et al. Ethosuximide, valproic acid, and lamotrigine in childhood absence epilepsy. N Engl J Med. 2010;362(9):790–9.
4. Tomson T, Battino D, Bonizzoni E, Craig J, Lindhout D, Perucca E, et al. Comparative risk of major congenital malformations with eight different antiepileptic drugs: a prospective cohort study of the EURAP registry. Lancet Neurol. 2018;17(6):530–8.
5. Gesche J, Hjalgrim H, Rubboli G, Beier CP. Risk factors of paradoxical reactions to antiseizure medication in genetic generalized epilepsy. Epilepsy Res. 2021;170:106547.
6. Thomas P, Valton L, Genton P. Absence and myoclonic status epilepticus precipitated by antiepileptic drugs in idiopathic generalized epilepsy. Brain. 2006;129(Pt 5):1281–92.

Examination Tips in Suspected First Presentation with Multiple Sclerosis

Richard J. Stark

1 Clinical Pearl

The neurological examination usually consists of a routine procedure (the "core examination") supplemented by extra elements which depend on the clinical picture. Deciding which extras to add in a particular case is one of the most important skills to learn. It means you have to think through the diagnostic possibilities before starting the neurological examination so that you can use the examination for hypothesis testing.

2 Clinical Case

A 24-year-old woman presents with a numb feeling in the left arm. It started in the fingers and extended over a few days to the hand and forearm. The hand feels a bit clumsy but is not weak. There is no definite past history of neurological symptoms, but a year earlier there was some mild visual blurring in one eye which settled in a few days and was not pursued.

You wonder if this might be a first presentation with demyelination and plan your examination accordingly.

Fundi appear normal, but there is a hint of an afferent pupillary defect in the left eye on the swinging flashlight test. You test for colour desaturation with a red pin, and colour seems "washed out" with the left eye. You check colour vision more thoroughly with Ishihara-style plates from a smart-phone app and confirm impaired colour vision on the left. Visual acuity is normal. Routine tests of pursuit eye movements seem normal, but on testing horizontal saccades there seems to be some

R. J. Stark (✉)
Neurology Department, Alfred Hospital, Melbourne, VIC, Australia

Department of Neurosciences, Monash University, Melbourne, VIC, Australia

R. Junckerstorff et al. (eds.), *Beyond Evidence-Based Medicine*,
https://doi.org/10.1007/978-981-99-4440-8_96

slowing of adduction of the right eye. There is no leading eye nystagmus. Checking oblique saccades confirms slowing of right eye adduction.

Power and reflexes in the limbs are normal but there is slight drift up and laterally of the outstretched left arm with eyes closed. There is some reduction of joint position sense and vibration sense in the left hand and some impairment of texture sensitivity but normal pain and temperature sensation. There is mild slowing of rapid alternating finger movements.

Lower limb examination and the rest of the neurological examination are normal.

You have documented some "dorsal column" sensory loss, relevant to the presenting complaint but also evidence suggestive of previous left optic neuritis and an internuclear ophthalmoplegia (INO). This is highly suggestive of a diagnosis of multiple sclerosis (MS). MRI is promptly arranged and shows typical features consistent with a diagnosis of MS.

3 Discussion

In any patient in whom the diagnosis of MS is being considered, you should look for signs of previous episodes which may have been asymptomatic or not interpreted as significant at the time. These would include checking for evidence of optic neuritis and INO and looking for subtle features of upper motor neuron or cerebellar dysfunction.

Tests that can be performed quickly at the bedside without much additional equipment are of great practical value [1].

Signs of old optic neuritis include:

(a) Pale optic discs (subtle changes may be difficult for the inexperienced)
(b) Impaired colour vision: this can be screened for quickly by testing for colour desaturation or more formally with Ishihara charts (more time consuming)
(c) Afferent pupillary defect (quick, effective, and well known, but subtle changes may be difficult to see)
(d) Subtle central or paracentral field defects (not easy to detect at the bedside by ordinary methods). Testing visual fields with a laser pointer can be helpful [2].

Testing for colour desaturation is quick and easy: hold up a red object such as the top of a hat-pin and cover each of the patient's eyes in turn. Ask whether the colour seems washed out or dulled in one eye compared with the other.

Clearly this detects asymmetrical colour desaturation. Its advantages are that it is quick and reasonably sensitive. It can be included in the examination with minimal loss of time even when the chance of a positive response is quite low. Naturally, a more detailed assessment for evidence of optic neuritis should be provoked by a positive response or a history suggesting that optic neuropathy is likely.

INO is found in patients with a lesion in the medial longitudinal fasciculus and is a relatively common finding in patients with MS. It is easy to detect when severe: there is incomplete adduction of one eye and leading eye nystagmus in the abducting eye. It can be more difficult to detect when mild. The earliest sign is usually slowing of adduction on saccadic (refixation) eye movements. This is fairly easy to recognise if you have seen it before but can be tricky for inexperienced examiners.

Of course, the speed of vertical saccades will be completely normal in patients with INO. One way to make differences in vertical and horizontal saccadic speed more apparent to the inexperienced is to ask the patient to perform an oblique saccade: they are asked to look from a high target on the right to a low target on the left for example. If there is slowing of adduction of the right eye but other movements are normal, the left eye will travel in a straight line and the right eye will follow a curve going downwards before it goes leftwards. Many will find the abnormal shape of the path of the eye easier to detect than the slowed speed.

In this case, the presentation with sensory symptoms means that detailed sensory testing is required. Checking for drift of the outstretched hands with the eyes closed is a very useful initial screening test and drift up or laterally is suggestive of proprioceptive dysfunction. Dorsal column sensation is typically tested with joint position sense and vibration sense. Another useful test to assess large fibre/dorsal column/parietal sensory function in the hand is texture sense [1]. This is quick and simple. The patient closes their eyes, and the examiner takes the patient's index finger and touches the pulp against the skin of the examiner's hand or his/her shirt or coat sleeve. The patient is given a series of these stimuli in succession and is asked to identify 'skin' or 'sleeve'.

This can be particularly helpful in patients with parietal sensory dysfunction (from a stroke, for example) and is less cumbersome and requires less concentration from the patient than graphaesthesia or stereognosis. But it is also a good sign of dorsal column dysfunction.

4 Take Home Messages

- If you suspect multiple sclerosis, you should actively look for subtle signs of previous episodes.

References

1. Stark RJ. Tips for trainees: some practical tips on clinical examination. Pract Neurol. 2020;20:489–93. http://pn.bmj.com/cgi/content/full/practneurol-2020-002659v1?ct.
2. Stark RJ. Clinical testing of visual fields using a laser pointer and a wall. Pract Neurol. 2013;13(4):258–9. (Published Online First: 26 April 2013). https://doi.org/10.1136/practneurol-2013-00056.

Migraine Aura: Typical and Atypical

Richard J. Stark

1 Clinical Pearl

The key to diagnosing migraine aura is the way it evolves over time during the attack.

2 Clinical Case

A 55-year-old man presents with a history of three episodes of visual disturbance in the past 3 months. Each episode starts with blurring or smudging of an area in the centre of his vision so that it is hard to read: the letters he is looking at are blurred but vision more peripherally is normal. Within 5 minutes the area of blurring has extended further to his left. There is a shimmery quality to the edge of the smudge. After another 5 minutes the smudge has become larger still, but he is starting to see more clearly in central vision. Over the next 15 minutes the left-most edge of the smudge gradually moves to the periphery of his vision with some irregular shimmery zigzags at the advancing edge. By this stage central vision is back to normal. After another 10 minutes his vision is normal again. When you ask about headache, he says there was a very mild headache for the next half hour but not enough to require any treatment.

There is no previous history of migraine or cardiovascular disease. Neurological and cardiac examination is normal.

R. J. Stark (✉)
Neurology Department, Alfred Hospital, Melbourne, VIC, Australia

Department of Neurosciences, Monash University, Melbourne, VIC, Australia

R. Junckerstorff et al. (eds.), *Beyond Evidence-Based Medicine*,
https://doi.org/10.1007/978-981-99-4440-8_97

You diagnose migraine aura without headache.

Two months later, he returns to see you because of an episode of left arm sensory disturbance. This was transient and there are no ongoing left arm symptoms. Again, neurological and cardiac examination is normal. You explore the detail of how the episode developed:

Scenario 1: The whole left arm became numb within a second or two. There was some numbness of the left side of the face too. Perhaps the left hand was very slightly clumsy. The episode lasted about 5–10 minutes and then the changes disappeared.

Scenario 2: The numbness started in the left thumb with a buzzing slightly electrical feeling. Within a few seconds it spread to involve the other fingers of the left hand and within 10 seconds involved the forearm. Within another 5 seconds the left shoulder was affected and then 5 seconds later the left side of the face. The symptoms then resolved so that the episode was over within a minute or so. The arm felt a bit heavy for the next 5 minutes.

Scenario 3: The numbness started in the left thumb. Within 5 minutes it spread to involve the other fingers of the left hand and after another 10 minutes involved the forearm. Within another 5 minutes the left shoulder was affected and then 10 minutes later the left side of the face. By this stage the hand was improving. The symptoms then resolved so that the episode was over within half an hour.

3 Discussion

This case raises a number of learning points.

3.1 *Late-Life Migraine Accompaniments*

Episodes of typical migrainous visual aura are very common in people in their 50s and beyond [1]. They are often not accompanied by headache. Their cause is speculative but the mechanism is almost certainly the process of spreading cortical depression. This has been extensively explored in animal models [2] and probably explains migraine aura. The key point is that a wave of altered activity spreads gradually over an area of cortex over a period of 15–30 minutes, and as it does so the clinical symptoms evolve gradually. In animals, the process can be triggered in a wide range of ways, mostly from irritating the cortical surface directly. In people with a strong genetic susceptibility to migraine, it is clearly triggered more easily and the process then, in turn, provokes or enhances a cascade of other processes resulting in pain, nausea and other features of a migraine attack. Patients who have never had a migraine until their 50s but then get painless visual aura symptoms are presumably less genetically predisposed but still susceptible to some degree. What triggers the attacks in such people? It is speculative, but it may be that circulating platelet microemboli could be a factor. The increased incidence of migraine with aura in those with patent foramen ovale could have a similar explanation.

3.2 Distinguishing Between Migraine Aura, TIA and Focal Seizure

The very typical history of evolving scintillating scotoma is highly suggestive of migraine aura. If the aura symptoms are not visual, the distinction is more difficult.

The history of evolution & progression of the symptoms is vital
Abrupt onset suggests TIA.
Evolution over seconds to a couple of minutes suggests focal seizure
Evolution over 5–30 minutes suggests migraine
Development of headache is helpful but not definitive
Ischaemia can trigger headache and so can seizures
Aura without headache is common
Nature of positive visual symptoms [3] *is helpful but not definitive*
Black & white suggests migraine, colour suggests seizure (but up to 40% of migraine auras have some coloured component)
Jagged edges suggest migraine, rounded edges suggest seizure
Complete hallucinatory images are not typically migrainous

In the case described above, based on the time-course of the evolution of symptoms, scenario 1 would suggest that TIA is likely, scenario 2 raises focal epilepsy as a likely cause while scenario 3 would be typical of migraine aura.

3.3 Distinguishing True Migraine Aura from Other "Aura-Like" Symptoms of Migraine

The International Classification of Headache Disorders (ICHD3) [4] is quite strict in defining aura as follows:

A. *At least two attacks fulfilling criteria B and C*
B. *One or more of the following fully reversible aura symptoms:*

    1. visual
    2. sensory
    3. speech and/or language
    4. motor
    5. brainstem
    6. retinal

C. *At least three of the following six characteristics:*

    1. at least one aura symptom spreads gradually over 5 minutes
    2. two or more aura symptoms occur in succession
    3. each individual aura symptom lasts 5–60 minutes
    4. at least one aura symptom is unilateral

5. at least one aura symptom is positive
6. the aura is accompanied, or followed within 60 minutes, by headache

D. *Not better accounted for by another ICHD-3 diagnosis*

In the case described, both the visual symptoms reported initially and the sensory symptoms in scenario 3 would meet criteria for migraine aura.

Patients with migraine often have enhanced sensitivity to a range of sensory stimuli. This may result in symptoms that might be considered "aura-like" but do not meet the diagnostic criteria for aura. For example, they may report distress from strong smells or have enhanced scalp sensitivity. Some will report an unusual visual symptom known as "visual snow" [5]. This is a continuous TV-snow like visual disturbance in the entire visual field. They may also report persistent palinopsia, photophobia, impaired night vision, excessive floaters, and other persisting visual symptoms. These are clearly quite different from true aura.

Vestibular migraine is a somewhat controversial term. The condition exists and is defined in ICHD3 Appendix [4]. At least half of episodes of vertigo must be associated with at least one of: migrainous headache, photophobia & phonophobia, or visual aura. By contrast many patients with migraine describe more persistent vestibular symptoms which are better termed PPPD (Persistent Postural Perceptual Dizziness). This condition's features include dizziness, unsteadiness, or non-spinning vertigo, typically aggravated by motion or moving visual stimuli. It can be thought of as a hypersensitivity to vestibular activation.

4 Take Home Messages

- Migraine aura typically spreads gradually over 5 minutes or more and lasts 5–60 minutes. TIA and focal seizures evolve more rapidly.

References

1. Fisher CM. Late-life migraine accompaniments as a cause of unexplained transient ischemic attacks. Can J Neurol Sci. 1980;7(1):9–17. PMID: 7388704.
2. Leao AAP. Spreading depression of activity in the cerebral cortex. J Neurophysiol. 1944;7(6):359–90.
3. Panayiotopoulos CP, Sharoqi IA, Agathonikou A. Occipital seizures imitating migraine aura. J R Soc Med. 1997;90(5):255–7. https://doi.org/10.1177/014107689709000506.
4. Headache Classification Committee of the International Headache Society. The International Classification of Headache Disorders, 3rd edition. Cephalalgia. 2018;38:1–211.
5. Schankin CJ, Maniyar FH, Digre KB, Goadsby PJ. 'Visual snow'—a disorder distinct from persistent migraine aura. Brain. 2014;137:1419–28. https://doi.org/10.1093/brain/awu050.

Acute Transient Amnesia

Richard J. Stark

1 Clinical Pearl

1. Transient global amnesia has a very characteristic presentation. Asking the same question repeatedly is a key feature.
2. Transient epileptic amnesia is less common but important to diagnose as it is treatable.

2 Clinical Case

A 60-year-old man went for a swim in the surf while on holidays. When he emerged, he seemed confused and asked his wife why they were at the beach. She replied to say that they were on holidays, but he asked the same question a minute or two later. It became clear that he could not recall anything that had happened in recent weeks. She took him to a local hospital where no abnormalities were found on neurological examination and a CT scan of brain was said to be normal. BP and ECG were normal. His memory returned so that he could recall events of recent weeks and going to the beach, but he was never able to recall the amnestic period (the time from emerging from the surf until his memory cleared).

They returned home after this event and present for review 2 days later.

At this stage there are no physical findings on neurological or cardiac examination and his memory seems fine. He performs well at the MMSE but still has no recollection of what occurred during the amnestic period.

Your more detailed questioning could reveal two alternative possibilities:

R. J. Stark (✉)
Neurology Department, Alfred Hospital, Melbourne, VIC, Australia

Department of Neurosciences, Monash University, Melbourne, VIC, Australia

R. Junckerstorff et al. (eds.), *Beyond Evidence-Based Medicine*,
https://doi.org/10.1007/978-981-99-4440-8_98

Scenario 1: He had never had a similar episode before. His wife gave a very clear history of repeated questioning along the lines "why are we here" during the event. The amnestic period was 6 hours and at the end of it, his memory for events of the previous weeks gradually reappeared. You suspect Transient Global Amnesia (TGA) and arrange MRI brain (which shows a small punctate area of diffusion restriction in the right hippocampus) and an EEG (which is normal).

Scenario 2: He had had similar episodes three times before over the previous 2 years. His wife gave a very clear history of repeated questioning along the lines "why are we here" during the event. The amnestic period was 45 min and at the end of it, his memory for events of the previous weeks gradually reappeared. His wife says that even between events there were some odd "glitches" in his memory. For example, they had been to Bali 5 years earlier on holiday and when she showed him some pictures from that trip 6 months ago, he said he really could not remember it. You suspect Transient Global Amnesia but note some atypical features and arrange MRI brain (which is normal) and an EEG (which is shows an occasional right temporal sharp wave).

3 Discussion

This case demonstrates many of the typical features of TGA.

Diagnostic criteria have been proposed by Hodges and Warlow [1] and are as follows:

1. Attacks must be witnessed.
2. There must be anterograde amnesia during the attack (usually evidenced with repetitive questioning).
3. Cognitive impairment must be limited to amnesia.
4. No clouding of consciousness or loss of personal identity.
5. No focal neurological signs or symptoms.
6. No epileptic features.
7. Attacks must resolve within 24 hours.
8. No recent head injury or active epilepsy.

The key clinical features [2] include complete or near complete loss of encoding new memories (anterograde amnesia) during the episode (as if the "record" button is not working) so that memory for the duration of the event will never reappear. This typically lasts 4–6 hours. In addition, during the event there is inability to recall events from the recent past (weeks to months, sometimes even years), retrograde amnesia, which returns over minutes to hours (often the oldest memories retuning first) at the end of the event. The amnesia is mainly for events (episodic memory) with relatively spared recall for facts such as name or birthdate (semantic memory).

The cause of TGA is not known but as it is frequently triggered by events such as exertion, immersion in cold water, stress, or sexual intercourse. Transient vasospasm has been suggested as a possible cause; vasospasm is not typically found on imaging, however. In some cases, a tiny punctate area of diffusion restriction is seen in the hippocampus (perhaps suggesting ischaemia) but unlike stroke, it is usually not seen immediately after the event but often after a couple of days' delay. Against a vascular cause, patients with TGA have no increase in risk of subsequent stroke or other cardiovascular events.

TGA recurs in only about 10% of cases: a history of recurrent episodes does not exclude the diagnosis but should raise the possibility of another cause.

One alternative diagnosis is transient epileptic amnesia [2, 3] (TEA). This is less common that TGA. The clues to this diagnosis are recurrent episodes, briefer than TGA (typically less than an hour) and sometimes other features to suggest temporal lobe epilepsy (such as olfactory hallucinations). Patients with TEA may display an unusual pattern of patchy auto-biographical amnesia forgetting episodes from earlier life that one would expect to be well-remembered. The EEG may show focal sharp activity (but not always) and the MRI might show focal pathology in the hippocampal region (but not always). Scenario 2 in the case above is suggestive of TEA.

Other causes of acute amnesia are usually easy to diagnose. In post-traumatic amnesia there will be a history of trauma. Stroke causing amnesia is usually associated with other neurological signs and a larger area of abnormality on MRI. Toxic or drug related amnesia is usually associated with fluctuating conscious state and other features of encephalopathy. Psychogenic amnesia should be a diagnosis reached with some caution; especially as stressful events might trigger TGA: with psychogenic amnesia there may be bizarre features such as inability to recall their own name.

4 Take Home Messages

- Details of the history are the key to accurate diagnosis.

References

1. Hodges JR, Warlow CP. Syndromes of transient amnesia: towards a classification. A study of 153 cases. J Neurol Neurosurg Psychiatry. 1990;53:834–43.
2. Miller TD, Butler CR. Acute-onset amnesia: transient global amnesia and other causes. Pract Neurol. 2022;22:201–8.
3. Butler CR, Zeman AZ. Recent insights into the impairment of memory in epilepsy: transient epileptic amnesia, accelerated long-term forgetting and remote memory impairment. Brain. 2008;131:2243–63.

Wasted First Dorsal Interosseous Muscle: What Does It Mean?

Richard J. Stark

1 Clinical Pearl

If a patient reports (or you notice) wasting of the first dorsal interosseous muscle of the hand, there are several possible causes. The most common by far is ulnar neuropathy. This is easily distinguished from most other possibilities by the sparing of the bulk of the thenar muscle group. Of course, a thorough examination should then confirm that other signs are consistent with this hypothesised diagnosis.

2 Clinical Case

A 70-year-old man with type 2 diabetes for many years has noticed in recent months some weakness of the right hand and points out loss of muscle bulk in the webspace between thumb and index finger, indicating the first dorsal interosseous muscle (FDI).

He has some mild numbness in both feet but no complaint of weakness in the lower limbs or left hand.

You suspect that this might be either an ulnar neuropathy or a manifestation of diabetic peripheral neuropathy but are keen to exclude other conditions such as motor neuron disease and plan your clinical examination accordingly.

R. J. Stark (✉)
Neurology Department, Alfred Hospital, Melbourne, VIC, Australia

Department of Neurosciences, Monash University, Melbourne, VIC, Australia

R. Junckerstorff et al. (eds.), *Beyond Evidence-Based Medicine*,
https://doi.org/10.1007/978-981-99-4440-8_99

3 Discussion

This case raises a number of learning points.

3.1 *Ulnar Neuropathy in Patients with Diabetes*

Diabetic peripheral neuropathy produces a susceptibility to compressive mononeuropathies. So, in addition to seeing length dependent changes of neuropathy starting in the feet, it is quite common to see a superimposed ulnar neuropathy from compression of the nerve at the elbow or perhaps carpal tunnel syndrome. It seems that diabetes reduces the nerve's resilience against minor compressive injury. Thus, in a patient like this we would not be surprised to find both signs of peripheral neuropathy (perhaps some wasting of the small muscles of the feet, reduced or absent ankle jerks and distal sensory loss in the feet) and clear signs of ulnar neuropathy. These features would also be apparent on nerve conduction studies with neuropathy in the lower limbs and focal slowing in the ulnar nerve at the elbow.

3.2 *Signs of Ulnar Neuropathy*

Peripheral nerve lesions respect the anatomical distribution of the nerve. It is important to know which muscles are supplied by the ulnar nerve and how to test them [1]. In the hand, the interossei, the hypothenar muscles, the ulnar two lumbricals and the adductor pollicis are supplied by the ulnar nerve but the other three muscles which make up the bulk of the thenar eminence (abductor pollicis brevis, flexor pollicis brevis and opponens pollicis) are not. So, one would expect wasting and weakness of the affected muscles but sparing of the three median innervated thenar muscles with little or no wasting of the thenar eminence.

In the forearm, the flexor digitorum profundus of the ulnar two digits will be involved but long flexors of the thumb, index finger and middle finger will not.

There are some special tests which may emphasise these differentiating features [2].

The Froment sign is well known as an indicator of ulnar neuropathy. It is an example of two muscles normally cooperating to complete an action. Weakness of one component produces an easily observable effect.

In this case, adductor pollicis (ulnar innervated) and flexor pollicis longus (FPL) (supplied by anterior interosseus branch of median nerve) combine when the patient is asked to grip an object forcibly between thumb and the adjacent side of index finger.

While many books advise using a piece of card as the object to grip, a simple way to do the test without any equipment is to ask the patient to hold the palms of the two hands together. The examiner then slides the ulnar border of his/her own hand under the patient's thumbs and over the radial aspect of the index fingers and asks the patient to grip the palm (Fig. 1).

Normally the thumbs adopt a semiflexed posture, but if there is an ulnar neuropathy on one side, the thumb on that side becomes more flexed than normal due to the unopposed action of FPL. However, if there is an anterior interosseous nerve (or high median nerve) palsy the affected thumb remains extended.

Another easily observed sign is the Wartenberg sign. If the interosseous muscle between the ring and little finger is weak (as it is with an ulnar neuropathy), the little finger tends to drift away from the ring finger so that a gap is visible between them at rest.

The "ulnar claw" refers to the posture of extension of the metacarpophalangeal joints and flexion of the interphalangeal joints in the little and ring fingers more than the index and middle fingers. It results from weakness of IP joint extension in the ulnar two digits as their lumbrical muscles are supplied by the ulnar nerve and there is unopposed action of flexor digitorum superficialis (which is supplied by the median nerve for all fingers).

Of course, one would search for sensory loss in the typical ulnar distribution too. In real-life clinical practice the edge of the sensory loss may not be so clearly down the midline of the ring finger as textbooks would suggest but reduction of sensation in the little finger when compared with the middle or index finger is typical.

Ulnar nerve compression at the elbow would typically not produce any definite reflex changes.

Sometimes the ulnar nerve is palpably thickened in the ulnar groove at the elbow. It only takes a moment to check on this. If you check for this often, you will have a good idea of how thick the nerve is normally.

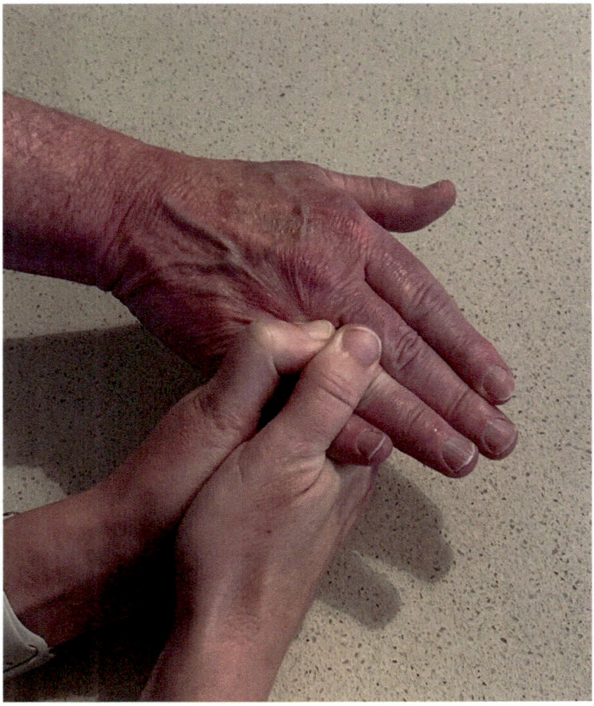

Fig. 1 Froment sign showing prominent flexion of the left thumb IP joint suggesting ulnar neuropathy

3.3 What Signs Would Raise the Question of Another Cause?

Peripheral neuropathy without superimposed compressive mononeuropathy would typically involve median and ulnar innervated muscles equally, so the thenar muscles such as abductor pollicis brevis will be involved to the same extent as FDI. Both hands would usually be affected. Sensory loss would be distal (glove) rather than in the distribution of a single nerve.

Lower trunk plexopathies (such as Pancoast syndrome) would also involve both median and ulnar innervated muscles.

Motor neuron disease often produces an unusual pattern of weakness, the "split hand syndrome" [3]. This refers to disproportionate weakness on the radial side of the hand (involving both FDI and the thenar group) compared with relative sparing of the hypothenar muscles. Other clues in favour of motor neuron disease would be the absence of sensory signs and the presence of brisk reflexes in the wasted limb.

Some unusual spinal disorders result in selective damage to the anterior horn cells of the lower cervical cord. T2 hyperintensities in this region may look like "snake eyes" on axial MRI images [4]. These conditions tend to cause a gradation of severity of motor loss over several myotomes (for example C8 & T1 severely affected, C7 moderately and C6 mildly affected) with little sensory change. This pattern may occur in Hirayama disease or when the cord is compressed resulting in ischaemic injury—the anterior horn cells seem unusually sensitive to this.

C8 or T1 radiculopathy would usually involve median and ulnar innervated muscles in various combinations, and so differ from the highly selective distribution of weakness seen in ulnar neuropathy.

4 Take Home Messages

- The commonest (but not the only) cause of wasted first dorsal interosseous muscle is ulnar neuropathy.

References

1. O'Brien M. Aids to the examination of the peripheral nervous system. 5th ed. Saunders Ltd.; 2010. ISBN: 9780702034473.
2. Goldman SB, Brininger TL, Schrader JW, Curtis R, Koceja DM. Analysis of clinical motor testing for adult patients with diagnosed ulnar neuropathy at the elbow. Arch Phys Med Rehabil. 2009;90(11):1846–52. https://doi.org/10.1016/j.apmr.2009.06.007. PMID: 19887207.
3. Corcia P, Bede P, Pradat P, et al. Split-hand and split-limb phenomena in amyotrophic lateral sclerosis: pathophysiology, electrophysiology and clinical manifestations. J Neurol Neurosurg Psychiatry. 2021;92:1126–30.
4. Foster E, Tsang BKT, Kam A, Stark RJ. Mechanisms of upper limb amyotrophy in spinal disorders. J Clin Neurosci. 2014;21:1209–14. https://doi.org/10.1016/j.jocn.2013.10.035.

Part XIV
Stroke

Waking with a Weak Hand: Cortical Stroke Versus Radial Palsy

Richard J. Stark

1 Clinical Pearl

Waking with a weak and clumsy hand could be the result of a cortical stroke or a "Saturday night palsy". Distinguishing between the two is aided by good examination technique, remembering the detail of the motor supply of the radial nerve, and knowing how subtle cortical dysfunction may present. The general principles are:

1. Peripheral nerve lesions respect the anatomical distribution of the nerve.
2. Cortical motor loss involves disproportionate loss of dexterity (beyond what would be expected from the degree of weakness) and does not respect peripheral nerve distributions.

2 Clinical Case

A 40-year-old man presents with clumsiness and weakness of his left hand. He had been drinking at a friend's house the previous night and slept on the friend's couch rather than drive home. He woke with the left-hand problem. He has a past history of hypertension and often omits his medication. There is a strong family history of ischaemic heart disease and stroke.

An emergency physician describes weakness of the left-hand worst in wrist and finger extension but also apparently involving finger abduction and causing a weak grip. Reflexes and sensation are reported to be normal. Neurological examination is normal except for the left upper limb.

Your examination could reveal two alternative sets of signs:

R. J. Stark (✉)
Neurology Department, Alfred Hospital, Melbourne, VIC, Australia

Department of Neurosciences, Monash University, Melbourne, VIC, Australia

R. Junckerstorff et al. (eds.), *Beyond Evidence-Based Medicine*,
https://doi.org/10.1007/978-981-99-4440-8_100

Scenario 1: The outstretched left arm is held in flexion at the wrist and fingers. Power in left wrist extension is Grade 1 as is power of extension of the metacarpophalangeal (MP) joints. Grip strength seems reduced as does finger abduction but when the wrist is supported in the neutral position, normal power in finger abduction and flexion can be demonstrated. When power is tested at the proximal interphalangeal (PIP) joints, it is found to be normal. Brachioradialis does not contract normally on the left (remember it is not easy to detect reduced power in brachioradialis—you have to look at it and feel it to see if it is contracting properly) but triceps power is normal. Rapid alternating finger movements are performed with some difficulty because of weakness. Reflexes are normal except that with the left brachioradialis/supinator jerk, activation of brachioradialis is not seen. Because the signs suggest radial nerve palsy, sensation is tested over the dorsal webspace between left thumb and index finger and is reduced in the typical distribution of the radial nerve.

Scenario 2: The outstretched left arm drifts slightly into pronation and into flexion at the fingers. Power in left wrist extension is Grade 3 as is power of extension of the MP joints. Grip strength seems reduced and finger abduction is Grade 1. When the wrist is supported in the neutral position, power in finger abduction and flexion is not improved. When power of extension is tested at the PIP joints, it is found to be Grade 2. Brachioradialis contracts normally on the left and in fact power at the elbow and shoulder are normal. Rapid alternating finger movements are performed very poorly with markedly impaired dexterity. Reflexes are normal and tone is normal except for an equivocal spastic catch with rapid supination. Because the signs suggest a possible upper motor neuron lesion, sensation testing includes graphaesthesia and stereognosis which are very slightly impaired. Because the signs are consistent with a cortical stroke, the patient is investigated and managed according to the stroke pathway and a cortical stroke is later confirmed on MRI imaging.

3 Discussion

This case raises a number of learning points [1].

3.1 Motor Signs of Radial Palsy

Presentation with wrist drop can sometimes cause surprising diagnostic difficulty, even when the history is highly suggestive of 'Saturday night palsy' of the radial nerve. Patients with wrist drop from radial nerve palsy may have difficulty activating intrinsic muscles of the hand such as interossei while the wrist is in flexion. This may raise the question of a more proximal lesion or even a cortical stroke. The apparent weakness of the intrinsics can usually be improved by supporting the wrist in a neutral position.

However, the most convincing clinical evidence that the radial nerve is at fault comes from comparison of power of extension at the MP joints with that at the IP joints. Extension of the MP joints is performed by the long extensors of the forearm (supplied by the radial nerve) while extension at the IP joints is done by lumbricals supplied by median and ulnar nerves.

This requires precise technique, stabilising by gripping just proximal to the joint to be tested and resisting the attempted extension just distal to the joint. The principle is: when testing power, test over one joint at a time.

Prominent weakness of MP joint extension with preserved power at IP joint extension is highly suggestive of radial nerve dysfunction: more proximal lesions do not produce this pattern.

Further support that the radial nerve is the culprit is provided by weakness of brachioradialis (again, the muscle must be observed and palpated during activation against resistance) with preserved power in other elbow flexors.

3.2 *Loss of Dexterity as an Indicator of Upper Motor Neurone (UMN) Dysfunction*

A very sensitive sign of UMN weakness in the upper limb is loss of dexterity. This can be tested in many ways, but a simple method is to ask the patient to place their index and ring fingers on the back of their other hand and to raise and lower them alternately as fast as they can (run on the spot with the fingers).

This is recommended as a routine part of the examination for every patient. Of course, slowing of rapid alternating movements may occur in other conditions such as bradykinesia of Parkinson's disease or as part of dysdiadokokinesia in cerebellar disorders. It is therefore a screening tool and the cause for slowing must be clarified by the rest of the examination.

Sometimes a patient will present with weakness largely confined to the hand and it may not be clear whether this is an upper motor neuron problem (such as a small cortical lesion or cervical cord abnormality) or a peripheral problem. If dexterity is disproportionately affected compared with power, this suggests UMN disorder.

3.3 *Checking for Pronator Drift*

It is helpful and efficient to start the motor examination with a screening test which might identify or suggest specific deficits. A useful method for the upper limbs is to look for pronator drift: this technique may reveal a range of motor and other abnormalities.

Method: Ask the patient to lift their arms in front to the horizontal, turn the palms upwards, close eyes and hold this position for a few seconds.

Overshoot and "bounce" as an arm is elevated may suggest ipsilateral cerebellar dysfunction.
Drift of the arm up or laterally suggests proprioceptive impairment proximally.
Drift of the arm down suggests weakness.
Drift down with prominent drift into pronation or into flexion of fingers or elbow suggests the weakness may be pyramidal in type.
Surprisingly severe drift of this type when weakness is mild suggests concurrent proprioceptive loss.
Fine irregular finger movements (pseudoathetosis) suggest proprioceptive loss in the fingers.

This information, obtained within a few seconds, while not definitively diagnostic, can direct the examiner to look carefully for signs relevant to the observed features.

3.4 Plan the Sensory Examination

The sensory examination is a powerful tool at testing hypotheses as the examination can be directed to the relevant diagnostic points. It is of very little value as a general and unfocussed data gathering exercise. Hence a key rule of the neurological examination is: "Never do a sensory examination until you know what you will find, or at least what you are looking for".

The nature of sensory testing will be very different if a cortical problem is suspected (graphaesthesia and stereognosis might be tested) compared with a peripheral nerve disorder. In the latter, the distribution of sensory loss is the key to localisation so the edges of any area of loss should be explored intelligently.

4 Take Home Messages

- Some anatomical knowledge, knowing what to look for and precise examination technique are the keys in this case.

Reference

1. Stark RJ. Tips for trainees: some practical tips on clinical examination. Pract Neurol. 2020;20:489–93. http://pn.bmj.com/cgi/content/full/practneurol-2020-002659v1?ct.

Acute Onset Painful Upper or Lower Extremity Limb Weakness Is Unlikely to Be Due to Stroke

Channa Senanayake and Shaloo Singhal

1 Clinical Pearl

Stroke is a common cause of sudden onset motor deficits. However, pain at the onset of stroke is rare. Presence of sudden pain associated with motor deficits should prompt consideration of other differential diagnoses.

2 Clinical Case

A 65-year-old right hand dominant female calls an ambulance after developing an acute painful weakness of the right arm. The ambulance notifies the receiving hospital about a potential stoke and on arrival to the emergency department, a "Code Stroke" is activated to allow for rapid evaluation of the patient by the stroke team. The patient is noted to be in new-onset atrial fibrillation. On assessment, the patient describes sudden onset pain and weakness of the right arm. On examination the right arm is markedly weak with no antigravity power proximally and marked weakness of all muscle groups of the hand. The patient appears distressed due to pain and the sensory examination reveals patchy light touch sensory loss. Further examination reveals no focal neurological deficits in the contralateral arm nor lower limbs or cranial nerves. The patient undergoes urgent multimodal stroke imaging (non-contrast Computed Tomography (CT) brain, CT angiogram and CT perfusion) which do not demonstrate any abnormalities. If caused by a stroke the significant right arm weakness is likely to result in permanent disability, thus thrombolysis is

C. Senanayake · S. Singhal (✉)
Department of General Medicine, Eastern Health, Melbourne, VIC, Australia

Stroke and Aging Research Group, School of Clinical Sciences, Monash University, Melbourne, VIC, Australia

R. Junckerstorff et al. (eds.), *Beyond Evidence-Based Medicine*,
https://doi.org/10.1007/978-981-99-4440-8_101

considered. Further examination is conducted after stroke imaging which reveals a pale right arm with prolonged capillary refill and the radial pulse is noted to be absent. The patient is subsequently diagnosed with acute ischaemia of right arm and undergoes an urgent CT angiogram of thoracic aorta, which demonstrates an acute thromboembolic occlusion of the right subclavian artery. The Electrocardiogram (ECG) demonstrates atrial fibrillation without acute ischaemic changes. The patient is referred to the vascular team for ongoing management.

3 Discussion

The differential diagnosis of isolated upper extremity weakness includes vascular, neurological, and traumatic causes.

Vascular aetiology is typically due to arterial occlusion but can also be due to extensive deep venous thrombosis. Arterial occlusion presentations are associated with the "six Ps" (pain, pallor, poikilothermia, pulselessness, paraesthesia, and paralysis). Arterial occlusion can be due to thromboembolism, dissection, hypercoagulability, atherosclerotic plaque, or aneurysm. CT angiogram is the investigation of choice for diagnosis and planning management. In the above clinical case, the presence of new onset atrial fibrillation favours thromboembolism. Deep venous thrombosis usually presents with a hot painful swelling of the limb associated with a raised D-dimer. Muscle power is relatively spared. A venous Doppler ultrasound of the limb is adequate to make the diagnosis.

Neurological causes of upper extremity weakness can be divided in to central and peripheral causes.

3.1 Central Causes

Central causes include stroke, spinal cord pathology and polyradiculopathy.

Isolated upper limb weakness due to stroke is a relatively rare stroke presentation. A study of 7643 stroke patients demonstrated that only 1.1% presented with isolated upper limb weakness [1]. Refer to the previous clinical pearl for a detailed discussion of cortical stroke.

Many intrinsic spinal cord pathologies and extrinsic compression of the spinal cord can lead to painful upper extremity weakness. Intrinsic lesions include demyelination, inflammation (myelitis) and neoplasms. Extrinsic pathologies include trauma, infection (epidural abscess), haemorrhage and degenerative disorders such as disc protrusions.

Polyradiculopathy typically presents with chronic, progressive symptoms however more acute presentations are possible. Spinal cord pathology and polyradiculopathy are associated with corresponding lower motor neuron signs at the level of the lesion and in the case of spinal cord lesions, upper motor neuron signs below the level of the lesion.

3.2 *Peripheral Causes*

Peripheral causes include Parsonage-Turner syndrome (neuralgic amyotrophy) and peripheral nerve lesions. Parsonage-Turner syndrome is characterised by rapid onset severe pain involving the shoulder and arm associated with weakness, sensory changes with examination demonstrating lower motor neuron signs. Diagnosis is clinical together with supportive evidence from nerve conduction studies and electromyography.

3.3 *Pain Due to Stroke Is Usually Delayed in Onset*

Stroke involving the spinothalamic or trigeminothalamic pathways can result in centrally mediated pain. These pathways are responsible for pain and temperature sensation. Common stroke types that result in damage to these pathways include thalamic stroke and the lateral medullary syndrome. Only 18% of thalamic strokes [2] and 14% of lateral medullary strokes [3] present with pain at the onset of stroke. Isolated upper extremity weakness with these stroke subtypes is highly unlikely.

The thalamus is a densely packed mass of grey matter containing nuclei that serve arousal, all major sensory domains except the sense of smell, motor function and aspects of language, cognition, mood and motivation [4]. Vascular lesions of the thalamus will produce sensorimotor and behavioural syndromes depending on the combination of nuclei damaged.

Lateral medullary syndrome results in damage to the vestibular nuclei (vomiting, vertigo, nystagmus), inferior cerebellar peduncle (ipsilateral incoordination), central tegmental tract (palatal myoclonus), lateral spinothalamic tract (contralateral loss of pain and temperature sensation of limbs and torso), spinal trigeminal tract (ipsilateral loss of pain and temperature sensation of the face), nucleus ambiguus (ipsilateral pharyngeal, laryngeal, and palatal paralysis), and descending sympathetic fibres (ipsilateral Horner's syndrome).

References

1. Topcuoglu MA, Rocha EA, Siddiqui AK, Mills BB, Silva GS, Schwamm LH, et al. Isolated upper limb weakness from ischemic stroke: mechanisms and outcome. J Stroke Cerebrovasc Dis. 2018;27(10):2712–9.
2. Nasreddine ZS, Saver JL. Pain after thalamic stroke: right diencephalic predominance and clinical features in 180 patients. Neurology. 1997;48(5):1196–9.
3. Andersen G, Vestergaard K, Ingeman-Nielsen M, Jensen TS. Incidence of central post-stroke pain. Pain. 1995;61(2):187–93.
4. Schmahmann JD. Vascular syndromes of the thalamus. Stroke. 2003;34(9):2264–78.

Thunderclap Headache Requires Urgent Investigation and Management

Channa Senanayake and Shaloo Singhal

1 Clinical Pearl

A "Thunderclap headache" refers to a sudden onset severe headache. The onset of headache and maximal intensity is reached suddenly, analogous to the cracking of thunder. Thunderclap headache is associated with serious intracranial pathologies. Early diagnosis and intervention are vital to maximise patient outcomes.

2 Clinical Case

A forty year-old male wakes in the morning at 5 am with severe headache. He takes paracetamol and ibuprofen, but the headache does not resolve after several hours. He has difficulty concentrating at work and concerned colleagues encourage him to go to hospital. On assessment in the Emergency Department (ED) he is alert, Glasgow Coma Scale (GCS) is 15, temperature 37.2 °C, heart rate 120 beats per minute, respiratory rate 24, and blood pressure 200/110 mmHg. He describes this headache as the worst of his life with sudden severe generalised pain reaching maximum intensity within seconds. He appears distracted and difficult to engage, denies visual changes, and answers appropriately in short sentences. There is no papilloedema and no focal neurological findings are noted on cranial nerve, upper limb, and lower limb examination. His headache responds to treatment with opiate analgesia and after 6 hours it gradually resolves. Routine blood tests are normal and a

C. Senanayake · S. Singhal (✉)
Department of General Medicine, Eastern Health, Melbourne, VIC, Australia

Stroke and Aging Research Group, School of Clinical Sciences, Monash University, Melbourne, VIC, Australia

R. Junckerstorff et al. (eds.), *Beyond Evidence-Based Medicine*,
https://doi.org/10.1007/978-981-99-4440-8_102

non-contrast Computed Tomography (CT) scan of his brain performed 12 hours after symptom onset is reported as normal. He is discharged home with instructions to return if the headache returns. The next day he returns with recurrent thunderclap headache. Examination finding are similar but this time he undergoes a non-contrast CT brain and CT angiogram. These investigations demonstrate a subarachnoid haemorrhage (SAH) and a 5 mm left anterior communicating artery aneurysm. Referral is made to neurosurgery and he undergoes urgent digital subtraction angiography and coiling of the aneurysm.

3 Discussion

Headache is common with a prevalence of approximately 90% in the general population [1]. Migraines and tension headaches make up the majority of headache presentations to health professionals. Thunderclap headache is comparatively rare with an incidence of 43 per 100,000 adults per year [1]. Any thunderclap headache even in a patient with a history of benign headaches such as migraines must be taken seriously. It is associated with medical emergencies, most commonly sub-arachnoid haemorrhage (SAH). Thunderclap headaches have an explosive onset and reaches a peak intensity within 1 min or less [2]. Careful history taking is important as "sudden onset headache" is a subjective term to both patients and physicians which can lead to diagnostic error. The mode of onset and severity can be determined by asking how quickly did the headache start? How severe is the headache? And how quickly did the headache peak? Approximately 50% of patients with a SAH report a thunderclap headache. Please see Table 1 for other causes of thunderclap headache.

Thunderclap headaches can be associated with a variety of other clinical signs often giving a clue to the underlying aetiology. Neck stiffness is associated with SAH and meningitis. In SAH the neck stiffness is caused by breakdown of blood products resulting in aseptic meningitis. This process takes time thus the onset of meningism in SAH is often delayed by hours. Transient vision loss may be a feature of SAH.

Ipsilateral Horner's syndrome, pulsatile tinnitus and ipsilateral tongue palsy is associated with internal carotid artery dissection. Surgical third nerve palsy which is a dilated pupil involving oculomotor palsy is commonly associated with a posterior communicating artery aneurysm. Patients with raised intracranial pressure may

Table 1 Alternative causes of thunderclap headache

Reversible vasoconstriction syndrome
Meningitis
Cerebral venous sinus thrombosis
Cervical artery dissection
Posterior reversible leukoencephalopathy

have papilloedema, raised blood pressure, and avoid lying flat. History of trauma is suggestive of arterial dissection and fever is associated with meningitis.

Resolution of thunderclap headache does not signify benign aetiology. As demonstrated in the above clinical case, patients often experience thunderclap headache days to weeks prior to SAH, the so-called sentinel headache, which heralds later presentation with major SAH. Sentinel headache maybe due to a smaller 'warning leak' or changes in the vessel wall of the aneurysm. A retrospective study by Linn et al demonstrated that sentinel thunderclap headache occurs in up to 25% of SAH patients [3]. Patients with Reversible Vasoconstriction Syndrome (RCVS) often present with recurrent thunderclap headache over days to weeks with resolution of headache in between episodes. RCVS is commonly seen in the post-partum period and after exposure to adrenergic or serotonergic drugs and cannabis. Patients with RCVS may provide a history of triggers such as orgasm, physical exertion, coughing, swimming, or emotional distress.

With respect to investigation of thunderclap headache, it is very important to recognise that a normal non-contrast CT brain does not rule out serious pathology.

The sensitivity of a non-contrast CT brain for SAH is 95.5–100% when performed within 6 hours of onset of the headache and reported by a consultant radiologist [4, 5]. The sensitivity declines when CT brain is performed greater than 6 hours after the onset of symptoms [6]. It is unclear whether CT brain performed within 6 hours is adequate to conclusively rule out SAH. When clinical suspicion is high or when more than 6 hours have elapsed from time of symptom onset, we recommend performing lumbar puncture (LP) with measurement of the opening pressure and examining the cerebrospinal fluid (CSF) for red blood cells (RBC) and xanthochromia. When RBCs are present in the CSF for greater than 2 hours, they begin to lyse leading to degradation of haemoglobin contained within cells. These degradation products are detected as xanthochromia. Thus, performing LP too early can lead to falsely negative xanthochromia. When cerebrospinal fluid is analysed after 12 hours, the sensitivity of xanthochromia for the detection of SAH is 100% [7].

RCVS is characterised by diffuse cerebral arterial vasospasm that typically resolves within 3 months. Non contrast CT brain is usually normal, however 25% of patients may have a convexity SAH. This is a SAH occurring in the sulcal spaces near the cerebral convexities and is not due to aneurysmal haemorrhage. Patients may also demonstrate cerebral infarcts. The diagnosis of RCVS requires cerebral arterial imaging with either CT angiography, magnetic resonance angiography or digital subtraction angiography. The diagnostic features are widespread beading of cerebral arteries. Vasoconstriction typically spreads from distal to proximal vessels which can be a dynamic process. The initial angiogram maybe normal in up to 21% of cases [8]. When clinical suspicion is high, a repeat CT angiogram or MRI performed within few days may provide evidence of vasoconstriction.

References

1. Ducros A, Bousser MG. Thunderclap headache. BMJ. 2013;346:e8557.
2. Headache Classification Committee of the International Headache Society (IHS). The International Classification of Headache Disorders, 3rd edition. Cephalalgia. 2018;38(1):1–211.
3. Linn FH, Wijdicks EF, van der Graaf Y, Weerdesteyn-van Vliet FA, Bartelds AI, van Gijn J. Prospective study of sentinel headache in aneurysmal subarachnoid haemorrhage. Lancet. 1994;344(8922):590–3.
4. Perry JJ, Sivilotti MLA, Emond M, Hohl CM, Khan M, Lesiuk H, et al. Prospective implementation of the Ottawa subarachnoid hemorrhage rule and 6-hour computed tomography rule. Stroke. 2020;51(2):424–30.
5. Perry JJ, Stiell IG, Sivilotti ML, Bullard MJ, Emond M, Symington C, et al. Sensitivity of computed tomography performed within six hours of onset of headache for diagnosis of subarachnoid haemorrhage: prospective cohort study. BMJ. 2011;343:d4277.
6. Backes D, Rinkel GJ, Kemperman H, Linn FH, Vergouwen MD. Time-dependent test characteristics of head computed tomography in patients suspected of nontraumatic subarachnoid hemorrhage. Stroke. 2012;43(8):2115–9.
7. Vermeulen M, Hasan D, Blijenberg BG, Hijdra A, van Gijn J. Xanthochromia after subarachnoid haemorrhage needs no revisitation. J Neurol Neurosurg Psychiatry. 1989;52(7):826–8.
8. Ducros A, Boukobza M, Porcher R, Sarov M, Valade D, Bousser MG. The clinical and radiological spectrum of reversible cerebral vasoconstriction syndrome. A prospective series of 67 patients. Brain. 2007;130(Pt 12):3091–101.

Subcortical Infarcts Can Have a Stuttering Course Leading to Progressive Worsening of Deficits

Channa Senanayake and Shaloo Singhal

1 Clinical Pearl

Patients with subcortical infarcts can have stuttering onset of symptoms and progress over a few minutes to hours and sometimes over days. They are often preceded by transient ischemic attacks with similar symptoms. Patients can have minor stroke deficits initially and may even be assessed for early discharge from hospital only to experience progressive deficits. Patients with minor stroke deficits, especially ones with lacunar stroke syndromes, should be warned about potential worsening of symptoms despite institution of adequate preventative therapies.

2 Clinical Case

A 65-year old man with poorly controlled type 2 diabetes mellitus and hypertension experiences transient right face, arm, and leg weakness lasting 20 min. He presents to hospital where he is assessed as having a transient ischaemic attack. He undergoes non contrast computed tomography (CT) of the brain which does not show any evidence of recent infarction or haemorrhage. He is commenced on aspirin and high dose atorvastatin. He is discharged home with early outpatient carotid ultrasound which does not demonstrate significant internal carotid artery stenosis. One week later he represents with similar symptoms of right face, arm, and leg weakness. He undergoes acute multi-modal stroke imaging consisting of non-contrast CT brain, CT angiogram and CT perfusion. Stroke imaging reveals no signs of recent

C. Senanayake · S. Singhal (✉)
Department of Neurology, Eastern Health, Melbourne, VIC, Australia

Stroke and Aging Research Group, School of Clinical Sciences, Monash University, Melbourne, VIC, Australia

R. Junckerstorff et al. (eds.), *Beyond Evidence-Based Medicine*,
https://doi.org/10.1007/978-981-99-4440-8_103

infarction or haemorrhage, no large vessel occlusion, and no perfusion deficit. His symptoms rapidly improve, and assessment reveals a National Institute of Health Stroke Scale (NIHSS) score of 1 for minor right facial droop. Due to the non-disabling features of stroke, he does not receive acute reperfusion therapy with alteplase. He is admitted for observation in hospital overnight and discharged the next day with a diagnosis of pure motor lacunar infarct. Several hours later he returns with worsening of his symptoms. On this occasion his stroke severity NIHSS score is 5 (right facial droop 2, right arm weakness 2, and dysarthria 1) and he is unable to walk. He undergoes acute multi-modal stroke imaging which again demonstrates no abnormalities. He is admitted to hospital for observation. Subsequent Magnetic Resonance Imaging (MRI) brain demonstrates left posterior limb of internal capsule lacunar infarct.

3 Discussion

3.1 Subcortical Infarcts Can Have a Stuttering Course and Recognition of This Stroke Subtype Is Important for Patient Management

Subcortical infarcts can initially present with minor stroke deficits. In the Harvard Stroke Registry, 20% of stroke patients progressed after onset either gradually (10%) or in a stepwise manner (10%) [1]. Subcortical infarcts are responsible for the highest proportion of patients that experience progression of symptoms in hospital [2]. Patients with subcortical infarcts are often diagnosed with a minor stroke (stroke with mild non-disabling symptoms) initially, and most will stabilise. However, clinicians should be aware that a small percentage of such patients may deteriorate further.

Subcortical infarcts are located in the deep white matter or in the brainstem. Acute infarcts can be up to 20 mm in diameter and chronic infarcts are typically 2–15 mm in diameter [3]. After infarction the lesions shrinks as a result of liquefaction necrosis. Subcortical infarcts occur due to occlusion of a single perforator branch of a large cerebral artery. Pathophysiological mechanisms of perforator vessel occlusion can vary from small vessel disease due to long standing risk factors such as hypertension, artery to artery embolisation (as is the case in internal carotid artery atherosclerosis), or a cardio-embolic source. Thus, these patients should undergo a thorough screen for potentially treatable rick factors, such as atrial fibrillation or carotid stenosis.

Subcortical infarcts can often be recognised by the pattern of stroke symptoms. Five typical syndromes have been described in the literature (Table 1). These are pure motor, pure sensory, ataxic hemiparesis, sensorimotor and dysarthria clumsy hand syndrome. Due to the subcortical or brainstem location of the infarct, they do

Table 1 The five types of subcortical infarcts

Stroke syndrome	Symptoms	Infarct location
Pure motor hemiparesis	Contralateral face, arm and leg weakness without cortical signs	Posterior limb of Internal Capsule
Pure Sensory	Contralateral numbness of face, arm and leg without cortical signs	Thalamus
Ataxic Hemiparesis	Contralateral limb ataxia and weakness without cortical signs	Internal capsule, Pons or corona radiata
Sensorimotor Stroke	Contralateral weakness and numbness and face, arm and leg without cortical signs	Thalamus and adjacent posterior limb of Internal Capsule
Dysarthria-clumsy hand syndrome	Contralateral facial weakness, dysarthria, dysphasia and dysmetria/ataxia of upper limb	Pons or Genu of Internal Capsule

not exhibit signs of cortical dysfunction such as aphasia, hemianopia, neglect, agnosia, or apraxia.

Pure motor is the most common lacunar syndrome which accounts for almost half of subcortical strokes [4]. Pure motor lacunar infarcts typically result in hemiparesis of the face, arm and leg without any sensory features.

The second most common syndrome accounting for 20% of cases is pure sensory [4]. The characteristic feature is pure numbness on one side of the body involving the face, arm and leg without motor features.

Ataxic hemiparesis is characterised by hemiparesis on one side of the body accompanied by ataxia of the same side that is out of proportion to the motor deficit. Patients with ataxic hemiparesis may also have nystagmus, dysarthria, and gait deviation to the affected side but, as with all lacunar syndromes, will lack cortical signs.

Sensorimotor syndrome is characterised by face, arm, and leg hemiparesis and numbness.

Finally, dysarthria clumsy hand syndrome is the least common syndrome [4]. Typical features include facial droop, dysarthria, dysphagia, and ipsilateral clumsiness of the hand.

3.2 CT Brain Can Be Normal in Acute Subcortical Infarction

Up to two thirds of acute subcortical infarcts are not detected on non-contrast CT brain [5]. Detection is lower when CT is performed closer to the time of onset of symptoms. Even modern multi-modal imaging techniques are insensitive with up to 50% of cases failing to be identified on CT perfusion [6]. Thus, diffusion weighted MRI imaging is often required to make an imaging diagnosis of a subcortical infarct. Risk factors for progression of symptoms include diabetes mellitus, the severity of motor deficits at onset and the size of infarct seen on MRI diffusion weighted imaging [7]. Key principles of patient management include early diagnosis and initiation of antiplatelets, close patient observation, as well as nuanced discussions with the patient regarding potential for neurological deterioration.

References

1. Mohr JP, Caplan LR, et al. The Harvard Cooperative Stroke Registry: a prospective registry. Neurology. 1978;28:754–62.
2. Steinke W, Ley SC. Lacunar stroke is the major cause of progressive motor deficits. Stroke. 2002;33(6):1510–6.
3. Regenhardt RW, Das AS, Lo EH, Caplan LR. Advances in understanding the pathophysiology of lacunar stroke: a review. JAMA Neurol. 2018;75(10):1273–81.
4. Schonewille WJ, Tuhrim S, Singer MB, Atlas SW. Diffusion-weighted MRI in acute lacunar syndromes. A clinical-radiological correlation study. Stroke. 1999;30(10):2066–9.
5. Hommel M, Besson G, Le Bas JF, Gaio JM, Pollak P, Borgel F, et al. Prospective study of lacunar infarction using magnetic resonance imaging. Stroke. 1990;21(4):546–54.
6. Benson JC, Payabvash S, Mortazavi S, Zhang L, Salazar P, Hoffman B, et al. CT perfusion in acute lacunar stroke: detection capabilities based on infarct location. AJNR Am J Neuroradiol. 2016;37(12):2239–44.
7. Nakamura K, Saku Y, Ibayashi S, Fujishima M. Progressive motor deficits in lacunar infarction. Neurology. 1999;52(1):29–33.

Limb Shaking Transient Ischaemic Attack Is Frequently Mistaken for Focal Epilepsy

Channa Senanayake and Shaloo Singhal

1 Clinical Pearl

In the field of neurology, the term 'positive symptoms' reflect an excess of normal function (e.g. clonic jerking, abnormal movements, visual scintillations), whereas 'negative symptoms' refer to an absence of normal function (e.g. paralysis, loss of sensation, hemianopia). Stroke mimics such as migraines and seizures usually present with 'positive' symptoms while stroke usually result in 'negative' symptoms. Notable exceptions include limb shaking transient ischemic attacks (TIA) and acute hemichorea or hemiballismus.

2 Clinical Case

A 50-year-old man presents to the emergency department for recurrent episodes of abrupt onset left upper limb shaking that started 2 weeks ago. He is a current smoker and has a history of type 2 diabetes mellitus, hypertension, and chronic kidney disease. He describes brief episodes of whole left upper limb involuntary jerking lasting a few seconds to a few minutes. The onset and course of each episode is not stereotyped, and they are not associated with impaired conscious state, jerking of other limbs or his face. The episodes have no specific trigger but happen more frequently when standing. The episodes always resolve spontaneously, and the left upper limb function returns to normal immediately after the episode. On examination his Glasgow Coma Score is 15 and his vital signs are within normal limits. His

C. Senanayake · S. Singhal (✉)
Department of Neurology, Eastern Health, Melbourne, VIC, Australia

Stroke and Aging Research Group, School of Clinical Sciences, Monash University, Melbourne, VIC, Australia

R. Junckerstorff et al. (eds.), *Beyond Evidence-Based Medicine*,
https://doi.org/10.1007/978-981-99-4440-8_104

blood sugar is also normal. Cranial nerves are intact, upper and lower limb tone, sensorimotor exam, coordination and deep tendon reflexes are normal. Routine blood tests including thyroid function and non-contrast Computed Tomography (CT) brain reveal no abnormalities. He is diagnosed with focal motor seizures and admitted to the neurology ward. He is commenced on levetiracetam 250 mg twice daily, but the episodes of shaking continue. Subsequent Electroencephalogram (EEG) demonstrates normal background without epileptiform discharges. Gadolinium enhanced Magnetic Resonance Imaging (MRI) brain does not reveal an epileptogenic focus or stroke. MRI time of flight sequences demonstrate low flow signal in the right internal carotid artery (ICA). The patient then undergoes a CT angiogram of the neck which confirms 90% stenosis of the right ICA. Diagnosis of limb shaking TIA is considered and antihypertensive therapy with hydrochlorothiazide is discontinued. This leads to symptomatic improvement, and he is referred to a vascular surgeon for consideration of a right carotid endarterectomy.

3 Discussion

3.1 Limb Shaking TIA Is an Underrecognised Stroke Presentation

Limb shaking TIA was first described by Miller Fisher in 1962 [1]. It is frequently misdiagnosed as a focal motor seizure [2]. Classical descriptions include non-rhythmic flailing or jerking of limbs (upper and/or lower limbs) contralateral to the stenotic ICA lesion. The episodes usually last for seconds to minutes with abrupt onset/offset and can occur several times per day. There is no Jacksonian march, which is seen in focal motor seizures, where there is gradual spreading muscle activity starting distally and then ascending proximally to the face. Todd's paresis is also absent which is a common syndrome that produces weakness of part of the body following a seizure. Additionally, impaired consciousness is notably absent. The exact pathophysiological cause of limb shaking TIA is unknown, however it is postulated to be due to hypoperfusion of the brain caused by ICA stenosis. This results in dysfunction of cortico-subcortical pathways connecting the thalamus, basal ganglia, and cerebellum that act to adjust postural tone and movement [3]. Recognition of this syndrome is vital as prompt institution of adequate preventative measures and where indicated, vascular surgery will result in lower subsequent stroke risk [2].

3.2 *Movement Disorders in Acute Stroke*

Movement disorders secondary to stroke are rare, occurring in 1–4% of cases [4]. Stroke can produce a wide range of movement disorders including hemichorea-hemiballismus, dystonia, tremor, asterixis and parkinsonism. Most occur over a period of months to years rather than acutely [5].

Occasionally, both ischaemic and haemorrhagic stroke can produce movement disorders on presentation. The most common acute onset movement disorder following stroke is hemichorea-hemiballismus syndrome [5]. Hemichorea and hemiballismus are often used interchangeably. It refers to continuous involuntary movement of usually one side of the body contralateral to the stroke. Hemiballismus is characterised by violent and random flailing of a limb due to proximal muscle activation. Hemichorea presents as continuous, semirhythmic jerking movements with proximal and distal muscle activation, although on occasion activity can be restricted to the distal part of the limb. Often following an acute stroke hemiballismus is seen first which then progresses to hemichorea [6].

The most frequently reported location of stroke for this disorder is the thalamus and the basal ganglia [6], however, sudden onset hemichorea-hemiballismus can be the presenting symptom of an acute parietal or insular cortex stroke.

It is important for clinicians to seek urgent stroke review in patients who present with an acute movement disorder, as the patient may be amenable to acute reperfusion therapies such as thrombolysis or endovascular clot retrieval [7].

References

1. Fisher CM. Concerning recurrent transient cerebral ischemic attacks. Can Med Assoc J. 1962;86:1091–9.
2. Tiseo C, Ornello R, Degan D, Notturno F. Not all intermittent shakings are epilepsy. Intern Emerg Med. 2017;12(5):705–8.
3. Yoon Y, Kim JS. Limb-shaking TIA: an asterixis. Neurology. 2013;81(10):931–2.
4. Ghika-Schmid F, Ghika J, Regli F, Bogousslavsky J. Hyperkinetic movement disorders during and after acute stroke: the Lausanne Stroke Registry. J Neurol Sci. 1997;146(2):109–16.
5. Suri R, Rodriguez-Porcel F, Donohue K, Jesse E, Lovera L, Dwivedi AK, et al. Post-stroke movement disorders: the clinical, neuroanatomic, and demographic portrait of 284 published cases. J Stroke Cerebrovasc Dis. 2018;27(9):2388–97.
6. Defebvre L, Krystkowiak P. Movement disorders and stroke. Rev Neurol (Paris). 2016;172(8-9):483–7.
7. Carbayo A, Sarto J, et al. Hemichorea as presentation of acute cortical ischemic stroke. Case series and review of the literature. J Stroke Cerebrovasc Dis. 2020;29(10):105150.

Contiguous Weakness of Upper and Lower Limbs Sparing the Face Is Unusual in Stroke

Channa Senanayake and Shaloo Singhal

1 Clinical Pearl

Physicians are advised to carefully inspect for stroke mimics when contiguous unilateral or bilateral upper and lower limb weakness is observed sparing the face. Contiguous unilateral upper and lower limb weakness due to stroke is rare and only seen in the case of medial medullary syndrome.

2 Clinical Case

An acute code stroke notification is activated requiring immediate stroke team attendance at a major metropolitan hospital. The Stroke Team receives handover from the ambulance crew of a 76-year old female who was last seen well 2 hours ago. Her apixaban had been ceased for 3 days for an elective colonoscope scheduled for tomorrow. Her daughter called the ambulance upon finding the patient collapsed on the ground complaining of neck pain and difficulty moving her right side. Rapid assessment is conducted to facilitate acute stroke interventions. The patient is agitated, confused and has a Glasgow Coma Score (GCS) of 14 (eyes 4, verbal 4 and motor 6). Inspection reveals a laceration and bruising to the right side of her forehead. She is afebrile, tachycardic with a heart rate of 135 beats per minute in atrial fibrillation, blood pressure is 130/70 mmHg, respiratory rate of 24 per minute, and blood sugar of 6.9 mmol per litre. She appears alert but answers incorrectly to age and month. She can obey the command "close your eyes" and grips and releases her

C. Senanayake · S. Singhal (✉)
Department of Neurology, Eastern Health, Melbourne, VIC, Australia

Stroke and Aging Research Group, School of Clinical Sciences, Monash University, Melbourne, VIC, Australia

R. Junckerstorff et al. (eds.), *Beyond Evidence-Based Medicine*,
https://doi.org/10.1007/978-981-99-4440-8_105

non-paretic hand. Extraocular movements are intact without nystagmus and her pupils appear equal. Visual fields appear intact to confrontation testing. Face motor function is spared however, motor function of the right arm and leg is severely impaired with grade 2 power (active movement with gravity eliminated) in all muscle groups. Sensory examination reveals numbness of the right upper and lower limb, sparing the face. There is no evidence of cortical dysfunction (no aphasia or inattention) nor dysarthria or incoordination. NIHSS (National Institute of Health Stroke Scale) score is 10. The patient undergoes multi-modal stroke imaging. Non contrast Computed Tomography (CT) brain does not demonstrate acute haemorrhage or infarct. CT angiogram reveals no large vessel occlusion and CT perfusion is normal. NIHSS of 10 meets the threshold of disabling symptoms and an alternative explanation other than stroke is not apparent. Normal stroke imaging is not a contraindication for thrombolytic therapy. The case is deemed as meeting criteria for thrombolysis and the patient is given an alteplase infusion. Soon afterwards, the patient experiences rapid deterioration with rapid progressive quadriparesis and haemodynamic instability. Urgent Magnetic Resonance Imaging (MRI) of her spinal cord demonstrates high cervical epidural haematoma causing spinal cord compression.

3 Discussion

3.1 Stroke Mimics Should Be Considered When Contiguous Upper and Lower Limb Weakness Sparing the Face Is Present

The Primary Motor Cortex (PMC) located in the precentral gyrus is responsible for planning and execution of voluntary movement. Topography of the motor cortex is arranged medial to lateral starting with leg muscles followed by the arm and then the face. The medial part of the motor cortex encoding leg muscles receives blood supply from the anterior cerebral artery (ACA) and the more lateral portions encoding the arm and face is supplied by the middle cerebral artery (MCA). Thus, ACA ischemia causes leg more than arm weakness and vice versa with MCA ischemia. ACA ischemia typically spares the most lateral aspect of the PMC. This area contains motor neurons encoding the face, tongue, and swallowing. Thus, it is not uncommon to see relative or complete sparing of facial muscles in ACA ischemia. The ACA supplies the sensory cortex for leg and foot as well as medial surface of the posterior frontal lobe, cingulate gyrus, medial inferior portion of frontal, parietal and temporal lobes. Involvement of these structures result in numbness of the leg and cortical symptoms such as abulia, dyspraxia and tactile aphasia.

Isolated ischaemia of the motor area encoding arm and leg muscles can result in pure motor weakness of one limb (e.g. in ACA infarction only the leg is weak with normal motor function of face and arm) [1]. However, this pattern of stroke will not cause simultaneous weakness of the arm and leg. Small infarctions of deeper structures involving descending motor and sensory tracts such as the corona radiata, internal capsule and brainstem typically due to lacunar infarcts can produce pure motor, pure sensory or sensorimotor strokes. However, as the motor and sensory tracts descend through subcortical and brainstem structures, tracts of the face, arm and leg are compacted into smaller areas. As a result, infarction of these areas tends to produce a pattern of weakness or sensory deficits involving the contralateral face, arm and leg.

Finally, medial medullary infarction, also known as Djerine syndrome, caused by occlusion of the anterior spinal artery [2] results in contralateral upper and lower limb weakness sparing the face. Bilateral medial medullary infarction can cause quadriparesis with relative sparing of facial muscles. Other medial medullary structures include hypoglossal nerve fibres and the medial lemniscus may be affected resulting in ipsilateral tongue weakness, contralateral loss of touch, proprioception, and vibration. Medial medullary syndromes are extremely rare stroke syndromes with an incidence of less than 0.5% [3]. Theoretically facial muscles can be spared due to the location of the facial motor nucleus in the ventrolateral pontine tegmentum rostrally to the medulla oblongata [3].

3.2 *Normal Multi-Modal Stroke Imaging Should Prompt Consideration of Stroke Mimics*

Thrombolytic therapy of stroke mimics can result in serious adverse effects as seen in this case. Although thrombolytic therapy with normal stroke multi-modal imaging is not uncommon, clinicians should strongly consider the possibility of stroke mimics. The sensitivity of CT perfusion imaging for ischaemic stroke is 63% [4]. However, CT perfusion is insensitive at diagnosing stroke mimics. Although stroke mimics such as seizures, migraines and brain tumours can produce characteristic abnormalities on CT perfusion, the overall sensitivity of CT perfusion for detection of stroke mimics is 22% [5]. In this case there were elements in the history and examination intimating potential spinal trauma such as neck pain and bruising. The patient most likely had a hemicord or Brown-Sequard syndrome initially due to a high cervical epidural haematoma resulting in ipsilateral upper and lower limb weakness. The clinician should be mindful that the NIHSS is a tool designed for assessment of stroke severity and it performs poorly in identifying stroke mimics. Further examination of this patient may have revealed ipsilateral absence of reflexes and contralateral pain and temperature loss. In the time constrained environment of an acute stroke assessment, where "time is brain", a detailed neurological examination maybe considered inconsequential. We would however suggest careful consideration of each individual case, and if discrepancies are present, further examination/ investigation for stroke mimics is well advised.

References

1. Hiraga A. Pure motor monoparesis due to ischemic stroke. Neurologist. 2011;17(6):301–8.
2. Yokota J, Amakusa Y, Tomita Y, Takahashi S. [The medial medullary infarction (Dejerine syndrome) following chiropractic neck manipulation]. No To Shinkei. 2003;55(2):121–5.
3. Toyoda K, Imamura T, Saku Y, Oita J, Ibayashi S, Minematsu K, et al. Medial medullary infarction: analyses of eleven patients. Neurology. 1996;47(5):1141–7.
4. Hana T, Iwama J, Yokosako S, Yoshimura C, Arai N, Kuroi Y, et al. Sensitivity of CT perfusion for the diagnosis of cerebral infarction. J Med Invest. 2014;61(1–2):41–5.
5. Prodi E, Danieli L, Manno C, Pagnamenta A, Pravata E, Roccatagliata L, et al. Stroke mimics in the acute setting: role of multimodal CT protocol. AJNR Am J Neuroradiol. 2022;43(2):216–22.

Part XV
Endocrinology

Never Withhold Basal Insulin in Patients with Insulin Deficiency

Jessie Teng and Ie-Wen Sim

1 Clinical Pearl

Never withhold basal insulin in patients with insulin deficiency including type 1 diabetes, LADA (Latent Autoimmune Diabetes in Adults) and pancreatic insufficiency (previous pancreatectomy, recurrent pancreatitis). Consider the diagnosis of LADA in adult patients with a new diagnosis of diabetes without any other features of metabolic syndrome or insulin resistance.

2 Clinical Case

A 28-year-old man was diagnosed with diabetes based on a fingerprick blood glucose of 26 mmol/L after presenting with unintentional weight loss, polyuria and polydipsia. His Body Mass Index (BMI) was 23 kg/m^2 and he did not have any other significant past or family medical history. He was commenced on metformin 500 mg daily.

Two days later, he was admitted to the hospital with diabetic ketoacidosis and treated with an insulin infusion. He was subsequently commenced on basal bolus insulin. He had hypoglycaemia following dinner and this was treated with oral glucose. His evening long-acting insulin was subsequently withheld. The next morning, he was found to have a fingerprick blood glucose of 20 mmol/L and ketones of 4 mmol/L.

J. Teng
St Vincent's Health and Eastern Health, Eastern Health Clinical School, Monash University, Melbourne, VIC, Australia

I.-W. Sim (✉)
Eastern Health and Monash Health, Monash University, University of Melbourne, Melbourne, VIC, Australia

R. Junckerstorff et al. (eds.), *Beyond Evidence-Based Medicine*,
https://doi.org/10.1007/978-981-99-4440-8_106

3 Discussion

Insulin deficiency causes the body to metabolise amino acids and lipids instead of glucose for energy, leading to ketosis and subsequently acidosis. Other factors contributing to ketosis include starvation (e.g. hyperemesis in pregnancy), an alcoholic binge and sepsis. Patients who have insulin deficiency develop diabetic ketoacidosis (DKA) rapidly once the effect of subcutaneous insulin wears off: this could be within 3–4 h for patients using insulin pumps as only rapid-acting insulin is delivered through the insulin pump.

Latent autoimmune diabetes of adults (LADA) is a slowly progressing form of autoimmune diabetes. Most patients are treated with oral hypoglycaemic agents for a few months but rapidly progress to requiring insulin therapy or develop ketoacidosis. People with LADA are usually slim and do not have other features of insulin resistance or metabolic syndrome. Diabetes autoantibody levels (e.g. anti-GAD antibodies, anti-IA2 antibodies and ZnT8 antibodies) should be tested [1].

4 Other Gems

- Some patients with type 1 diabetes (T1DM) also have obesity and insulin resistance, and may be on metformin as an insulin sensitiser
- Patients who have exocrine pancreatic insufficiency (e.g. on Creon, a pancreatic enzyme replacement therapy) often have insulin deficiency
- Patients with T1DM on an insulin pump use continuous quick-acting insulin as their basal insulin. Hence, if there is pump failure or issues with the insulin delivery line, they rapidly become ketotic
- If patients with T1DM on insulin pumps present with hyperglycaemia despite multiple insulin boluses via their pump, this is a sign of pump failure. They need subcutaneous insulin injections or intravenous insulin infusion if ketoacidotic
- For patients with DKA transitioning off intravenous insulin, allow at least 1 hour overlap between discontinuation of intravenous insulin and administration of subcutaneous insulin to prevent recurrence of hyperglycaemia or ketoacidosis during the transition period
- Immune check-point inhibitors (usually Programmed Death 1 receptor (PD-1) or Programmed Death Ligand 1 (PD-L1) inhibitors) can lead to insulin deficiency presenting as new-onset diabetes or worsening of pre-existing type 1 diabetes. Consider checking fingerprick ketones or assessing innate insulin secretion by measuring paired serum glucose and C-peptide levels
- In Australia, patients with T1DM can access continuous glucose monitors with low glucose alarms subsidised by the National Diabetes Service Scheme (NDSS)

Reference

1. Fourlanos S, Dotta F, Greenbaum C, Palmer J, Rolandsson O, Colman P, Harrison L. Latent autoimmune diabetes in adults (LADA) should be less latent. Diabetologia. 2005;48(11):2206–12.

Osteoporosis Treatment Following Minimal Trauma Fractures

Ie-Wen Sim and Jessie Teng

1 Clinical Pearl

Do not delay osteoporosis treatment for patients with minimal trauma fractures

2 Clinical Case

A 78-year-old woman was admitted with left femoral neck fracture after slipping on wet pavement. She recovered well post-operatively and was found to have a vitamin D level of 42 nmol/L while taking oral vitamin D 1000 IU daily. Her vitamin D dose was increased, and she was advised to have formal dental review with her dentist and to have an outpatient bone density scan. She was subsequently referred to the Metabolic Bone Clinic.

Prior to her clinic appointment, she sustained a left radial fracture after another fall in her garden and was commenced on 6-monthly denosumab injections with her GP for treatment of osteoporosis. She tolerated the injections well without any adverse effects. Eighteen months later, she had a prolonged hospital admission with pneumonia requiring a period of inpatient rehabilitation. Her denosumab injection was missed and she developed new vertebral fractures during her admission.

I.-W. Sim (✉)
Eastern Health and Monash Health, Monash University, University of Melbourne, Melbourne, VIC, Australia

J. Teng
St Vincent's Health and Eastern Health, Eastern Health Clinical School, Monash University, Melbourne, VIC, Australia

R. Junckerstorff et al. (eds.), *Beyond Evidence-Based Medicine*,
https://doi.org/10.1007/978-981-99-4440-8_107

3 Discussion

Osteoporosis is characterised by low bone mass and disruption of bone microarchitecture, leading to increased risk of fractures. The risk of a second major osteoporotic fracture is highest immediately after the first fracture. Diagnosis of osteoporosis is based on the presence of fracture after minimal trauma ***or*** by detecting low bone mineral density. Up to 50% of women with vertebral fractures have normal bone mineral density by Dual Energy X-ray Absorptiometry (DEXA) [1].

Delay in initiating osteoporosis treatment is associated with increased fractures. Ideally, patients should have osteoporosis treatment commenced prior to discharge after presenting with a minimal trauma fracture. Unless clinical risk of osteomalacia is high, vitamin D levels can be boosted by an oral loading dose or given parenterally. The risk of osteonecrosis of the jaw is low in the osteoporosis setting, and a review of dental symptoms and a visual assessment of oral health will usually suffice for patients prior to commencing anti-resorptive therapy. Table 1 lists the current osteoporosis drugs available in Australia [2].

Denosumab (Prolia) is a common choice for osteoporosis management primarily due to its simple subcutaneous administration and that it need only be given every 6 months. However, the rapid offset of denosumab means that its potent anti-resorptive action wears off quickly if a subsequent dose is delayed. Delay in denosumab administration has been associated with rebound loss of bone mineral density and new incident vertebral fractures, which are often multiple [3]. Denosumab should **not** be ceased or delayed, even for acute illness or dental review. If denosumab needs to be discontinued, specialist management is indicated, with patients requiring careful transition to an alternative osteoporosis therapy.

Table 1 Current available therapies for osteoporosis

Drug	Common adverse events
Oral bisphosphonates	Upper gastrointestinal effects (gastro-oesophageal reflux, erosive oesophagitis)
Intravenous bisphosphonates	Hypocalcaemia Flu-like illness following infusion (acute phase reaction)
Denosumab	Hypocalcaemia Injection-site reactions Atraumatic vertebral fractures following discontinuation
Raloxifene	Hot flushes Venous thromboembolism
Teriparatide	Hypercalcaemia Injection-site reactions
Romosozumab	Injection-site reactions

4 Other Gems

- Falls prevention is an important component of osteoporosis management.
- Denosumab is not ideal for younger patients given the need for ongoing therapy.
- Atypical femoral fractures (AFFs) are uncommon but need to be considered based on history (typically the patient reports a crack prior to falling) and radiological appearance of the fractures. Risk of AFF is increased with longer duration of anti-resorptive therapy and being of Asian ethnicity. In patients on long term anti-resorptive therapy, patients should be asked about groin or thigh pain during review.
- Given the small risk of atypical femoral fracture, treatment intermission (drug holiday) from antiresorptive therapy can be considered if absolute fracture risk is low. Treatment intermission is NOT indicated in patients on denosumab, nor in patients with high risk of fragility fracture, e.g. ongoing glucocorticoid therapy or Bone Mineral Density (BMD) < −2.5.

References

1. Greenspan SL, von Stetten E, Emond SK, Jones L, Parker RA. Instant vertebral assessment: a noninvasive dual X-ray absorptiometry technique to avoid misclassification and clinical mismanagement of osteoporosis. J Clin Densitom. 2001;4:373–80.
2. https://www.nps.org.au/australian-prescriber/articles/treating-osteoporosis-risks-and-management#t2
3. Symonds C, Kline G. Warning of an increased risk of vertebral fracture after stopping denosumab. CMAJ. 2018;190(16):E485–6. https://doi.org/10.1503/cmaj.180115. PMID: 29685907; PMCID: PMC5915244.

Euglycaemic Ketoacidosis with Sodium Glucose Co-Transport 2 (SGLT2) Inhibitors

Jessie Teng and Ie-Wen Sim

1 Clinical Pearl

Screen for euglycaemic ketoacidosis in all hospital inpatients taking Sodium Glucose Co-Transport 2 (SGLT-2) inhibitors

2 Clinical Case

A 56-year-old woman with type 2 diabetes was admitted for elective colonoscopy for investigation of iron-deficiency anaemia. Pre-procedure fingerprick blood glucose level was 7.5 mmol/L. Post-procedure, she developed significant nausea and vomiting. She was found to have ketoacidosis with fingerprick blood glucose 5.4 mmol/L, fingerprick ketones 4.5 mmol/L and pH 7.1 (normal range 7.35–7.45) requiring an intravenous insulin and dextrose infusion. Medication history further elucidated that she was on metformin and dapagliflozin for glycaemic control.

J. Teng
St Vincent's Health and Eastern Health, Eastern Health Clinical School, Monash University, Melbourne, VIC, Australia

I.-W. Sim (✉)
Eastern Health and Monash Health, Monash University, University of Melbourne, Melbourne, VIC, Australia

R. Junckerstorff et al. (eds.), *Beyond Evidence-Based Medicine*,
https://doi.org/10.1007/978-981-99-4440-8_108

3 Discussion

SGLT-2 inhibitors (empagliflozin, dapagliflozin) are an important class of diabetes medications but have been associated with increased urogenital infections and euglycaemic ketoacidosis. Due to their cardioprotective and renoprotective effects, SGLT-2 inhibitors are increasingly being prescribed in non-diabetic patients with cardiac failure or kidney disease. The proposed mechanism of SGLT-2 inhibitor-associated ketoacidosis implicates glucosuria leading to decreased plasma glucose and decreased insulin release. Carbohydrate deficiency, insulinopenia, and increased glucagon release leads to upregulation of lipolysis and ketogenesis [1].

All patients on a SGLT-2 inhibitor should have a fingerprick blood glucose and ketone check on hospital admission to exclude euglycaemic ketoacidosis. Patients are advised to withhold SGLT-2 inhibitors if they are unwell with reduced oral intake, or for at least 72 h prior to fasting for a procedure. For unwell patients requiring admission, SGLT-2 inhibitors are ceased temporarily until they recover and resume normal oral intake.

4 Other Gems

- The choice of diabetes therapy for patients with T2DM should be tailored to the patient's medical co-morbidities [2]
- Glycaemic targets should be based on patient comorbidities, age and risk of hypoglycaemia

References

1. Hamblin P, Wong R, Ekinci E, et al. SGLT2 inhibitors increase the risk of diabetic ketoacidosis developing in the community and during hospital admission. J Clin Endocrinol Metab. 2019;104(8):3077–87.
2. Australian Diabetes Society Treatment Algorithm for T2DM: https://treatment.diabetessociety.com.au/plan/

Free T4 Levels and Pituitary Disorders

Jessie Teng and Ie-Wen Sim

1 Clinical Pearl

Measure paired TSH and fT4 levels in patients with known or suspected pituitary disorders.

2 Clinical Case

A 35-year-old woman presents to hospital with a severe headache for several days, 2 months post-partum. CT-brain confirmed diagnosis of pituitary apoplexy with features of mild subacute haemorrhage. Morning cortisol level and thyroid function tests were ordered to assess pituitary hormone sufficiency, with the following results:

Cortisol 150 nmol/L (reference range 100–650 nmol/L).

Thyroid Stimulating Hormone (TSH) 4.2mIU/L (reference range 0.5–5).

She is commenced on oral hydrocortisone 20 mg bd and referred to the Endocrinology Clinic. A week later she presents to her General Practitioner (GP) with lethargy, low mood, joint aches and is found to mildly hyponatraemic. Repeat thyroid function tests demonstrates a TSH of 3.8mIU/L. Two weeks later, she presents to the Emergency Department (ED) significantly unwell with progressive hyponatraemia and bradycardia. Paired TSH and free T4 (fT4) levels are ordered, showing significant secondary hypothyroidism.

J. Teng
Endocrinologist, St Vincent's Health & Eastern Health, Eastern Health Clinical School, Monash University, Clayton, VIC, Australia

I.-W. Sim (✉)
Endocrinologist & Andrologist, Eastern Health & Monash Health, Monash University, University of Melbourne, Clayton, VIC, Australia

R. Junckerstorff et al. (eds.), *Beyond Evidence-Based Medicine*,
https://doi.org/10.1007/978-981-99-4440-8_109

TSH- 2.4mIU/L (reference range 0.5–5).
fT4- **3.4** pmol/L (reference range 10–25).

3 Discussion

The pituitary gland secretes a range of hormones including Adrenocorticotropic Hormone (ACTH), TSH, Luteinizing Hormone (LH), Follicle Stimulating Hormone (FSH), Growth Hormone (GH) and prolactin from the anterior pituitary gland, as well as oxytocin and arginine vasopressin (AVP) from the posterior pituitary gland. AVP deficiency (previously known as cranial diabetes insipidus) may present as polyuria, with diagnosis determined by assessment of fluid balance and serum sodium and osmolality.

Anterior pituitary hormones can be measured routinely, but assessment of adequacy of these hormones needs to be interpreted based on the end-hormone levels. In pituitary patients with secondary hypothyroidism, the pituitary gland is unable to mount a TSH response to low fT4/fT3 levels. In this case, TSH levels were inappropriately within the normal reference range, for the degree of hypothyroidism (low fT4 and fT3 levels). In Australia, most pathology labs will only run TSH levels if 'thyroid function tests' are requested. For patients with pituitary pathologies or suspected pituitary pathologies, free T4 level needs to be specifically requested, with clinical indication of 'pituitary patient' specified on the request form.

4 Other Gems

- ACTH levels need to be collected in an EDTA tube on ice, plasma separated, and frozen immediately
- Serum cortisol levels fluctuate throughout the day due to diurnal variation and adequate levels need to be interpreted based on time of day and the patient's usual sleep-wake cycle (e.g. people who work night shifts)
- For patients with suspected pituitary dysfunction who are acutely unwell and hypothyroid, administer intravenous hydrocortisone prior to thyroxine replacement because in a patient with adrenal insufficiency, correcting hypothyroidism can increase the metabolism of cortisol and thus may precipitate an adrenal crisis.
- For patients with primary hypothyroidism, adequacy of thyroxine replacement is assessed on normal range TSH levels, 6–8 weeks post-thyroxine commencement or dose adjustments.
  - fT4 levels are usually mildly elevated when blood samples are collected post-dose reflecting absorption of thyroxine

  - E.g. for a patients on thyroxine 100mcg daily with TSH 3.5mIU/L (reference range 0.5–5) and fT4 of 27 pmol/L (reference range 10–25), her dose of thyroxine does not need to be adjusted

- For patients with secondary hypothyroidism, adequacy of thyroxine replacement is assessed on normal range fT4 and fT3 levels. These patients often have low or undetectable TSH levels, and thyroxine dosing should **NOT** be titrated according to TSH.

The Testes Are the Most Accessible Endocrine Organ

Ie-Wen Sim and Jessie Teng

1 Clinical Pearl

The testes are the most accessible endocrine organ.

2 Clinical Case

A 35-year-old man presents with acute onset lower back pain. An x-ray of the lumbar spine demonstrates 30% loss of height of the L3 vertebra, consistent with a compression fracture. The patient does not report any previous fragility fractures however, subsequent bone densitometry is consistent with severe osteoporosis (lumbar spine T-score − 3.5 [Z-score − 3.2], femoral neck T-score − 2.8 [Z-score − 2.5]).

A secondary osteoporosis screen demonstrates primary hypogonadism, including a serum total testosterone of 3.2 nmol/L, accompanied by elevated serum gonadotrophins (FSH 52 IU/L reference range 1–9 IU/L, LH 37 IU/L reference range 1–9 IU/L). Further medical history includes a previous diagnosis of Attention Deficit Hyperactivity Disorder (ADHD), manifested by significant learning difficulties while at school. Gonadal examination reveals small 2 mL testes bilaterally.

I.-W. Sim (✉)
Endocrinologist & Andrologist, Eastern Health & Monash Health, Monash University, Clayton, VIC, Australia

University of Melbourne, Clayton, VIC, Australia

J. Teng
Endocrinologist, St Vincent's Health & Eastern Health, Eastern Health Clinical School, Monash University, Clayton, VIC, Australia

R. Junckerstorff et al. (eds.), *Beyond Evidence-Based Medicine*,
https://doi.org/10.1007/978-981-99-4440-8_110

Karyotype testing confirms a diagnosis of Klinefelter syndrome, which could explain his learning difficulties, as well as his primary hypogonadism. After counselling regarding fertility options, he is commenced on testosterone replacement. Intravenous zoledronic acid is also administered to reduce the risk of future fragility fractures.

3 Discussion

Hypogonadism is a potential contributing cause of osteoporosis. Hypogonadism should be considered in men diagnosed with osteoporosis, especially when diagnosed at less than 50 years of age [1]. Other common secondary causes of osteoporosis include primary hyperparathyroidism, thyroid dysfunction, malabsorption, myeloma, as well as tobacco use and heavy alcohol consumption.

The clinical features of Klinefelter syndrome include behaviour and cognitive features that are specific to the syndrome, in addition to the clinical features of androgen deficiency [1, 2]. Men with Klinefelter syndrome often have a history of learning difficulty, delayed speech, and/or psychiatric disturbance and many men will have primary infertility [1, 2]. Accurate measurement of testicular volume during routine physical examination will improve detection of Klinefelter syndrome, and ameliorate the sequelae associated with the syndrome [1].

Klinefelter syndrome refers to the presence of two or more X chromosomes in men, with the most common karyotype being 47, XXY. Klinefelter syndrome occurs in 1–2 per 1000 men and is the commonest congenital cause of primary testicular failure in men [2]. Unfortunately, only approximately one quarter of men are ever diagnosed. Men with Klinefelter syndrome benefit from testosterone replacement therapy.

Infertility is common in men with Klinefelter syndrome. Even though azoospermia is common, it may be possible to harvest spermatozoa in over half of these men through micro-dissection testicular sperm extraction (micro-TESE), potentially allowing these men to have biological children [1]. Discussion regarding fertility aspirations should occur prior to the commencement of testosterone therapy due to the potential contraceptive effects of exogenous androgens.

4 Other Gems

- Testicular examination is an essential part of the assessment of a patient's gonadal status, with small testes being the only reliable clinical sign of hypogonadism.
- Fertility aspirations must be considered prior to commencement of testosterone therapy, as testosterone suppresses serum gonadotrophins and reduces semen parameters in most men

- Screening for secondary causes of osteoporosis is indicated in patients where the Z-score is ≤ -2.0

References

1. Shiraishi K, Matsuyama H. Klinefelter syndrome: from pediatrics to geriatrics. Reprod Med Biol. 2019;18:140–50.
2. Groth K, Skakkebæk A, Høst GC, Bojesen A. Klinefelter syndrome—a clinical update. J Clin Endocrinol Metab. 2013;98(1):20–30.

Part XVI
Rheumatology

Premenopausal Females Don't Get Gout

Jessica Fairley and Indi Rasaratnam

1 Clinical Pearl

Premenopausal females don't get gout: oestrogen is uricosuric.

2 Clinical Case

A previously well 35-year-old woman presents with a painful, red, swollen and warm left foot with exquisite tenderness centred at the big toe metatarsophalangeal (MTP) joint. The referring physician wonders if this is her first episode of gout. She is found to have a new pansystolic murmur at the apex radiating to the axilla consistent with mitral regurgitation. Subacute bacterial endocarditis (SBE) is considered with all three blood cultures subsequently growing *Streptococcus mitis*. She had a complicated dental extraction 3 weeks prior. She subsequently developed severe mid-thoracic back pain. MRI confirmed features suggestive of T6 and left first MTP joint osteomyelitis/septic arthritis. Aspiration of the left first MTP joint

J. Fairley
Alfred Health, Melbourne, VIC, Australia

The University of Melbourne, Melbourne, VIC, Australia

I. Rasaratnam (✉)
Alfred Health and Epworth Healthcare, Melbourne, VIC, Australia

Epworth Medical School, Monash University, Melbourne, VIC, Australia

Undergraduate and Postgraduate Medical Education, Central Clinical School, Monash University and Alfred Health, Melbourne, VIC, Australia

R. Junckerstorff et al. (eds.), *Beyond Evidence-Based Medicine*,
https://doi.org/10.1007/978-981-99-4440-8_111

revealed no crystals but grew *Streptococcus mitis*. Trans-oesophageal echocardiogram confirmed friable vegetations at the mitral valve leaflet. SBE complicated by septic emboli is confirmed as the cause of this woman's musculoskeletal symptoms.

3 Discussion

Gout is the most common form of inflammatory arthritis, affecting approximately 3–5% of people in high-income countries [1, 2]. Gout typically presents as an acute monoarthritis characterised by intense swelling and pain, erythema and loss of function in the absence of a history of trauma [3]. Gout may also present as a chronic arthritic process characterised by radiographic erosions [4], and tophaceous deposits. Tophi may occur in skin or soft tissues, causing ligamentous disruption [5], tenosynovitis [6] and even nerve entrapment including carpal tunnel syndrome [7]. Typical risk factors include male gender, older age, renal impairment, obesity and dietary factors including alcohol intake and high-fructose soft-drinks [8–10].

Gout occurs due to prolonged hyperuricaemia. The low solubility of monosodium urate (MSU) results in crystal deposition in joints and soft tissues [8]. Hyperuricaemia is common, occurring in up to 10% of adults, and does not always equate to a diagnosis of gout [11]. Hyperuricaemia is often multifactorial, related to a combination of impaired uric acid excretion and excess uric acid intake or production. The kidneys excrete approximately 70% of uric acid [8], meaning that impaired renal function is a significant risk factor for hyperuricaemia and gout. Certain medications, including thiazide diuretics, also reduce renal uric acid excretion [12]. The gastrointestinal tract is responsible for the remainder of uric acid excretion [8]. Increased uric acid production can result from increased purine catabolism [8] which can occur in the context of high cell turnover (e.g., haematologic malignancy), and certain dietary factors (diets high in purine-rich foods, beer and high-fructose soft-drinks) [12]. Certain genetic polymorphisms may also alter purine production and reduce renal uric acid excretion [8, 12].

Gout is rarely observed in premenopausal women [13]. In one cohort study, gout only occurred in premenopausal women with another significant risk factor including renal failure, obesity, diabetes or cardiac failure [13]; most patients had multiple risk factors. This is because oestrogen is thought to stimulate urinary uric acid excretion and thus prevents development of hyperuricaemia [13, 14]. Menopause has been associated with a rise in serum uric acid levels, while hormone replacement therapy has been associated with lower serum uric acid [14].

Accordingly, as in the case described, a diagnosis of gout should always be thoroughly interrogated in a premenopausal woman without other risk factors.

4 Other Gems

- A normal serum uric acid does not preclude diagnosis of gout in the correct clinical setting; acute inflammation is also uricosuric. Thus, in the context of an acute attack of gout, uric acid levels may be inappropriately normal due to the uricosuric effect of acute inflammation.
- A history of gout, or presence of monosodium urate crystals on joint aspiration does NOT preclude a diagnosis of septic arthritis: gout and septic arthritis may co-exist.
- Asymptomatic hyperuricaemia is common and does not always equate to a diagnosis of gout. Hyperuricaemia does not require treatment in the absence of symptoms of gout or another complication of hyperuricaemia (urolithiasis or acute uric acid nephropathy).
- Uric acid may act as an antioxidant in neurodegenerative diseases, thus treating hyperuricaemia without a clear indication is not advised.

References

1. Ting K, Gill TK, Keen H, Tucker GR, Hill CL. Prevalence and associations of gout and hyperuricaemia: results from an Australian population-based study. Intern Med J. 2016;46(5):566–73.
2. Zhu Y, Pandya BJ, Choi HK. Prevalence of gout and hyperuricemia in the US general population: the National Health and Nutrition Examination Survey 2007-2008. Arthritis Rheum. 2011;63(10):3136–41.
3. Neogi T, Jansen TL, Dalbeth N, et al. 2015 Gout classification criteria: an American College of Rheumatology/European League Against Rheumatism collaborative initiative. Ann Rheum Dis. 2015;74(10):1789–98.
4. Dalbeth N, Stamp L. Hyperuricaemia and gout: time for a new staging system? Ann Rheum Dis. 2014;73(9):1598–600.
5. Ohishi T, Koide Y, Takahashi M, Miyata R, Kushida K. Scapholunate dissociation caused by gouty arthritis of the wrist. Case report. Scand J Plast Reconstr Surg Hand Surg. 2000;34(2):189–91.
6. Aslam N, Lo S, McNab I. Gouty flexor tenosynovitis mimicking infection: a case report emphasising the value of ultrasound in diagnosis. Acta Orthop Belg. 2004;70(4):368–70.
7. Chen CK, Chung CB, Yeh L, et al. Carpal tunnel syndrome caused by tophaceous gout: CT and MR imaging features in 20 patients. AJR Am J Roentgenol. 2000;175(3):655–9.
8. Maiuolo J, Oppedisano F, Gratteri S, Muscoli C, Mollace V. Regulation of uric acid metabolism and excretion. Int J Cardiol. 2016;213:8–14.
9. Roddy E, Mallen CD, Doherty M. Gout. BMJ. 2013;347:f5648.
10. Evans PL, Prior JA, Belcher J, Mallen CD, Hay CA, Roddy E. Obesity, hypertension and diuretic use as risk factors for incident gout: a systematic review and meta-analysis of cohort studies. Arthritis Res Ther. 2018;20(1):136.
11. Dincer HE, Dincer AP, Levinson DJ. Asymptomatic hyperuricemia: to treat or not to treat. Cleve Clin J Med. 2002;69(8):594, 7, 600-2 passim.
12. de Oliveira EP, Burini RC. High plasma uric acid concentration: causes and consequences. Diabetol Metab Syndr. 2012;4:12.
13. Kumar S, Gupta R, Suppiah R. Gout in women: differences in risk factors in young and older women. N Z Med J. 2012;125(1363):39–45.
14. Hak AE, Choi HK. Menopause, postmenopausal hormone use and serum uric acid levels in US women—the Third National Health and Nutrition Examination Survey. Arthritis Res Ther. 2008;10(5):R116.

Beware of Red Flags in Patients Presenting with Polymyalgia Rheumatica

Jessica Fairley and Indi Rasaratnam

1 Clinical Pearl

Beware of atypical features and red flags in a patient presenting with 'typical' polymyalgia rheumatica, especially a history of malignancy.

2 Clinical Case

An eighty-year-old woman presents with a 4-week history of neck, bilateral shoulder and pelvic girdle pain with early morning and inactivity stiffness. She has no symptoms of temporal arteritis. Her inflammatory markers were raised with an erythrocyte sedimentation rate (ESR) of 70 mm/hr. (range 1–10 mm/h) and a C-reactive protein (CRP) of 40 mg/L (range 0–5 mg/L). Her alkaline phosphatase (ALP) was noted to be raised at 240 U/L (normal <110 U/L). A clinical diagnosis of Polymyalgia Rheumatica (PMR) was made. Her response to prednisolone 15 mg mane was rapid with marked improvement in her inflammatory markers within 2 weeks of prednisolone therapy. However, a few weeks later she complained of nocturnal pain and pain on weight bearing in her right hip and thigh, which did not

J. Fairley
Alfred Health, Melbourne, VIC, Australia

The University of Melbourne, Melbourne, VIC, Australia

I. Rasaratnam (✉)
Alfred Health and Epworth Healthcare, Melbourne, VIC, Australia

Epworth Medical School, Monash University, Melbourne, VIC, Australia

Undergraduate and Postgraduate Medical Education, Central Clinical School, Monash University and Alfred Health, Melbourne, VIC, Australia

R. Junckerstorff et al. (eds.), *Beyond Evidence-Based Medicine*,
https://doi.org/10.1007/978-981-99-4440-8_112

respond to an escalation of the dose of prednisolone. In view of a distant history of breast cancer in 2006 (deemed to be cured and discharged from oncology care), MRI right hip was undertaken and revealed features suggestive of bony metastasis at the right head, neck and shaft of femur. A subsequent total body bone scan confirmed widespread bony metastasis. It was felt she has had both diagnoses of PMR and metastatic breast cancer. The raised ALP can occur in both diagnoses, though higher than expected for just PMR alone.

3 Discussion

PMR is an inflammatory rheumatic disease which occurs in older cohorts [1, 2]. The presentation of PMR can be highly varied, and there is no definitive diagnostic test to confirm this diagnosis [1, 2]. Accepted classification criteria suggest key features to be bilateral shoulder and hip girdle symptoms, prolonged morning stiffness, age 50 years or older and elevated CRP and ESR [1]. A rapid corticosteroid response is also considered a hallmark of PMR [1]. In PMR, ultrasound imaging may reveal bilateral shoulder abnormalities (including subacromial bursitis, bicipital tenosynovitis or a glenohumeral joint effusion), or abnormalities in one shoulder and one hip (e.g., joint effusion or trochanteric bursitis) [1].

When diagnosing PMR, classification criteria recommend that the clinician must consider and exclude a better alternative cause of the patient's clinical presentation [1]. This is because multiple conditions can mimic PMR; in one cohort of patients 50 years or older with new onset bilateral shoulder pain in the previous 12 weeks, non-PMR diagnoses included rheumatoid arthritis (29%), other seronegative arthritis (12%), connective tissue disease or vasculitis (5%), shoulder conditions (31%), chronic pain (15%), infection (3%) and previously undiagnosed malignancy (2%) [1]. In particular, rheumatoid arthritis (RA) or other inflammatory arthritis may have a "polymyalgic" onset that is highly suggestive of PMR [1, 3]. In RA, peripheral joint synovitis is more common than in PMR, and serologic testing may identify typical autoantibodies (rheumatoid factor and cyclic citrullinated protein (CCP)) [1].

In an older patient, however, presenting with raised inflammatory markers and bilateral hip and shoulder girdle pain, the differential diagnosis of malignancy or a paraneoplastic process must also be considered. A careful history should be taken to identify risk factors for malignancy (e.g., past history, or strong family history), atypical features (e.g., weight loss, fevers or night sweats) or a lack of rapid corticosteroid response. Further imaging can then be considered. Certain imaging modalities may in fact help to suggest a diagnosis of PMR, particularly positron emission tomography/computed tomography (PET/CT) scanning. In PMR, ^{18}F-FDG PET/CT scanning may demonstrate periarticular hip or shoulder avidity, iliopectinal bursitis or sternoclavicular joint uptake [4]. Furthermore, PET-CT scanning may help to identify features of large vessel vasculitis/giant cell arteritis (GCA) and exclude a malignancy. GCA may occur in 15–20% of people with PMR, and must be promptly identified to prevent serious complications including visual loss [2].

4 Other Gems

- Any patient presenting with suspected PMR must be evaluated for symptoms of giant cell arteritis, including headache, visual loss, jaw claudication and scalp tenderness. Different corticosteroid dosing regimens and other agents are available for management of GCA.
- CRP levels may change more quickly than ESR.
- Certain treatments for GCA, e.g., tocilizumab and interleukin-6 (IL-6) inhibitors, may prevent a rise in CRP levels, thus negating its utility as a biomarker for infection or inflammation. This must be considered in patients presenting with suspected infective/inflammatory diseases on IL-6 inhibition.
- ESR levels may be elevated with age, obesity, anaemia and paraproteinaemia. This is particularly true if there is a discordance between CRP and ESR levels, e.g., a normal CRP and moderately raised ESR.
- PMR may cause a mildly increased alkaline phosphatase on liver function testing.

References

1. Dasgupta B, Cimmino MA, Kremers HM, et al. 2012 Provisional classification criteria for polymyalgia rheumatica: a European League Against Rheumatism/American College of Rheumatology collaborative initiative. Arthritis Rheum. 2012;64(4):943–54.
2. Salvarani C, Cantini F, Boiardi L, Hunder GG. Polymyalgia rheumatica and giant-cell arteritis. N Engl J Med. 2002;347(4):261–71.
3. Gonzalez-Gay MA, Garcia-Porrua C, Salvarani C, Olivieri I, Hunder GG. The spectrum of conditions mimicking polymyalgia rheumatica in Northwestern Spain. J Rheumatol. 2000;27(9):2179–84.
4. Rehak Z, Sprlakova-Pukova A, Kazda T, Fojtik Z, Vargova L, Nemec P. (18)F-FDG PET/CT in polymyalgia rheumatica-a pictorial review. Br J Radiol. 2017;90(1076):20170198.

Methotrexate is Not Contraindicated in Rheumatoid Arthritis (RA) Patients with Interstitial Lung Disease (ILD)

Jessica Fairley and Indi Rasaratnam

1 Clinical Pearl

Methotrexate is not contraindicated in RA patients with ILD.

2 Clinical Case

A 76-year-old man with anti-cyclic citrullinated peptide (CCP) antibody and rheumatoid factor positive Rheumatoid Arthritis has persistent active disease involving the small joints of his hands, feet and both wrists. He has been on hydroxychloroquine 200 mg daily, salazopyrin 1.5 g twice daily and prednisolone 7.5 mg mane. He is an ex-smoker. Examination confirmed synovitis of both wrists and all metacarpophalangeal (MCP), proximal interphalangeal (PIP) and metatarsophalangeal (MTP) joints in both hands and feet. He was noted to have bi-basal lung crackles. X-ray of hands and feet confirmed erosions at the right and left second and third MCPs, PIPs and fifth MTPs. Chest x-ray and subsequent high resolution CT scan confirmed mild interstitial lung disease (ILD). Methotrexate was considered as the

J. Fairley
Alfred Health, Melbourne, VIC, Australia

The University of Melbourne, Melbourne, VIC, Australia

I. Rasaratnam (✉)
Alfred Health and Epworth Healthcare, Melbourne, VIC, Australia

Epworth Medical School, Monash University, Melbourne, VIC, Australia

Undergraduate and Postgraduate Medical Education, Central Clinical School, Monash University and Alfred Health, Melbourne, VIC, Australia

R. Junckerstorff et al. (eds.), *Beyond Evidence-Based Medicine*,
https://doi.org/10.1007/978-981-99-4440-8_113

next disease-modifying anti-rheumatic drug of choice. However, concern was raised given its association as a cause of ILD.

3 Discussion

Occurring in around 1% of people worldwide, rheumatoid arthritis (RA) is one of the most common inflammatory arthritides [1]. RA is complicated by fibrosing ILD in 4–7% of patients [2], and is associated with reduced survival [1]. Methotrexate is the first-line disease-modifying anti-rheumatic drug (DMARD) in RA [3], and remains the backbone of many treatment regimens in combination with other synthetic and biologic DMARDs.

Methotrexate can also be associated with an inflammatory pneumonitis, which may occur in around 1% of RA patients commencing methotrexate [4]. The mechanism of methotrexate pneumonitis is poorly understood [5]. Risk factors include older age, seropositivity for rheumatoid factor and anti-CCP antibodies, diabetes mellitus, renal dysfunction, male gender, pre-existing lung disease and certain genetic and environmental factors [5]. Methotrexate pneumonitis may present with dry cough, dyspnoea and fever [5, 6], and generally occurs within the first 12 months' of treatment [7] while RA-ILD may have a more subacute onset [8]. Those treated with methotrexate do not appear to be at increased risk of mortality from lung disease [9]. Treatment for methotrexate pneumonitis requires immediate cessation of methotrexate, and depending on severity, corticosteroids or other immunosuppressants. Overall prognosis appears to be good although methotrexate may lead to adverse outcome [5].

Methotrexate does not appear to be associated with risk of progressive fibrosing ILD [8, 10], with similar rates of ILD seen in those treated with methotrexate to general RA populations. Recent advances in high-resolution computed tomography (HRCT) have allowed more careful definition of patterns of ILD and differentiation between fibrotic ILD and methotrexate pneumonitis [5, 8]. Methotrexate pneumonitis may be characterised by diffuse, bilateral ground-glass change on HRCT rather than the usual interstitial pneumonia (UIP) or fibrotic non-specific interstitial pneumonia (NSIP) pattern of RA-ILD [8]. Treatment of RA-ILD generally involves corticosteroids and addition of other immunosuppressants [5]. Rituximab in particular may be associated with stabilisation of RA-ILD in up to 50% [11]. Overall, the cornerstone of management of RA-ILD is to control underlying RA [12].

4 Other Gems

- Extra-articular manifestations of RA, including ILD, scleritis and rheumatoid nodules generally occur in patients who are seropositive for rheumatoid factor and anti-CCP antibodies.

- Early treatment of RA may be associated with better long-term disease control and lower long-term risk of extra-articular manifestations.
- The most common serious toxicities of methotrexate requiring cessation is pneumonitis, hepatotoxicity and cytopenias, particularly anaemia and neutropenia.
- Gastrointestinal toxicity with methotrexate is generally mild and improves over the first month of treatment. Subcutaneous injection of methotrexate may help reduce gastrointestinal upset.
- Methotrexate should be taken with folic acid supplementation to minimise toxicity.
- Methotrexate must be taken WEEKLY – severe toxicity can result with daily dosing. If methotrexate toxicity is suspected, supplementation with folinic acid (calcium folinate) can be prescribed at a dose to 15 mg 6-hourly for 72 h.
- Methotrexate interacts with some prescription and non-prescription medications, particularly trimethoprim (risk of bone marrow suppression) and alcohol (risk of hepatotoxicity).
- Methotrexate is teratogenic and care must be taken to ensure women of child-bearing age are using adequate contraception. Methotrexate must be ceased for 3 months prior to pregnancy.

References

1. Smolen JS, Aletaha D, Barton A, et al. Rheumatoid arthritis. Nat Rev Dis Primers. 2018;4:18001.
2. Bongartz T, Nannini C, Medina-Velasquez YF, et al. Incidence and mortality of interstitial lung disease in rheumatoid arthritis: a population-based study. Arthritis Rheum. 2010;62(6):1583–91.
3. Smolen JS, Landewe RBM, Bijlsma JWJ, et al. EULAR recommendations for the management of rheumatoid arthritis with synthetic and biological disease-modifying antirheumatic drugs: 2019 update. Ann Rheum Dis. 2020;79(6):685–99.
4. Sathi N, Chikura B, Kaushik VV, Wiswell R, Dawson JK. How common is methotrexate pneumonitis? A large prospective study investigates. Clin Rheumatol. 2012;31(1):79–83.
5. Fragoulis GE, Nikiphorou E, Larsen J, Korsten P, Conway R. Methotrexate-Associated Pneumonitis and Rheumatoid Arthritis-Interstitial Lung Disease: Current Concepts for the Diagnosis and Treatment. Front Med (Lausanne). 2019;6:238.
6. Atzeni F, Boiardi L, Salli S, Benucci M, Sarzi-Puttini P. Lung involvement and drug-induced lung disease in patients with rheumatoid arthritis. Expert Rev Clin Immunol. 2013;9(7):649–57.
7. Saravanan V, Kelly CA. Reducing the risk of methotrexate pneumonitis in rheumatoid arthritis. Rheumatology (Oxford). 2004;43(2):143–7.
8. Dawson JK, Quah E, Earnshaw B, Amoasii C, Mudawi T, Spencer LG. Does methotrexate cause progressive fibrotic interstitial lung disease? A systematic review. Rheumatol Int. 2021;41(6):1055–64.
9. Conway R, Low C, Coughlan RJ, O'Donnell MJ, Carey JJ. Methotrexate and lung disease in rheumatoid arthritis: a meta-analysis of randomized controlled trials. Arthritis Rheumatol. 2014;66(4):803–12.
10. Ibfelt EH, Jacobsen RK, Kopp TI, et al. Methotrexate and risk of interstitial lung disease and respiratory failure in rheumatoid arthritis: a nationwide population-based study. Rheumatology (Oxford). 2021;60(1):346–52.

11. Md Yusof MY, Kabia A, Darby M, et al. Effect of rituximab on the progression of rheumatoid arthritis-related interstitial lung disease: 10 years' experience at a single centre. Rheumatology (Oxford). 2017;56(8):1348–57.
12. Sparks JA, He X, Huang J, et al. Rheumatoid arthritis disease activity predicting incident clinically apparent rheumatoid arthritis-associated interstitial lung disease: a prospective cohort study. Arthritis Rheumatol. 2019;71(9):1472–82.

Beware of the Indeterminate Interferon-Gamma Release Assay (IGRA) Tuberculosis Test

Jessica Fairley and Indi Rasaratnam

1 Clinical Pearl

Beware of the indeterminate Interferon-Gamma Release Assay (IGRA) tuberculosis (TB) test in a patient on immunosuppressive and immunomodulatory therapies.

2 Clinical Case

A 52-year-old woman of Indian ethnicity with longstanding seropositive rheumatoid arthritis is seen for review of disease modifying anti-rheumatic therapy (DMARD). She continues to have active synovitis in more than 20 small and large joints despite being on Methotrexate 20 mg weekly subcutaneously, Hydroxychloroquine 200 mg daily and Salazopyrin 1.5 g twice daily. She has previously been intolerant of Leflunomide 20 mg daily. As a pre-requisite for consideration of biologic DMARD therapy, she had a QuantiFERON-TB Gold (QFG) test that was "indeterminate" despite a good mitogen response. This result was reproduced on two further tests. She had no known exposure to TB and careful review of chest x-ray and subsequent CT chest did not reveal any evidence of previous TB

J. Fairley
Alfred Health, Melbourne, VIC, Australia

The University of Melbourne, Melbourne, VIC, Australia

I. Rasaratnam (✉)
Alfred Health and Epworth Healthcare, Melbourne, VIC, Australia

Epworth Medical School, Monash University, Melbourne, VIC, Australia

Undergraduate and Postgraduate Medical Education, Central Clinical School, Monash University and Alfred Health, Melbourne, VIC, Australia

R. Junckerstorff et al. (eds.), *Beyond Evidence-Based Medicine*,
https://doi.org/10.1007/978-981-99-4440-8_114

exposure. An Infectious Diseases opinion was sought and treatment for latent TB was suggested given her country of birth and where she spent her childhood and as a result, potential exposure to TB. However, she declined treatment with Isoniazid. After a 3-month period of tapering of her immunosuppression, her QFG test returned a negative (as opposed to indeterminate) result on three separate occasions. She subsequently commenced treatment with a tumour necrosis factor inhibitor and has remained in remission with withdrawal of all DMARDs except Methotrexate 10 mg weekly.

3 Discussion

Immunosuppressive treatments, particularly biologic agents and chemotherapies can reactivate latent infections in susceptible patients and so all patients require screening prior to commencing immunosuppressive therapies [1]. Patients should be screened for latent TB, Strongyloides and Hepatitis B and C infection [1]. After a period of antimicrobial therapy and appropriate monitoring, immunosuppressive medications can often be safely administered, but to do so without appropriate antimicrobial therapy may risk severe and life-threatening reactivations [2]. In the era of the COVID-19 pandemic, where biologic agents including tocilizumab and baricitinib have been used in severely unwell patients in combination with high-dose corticosteroids, consideration has to be given to pre-treatment screening for latent infections to avoid reactivation [3].

The QFG test is an interferon-γ release assay (IGRA) used to screen for latent TB infection [4]. IGRAs measure interferon (IFN)-γ release by antigen specific T-cells in response to stimulation by antigens from mycobacterium tuberculosis [4], with results reported as positive, negative or indeterminate. T-cell-mediated mitogen responses and IFN-γ secretion may be impaired with immunosuppressive drug use, leading to an indeterminate QFG result [5]. In particular, QFG results may be indeterminate in the context of high-dose corticosteroids (especially more than 20 mg prednisolone equivalent/day) [3, 5], lymphopenia [3] and unwell patients with disease flares and active inflammation [3, 5]. Accordingly, screening for latent infections should ideally be undertaken prior to commencement of any immunomodulatory or immunosuppressive treatments.

4 Other Gems

- While generally considered immunomodulatory rather than immunosuppressive, hydroxychloroquine has been associated with indeterminate QFG results [6], possibly by reducing IFN-γ levels [7] but further studies are required to confirm these findings.

- Patients with chronic Hepatitis B infection can have catastrophic reactivation with anti-CD-20 therapies (e.g. rituximab), and so screening for hepatitis B must include hepatitis B surface antigen and antibodies, and core antibodies (HBsAg, HBsAb and HBcAb). With specialist advice, these medications can often be safely used after initiating antiviral therapy (e.g. entecavir).
- In most cases, treatment for latent tuberculosis can be given for one month prior to initiating biologic therapies.
- Many immunomodulatory drugs, particularly biologic agents, are given infrequently (e.g. on a weekly, fortnightly, monthly or even annual basis) and can easily be forgotten as part of a regular medication history.
- High-dose corticosteroids are highly immunosuppressive, but the risk of opportunistic infection often depends on the underlying disease process. For example, patients with anti-neutrophil cytoplasmic antibody (ANCA)-associated vasculitis are at high risk of *Pneumocystis jirovecii* infection, while those with giant cell arteritis appear to be at lower risk.
- Immunosuppressed patients should not be given live vaccinations. Consideration should be given to optimising vaccination status prior to immunosuppression where possible.
- Immunosuppression not only increases the risk of opportunistic infections, but also non-infectious complications such as malignancy. In Australia, skin cancer screening is particularly important, and patients should be reminded to keep up to date with age-appropriate malignancy screening.
- Patients with inflammatory diseases may be at increased risk of cardiovascular disease including accelerated atherosclerosis, often as a complication of active inflammation and medication regimens. For example, rheumatoid arthritis may confer a similar cardiovascular risk as type 2 diabetes mellitus. Regular cardiovascular risk factor screening is recommended.

References

1. Singh JA, Saag KG, Bridges SL Jr, et al. 2015 American College of Rheumatology Guideline for the treatment of rheumatoid arthritis. Arthritis Rheumatol. 2016;68(1):1–26.
2. Matsue K, Kimura S, Takanashi Y, et al. Reactivation of hepatitis B virus after rituximab-containing treatment in patients with CD20-positive B-cell lymphoma. Cancer. 2010;116(20):4769–76.
3. Solanich X, Fernandez-Huerta M, Basaez C, et al. Clinical significance of indeterminate QuantiFERON-TB gold plus assay results in hospitalized COVID-19 patients with severe hyperinflammatory syndrome. J Clin Med. 2021;10(5):918.
4. Shafeque A, Bigio J, Hogan CA, Pai M, Banaei N. Fourth-generation QuantiFERON-TB gold plus: what is the evidence? J Clin Microbiol. 2020;58(9):10.
5. Hakimian S, Popov Y, Rupawala AH, Salomon-Escoto K, Hatch S, Pellish R. The conundrum of indeterminate QuantiFERON-TB Gold results before anti-tumor necrosis factor initiation. Biologics. 2018;12:61–7.

6. Gaffney RG, Werth VP. Evaluating results of an interferon-gamma release assay in patients with autoimmune disease who are taking hydroxychloroquine. J Am Acad Dermatol. 2019;80(4):1162–4.
7. van den Borne BE, Dijkmans BA, de Rooij HH, le Cessie S, Verweij CL. Chloroquine and hydroxychloroquine equally affect tumor necrosis factor-alpha, interleukin 6, and interferon-gamma production by peripheral blood mononuclear cells. J Rheumatol. 1997;24(1):55–60.

In Cases of Unexplained Elevated ALT and AST, Don't Forget to Check a CK

Jessica Fairley and Indi Rasaratnam

1 Clinical Pearl

In cases of unexplained elevated ALT and AST, don't forget to check a CK.

2 Clinical Case

A 45-year-old woman with a ten-year history of seropositive rheumatoid arthritis is noted to have raised transaminases. Both alanine aminotransferase (ALT) and aspartate aminotransferase (AST) were over three times the upper limit of normal. This was attributed to the escalation of her methotrexate dose three months prior to reach her current state of low disease activity. The three-monthly blood tests done to monitor for methotrexate toxicity revealed a microcytic hypochromic anaemia subsequently confirmed to be an iron deficiency anaemia. Endoscopy revealed a caecal carcinoma. On admission to hospital for surgical resection of the tumour, it was noted that she had Gottron's papules overlying the metacarpophalangeal and proximal interphalangeal joints. No muscle pain or weakness was identified. Creatine kinase (CK) was elevated at 800 IU/L and MRI of the thigh muscles revealed

J. Fairley
Alfred Health, Melbourne, VIC, Australia

The University of Melbourne, Melbourne, VIC, Australia

I. Rasaratnam (✉)
Alfred Health and Epworth Healthcare, Melbourne, VIC, Australia

Epworth Medical School, Monash University, Melbourne, VIC, Australia

Undergraduate and Postgraduate Medical Education, Central Clinical School, Monash University and Alfred Health, Melbourne, VIC, Australia

R. Junckerstorff et al. (eds.), *Beyond Evidence-Based Medicine*,
https://doi.org/10.1007/978-981-99-4440-8_115

oedema in the vastus lateralis and medialis. Cancer-related dermatomyositis was diagnosed. Most interestingly within 3 months of surgery, there was spontaneous resolution of the rash and normalisation of the CK, ALT and AST. The methotrexate dose had not been adjusted. The raised transaminases reflected the raised CK and myositis, rather than a liver pathology.

3 Discussion

Raised liver enzymes, particularly ALT and AST are generally considered to be markers of hepatocellular injury [1]. Hepatitis and raised liver enzymes may be caused by drugs including alcohol and complementary medications, viral infections, biliary obstruction, infiltrative processes, or non-alcoholic steatohepatitis [1]. However, where investigation of other potential contributors is unsuccessful and other liver enzymes (e.g., gamma-glutamyl transferase (GGT) and alkaline phosphatase (ALP) are normal, a non-hepatic aetiology should be considered.

One possible aetiology of an isolated rise in ALT and AST are skeletal muscle pathologies [2]. Skeletal muscle damage is generally characterised by a rise in muscle enzymes, particularly creatine kinase (CK) [2]. Muscle damage may be mediated by a toxic effect of drugs (e.g., statins), rhabdomyolysis, intense exercise, metabolic abnormalities, immune-mediated myositis, and necrotising myopathies [3]. The degree of CK elevation, temporal evolution of the condition, history of relevant medication use (e.g., commencement of statins or other myotoxins) and other clinical features (particularly rash, arthralgia, and other features of autoimmune disease e.g., Raynaud phenomenon) can give clues to a potential aetiology [3].

Levels of ALT and AST have been shown to be closely correlated with CK levels in inflammatory myopathies [2]. Aminotransferases exist in skeletal muscle and are released into the circulation along with CK in skeletal muscle injury [2, 4]. Accordingly, in the appropriate clinical context, raised ALT and AST may not indicate primary hepatic pathology and can be closely monitored [2]. ALT and AST levels should reduce as the CK normalises [2]. In the context of immune-mediated muscle pathology where immunosuppressive agents may be required to control disease, it is important to identify true hepatic injury. Many immunosuppressive agents confer significant risk of hepatotoxicity requiring close monitoring of liver enzymes with initiation.

4 Other Gems

- Statins can be associated with a range of muscle toxicities, ranging from myalgia, mildly elevated CK and immune-mediated necrotising myopathy. While statin-induced immune-mediated necrotising myopathy, characterised by anti-HMGCR-antibodies, is extremely rare and requires complete withdrawal of statin therapy, non-specific muscle symptoms are common and often don't require statin cessation. A systematic review and meta-analysis identified a similar frequency of non-specific muscle symptoms in statin-treated patients and controls [5].

- Immune-mediated myopathies commonly have a subacute and painless onset, with weeks to months of progressive weakness, fatigue and muscle wasting.
- Acute rhabdomyolysis often presents rapidly, without muscle wasting and with myalgia. Acute rhabdomyolysis can complicate autoimmune myositis but is uncommon.
- Rhabdomyolysis may be associated with electrolyte abnormalities and acute renal failure, so close monitoring of biochemistry is required.
- Raised muscle enzymes and myositis can occur with a variety of viral infections, including influenza.
- Failure of the CK to normalise with conservative management (e.g., rehydration or cessation of culprit medication) is often a clue to persistent muscle inflammation in autoimmune myopathies.
- Skeletal muscle pathologies may also be characterised by a raised troponin level; troponin T may be secreted by skeletal muscle while troponin I is more specific for myocardial involvement. Given the myocardium may be affected by any muscle pathology, care must be taken to exclude myocarditis or other cardiac muscle pathology with any elevation of cardiac enzymes.
- Skeletal muscle pathology may also be characterised by respiratory and gastrointestinal muscle weakness. Respiratory failure and dysphagia are associated with severe disease and may warrant escalation of treatment, so patients must be asked specifically about these complications. Neck flexion weakness may be a predictor of respiratory muscle weakness in myositis.
- Autoimmune myositis may be paraneoplastic; in some cases, onset of skeletal muscle disease may occur prior to clinical malignancy and thus act as an "early warning" sign. Certain myositis specific antibodies are associated with higher risk of malignancy and warrant more aggressive malignancy screening, particularly anti-transcription intermediary factor 1 (TIF-1)-gamma and anti-nuclear matrix protein (NXP-2) antibodies.

References

1. Kwo PY, Cohen SM, Lim JK. ACG clinical guideline: evaluation of abnormal liver chemistries. Am J Gastroenterol. 2017;112(1):18–35.
2. Mathur T, Manadan AM, Thiagarajan S, Hota B, Block JA. Serum transaminases are frequently elevated at time of diagnosis of idiopathic inflammatory myopathy and normalize with creatine kinase. J Clin Rheumatol. 2014;20(3):130–2.
3. Schmidt J. Current Classification and Management of Inflammatory Myopathies. J Neuromuscul Dis. 2018;5(2):109–29.
4. Bohlmeyer TJ, Wu AH, Perryman MB. Evaluation of laboratory tests as a guide to diagnosis and therapy of myositis. Rheum Dis Clin N Am. 1994;20(4):845–56.
5. Ganga HV, Slim HB, Thompson PD. A systematic review of statin-induced muscle problems in clinical trials. Am Heart J. 2014;168(1):6–15.

Antinuclear Antibody Interpretation

Krita Sridharan, Jacinta Cheng, and Anne Powell

1 Clinical Pearl

A negative Antinuclear antibody (ANA) can effectively rule out a diagnosis of systemic lupus erythematosus. However, a positive ANA may not be significant and should not be repeated.

2 Clinical Case

A 41-year-old female from Cambodia presents to the hospital acutely unwell. She is febrile, tachycardic and hypoxaemic. Investigations reveal a pancytopenia. A CT chest is performed, revealing widespread opacities and a small pericardial effusion. She is delirious and is unable to provide a history, however collateral history from her husband reveals she has been experiencing constitutional symptoms of fevers, fatigue and arthralgias over the past few months. The patient is admitted to the intensive care unit for a period of monitoring. She is treated empirically with piperacillin-tazobactam and vancomycin, with minimal improvement in her condition. The rheumatology team is consulted given the multi-system nature of her presentation, as to whether she could have a diagnosis of systemic lupus erythematosus (SLE). The following investigations were completed early in the admission (Table 1):

Based on the clinical scenario and negative ANA, the rheumatologist advises that SLE is unlikely. The infectious disease team is subsequently consulted, and after further workup, a diagnosis of disseminated tuberculosis is made. The patient is

K. Sridharan (✉) · J. Cheng · A. Powell
Alfred Health and Monash University, Melbourne, VIC, Australia

R. Junckerstorff et al. (eds.), *Beyond Evidence-Based Medicine*,
https://doi.org/10.1007/978-981-99-4440-8_116

Table 1 Summary of the patient's blood tests

Investigation	Patient value	Reference value
Erythrocyte sedimentation rate (ESR)	**26**	1–10 mm/h
C-reactive protein (CRP)	**258**	0–5 mg/L
ANA	Negative	N/A
Anti-double stranded DNA antibody (Anti-dsDNA Ab)	Negative	N/A
Anti-Smith antibody	Negative	N/A
Lupus anticoagulant	Negative	N/A
Beta-2 glycoprotein antibody	Negative	N/A
Anti-cardiolipin antibody	Negative	N/A
Complement C3	**0.52**	0.76–1.87 g/L
Complement C4	0.29	0.11–0.38 g/L
Rheumatoid factor	<10	<29 IU/mL
Anti-cyclic citrullinated peptide (CCP) antibody	<1	<5 u/mL

then appropriately treated with anti-mycobacterial agents and makes a slow recovery.

3 Discussion

SLE is a multi-system condition that can present in a myriad of ways. Patients may present with a subacute course but may also present acutely unwell with multi-organ failure. It is crucial in these cases for the diagnosis to be made accurately and alternative diagnoses excluded. Had a diagnosis of SLE been incorrectly made in this vignette and the patient treated with immunosuppressive therapy, the patient's clinical state would have deteriorated.

The ANA is a key part of the diagnosis of SLE. The 2019 EULAR/ACR criteria for SLE requires a positive ANA as entry criteria into the diagnostic algorithm [1]. This is because a negative ANA has an excellent negative predictive value for SLE, reported to be about 99% [2]. It is important to note that ANA positivity has a low positive predictive value for SLE, reported to be around 11% [3]. A positive ANA may be due to other causes, including non-autoimmune conditions. Therefore, the clinical context needs to be taken into consideration to determine a pre-test probability. Indirect immunofluorescence is the method of choice to detect ANA. The titre and pattern should be considered when making a diagnosis. The titre is the concentration of antibody in a patient's serum, and is determined by serial dilutions, from a dilution of 1:40 up to 1: 2560. A higher titre suggests a higher significance. Generally, a titre of 1:320 or more is considered clinically significant [4]. The patterns most often observed with SLE are homogenous and speckled. Other antibodies such as anti-dsDNA and anti-Smith are also helpful as these are highly specific for SLE, and when these are present are highly suggestive of the diagnosis.

In our case of an unwell patient with evidence of multi-system disease, a diagnosis of SLE was clinically suspected however successfully excluded based on a negative ANA. It is important to note that a positive ANA can be seen in infection. Repeating the ANA is not recommended [5], nor is repeating the extractable nuclear antigen antibody (ENA) as it rarely changes the working diagnosis [6].

4 Other Gems

- There is no utility in repeat ANA testing, and a change in ANA titre is not associated with disease activity.
- Conversely, anti-dsDNA levels can be monitored as a sign of disease activity in SLE.
- While a negative ANA can exclude SLE, it may not exclude other autoimmune conditions such as rheumatoid arthritis, seronegative spondyloarthropathies, inflammatory myositis, vasculitides, and Sjogren's syndrome [7].
- A CRP that is disproportionately elevated compared to ESR suggests an infectious cause to be more likely than a rheumatological cause of illness.

References

1. Aringer M, Costenbader K, Daikh D, et al. 2019 European League Against Rheumatism/American College of Rheumatology classification criteria for systemic lupus erythematosus. Arthritis Rheumatol. 2019;71(9):1400–12. https://doi.org/10.1002/art.40930.
2. Hissaria P, Broadfoot A, Baumgart KW. Revisiting the antinuclear antibody test with emphasis on a new pattern: anti-DFS70 antibody. Med J Aust. 2019;210(2):69–71. https://doi.org/10.5694/mja2.12103.
3. Slater CA, Davis RB, Shmerling RH. Antinuclear antibody testing. A study of clinical utility. Arch Intern Med. 1996;156(13):1421–5. https://doi.org/10.1001/archinte.1996.00440120079007.
4. Tan EM, Feltkamp TE, Smolen JS, et al. Range of antinuclear antibodies in 'healthy' individuals. Arthritis Rheumatol. 1997;40(9):1601–11. https://doi.org/10.1002/art.1780400909.
5. Yeo AL, Le S, Ong J, et al. Utility of repeated antinuclear antibody tests: a retrospective database study. Lancet Rheumatol. 2020;2(7):E412–7. https://doi.org/10.1016/S2665-9913(20)30084-9.
6. Yeo AL, Leech M, Ojaimi S, et al. Utility of repeat extractable nuclear antigen antibody testing—a retrospective audit. Rheumatology. 2022;62(3):1248. https://doi.org/10.1093/rheumatology/keac437.
7. O'Sullivan M, McLean-Tooke A, Loh RK. Antinuclear antibody test. Aust Fam Physician. 2013;42(10):718–21.

Cryoglobulinaemia

Krita Sridharan, Jacinta Cheng, and Anne Powell

1 Clinical Pearl

In an unwell patient where the vasculitic screen shows a positive rheumatoid factor, it is important to check serum cryoglobulins.

2 Clinical Case

A 59-year-old man presents to the hospital unwell with severe acute kidney injury. He describes a few months history of constitutional symptoms including fatigue, sweats and arthralgias. On examination he has a purpuric rash over his lower legs. Urinalysis demonstrates an active sediment with presence of dysmorphic red blood cells and red cell casts, as well as moderate proteinuria. Vasculitis is suspected and the following investigations were completed (Table 1).

Serum cryoglobulins results came back positive several days later, with a cryocrit of 23% (reference value <0.5%).

The diagnosis is made of mixed cryoglobulinaemic vasculitis secondary to hepatitis C infection. A renal biopsy confirms a membranoproliferative glomerulonephritis. The patient is treated with antiviral therapy and a short period of immunosuppression with corticosteroids and rituximab. His renal function improves dramatically following this and he continues to a recovery.

K. Sridharan (✉) · J. Cheng · A. Powell
Alfred Health and Monash University, Melbourne, VIC, Australia

R. Junckerstorff et al. (eds.), *Beyond Evidence-Based Medicine*,
https://doi.org/10.1007/978-981-99-4440-8_117

Table 1 Summary of the patient's blood tests

Investigation	Patient value	Reference value
Erythrocyte sedimentation rate (ESR)	**58**	1–10 mm/h
C-reactive protein (CRP)	**18**	0–5 mg/L
Antinuclear antibody (ANA)	**1:1280, homogenous pattern**	<1:160
Anti-double stranded DNA antibody	Negative	N/A
Anti-Smith antibody	Negative	N/A
Complement C3	0.78	0.76–1.87 g/L
Complement C4	**0.06**	0.11–0.38 g/L
Rheumatoid factor	**62**	<29 IU/ml
Anti-cyclic citrullinated peptide (Anti-CCP) antibody	<1	<5 u/mL
Extractable nuclear antigen (ENA)	Negative	N/A
Perinuclear anti-neutrophil cytoplasmic antibodies (p-ANCA)	Negative	N/A
Cytoplasmic anti-neutrophil cytoplasmic antibodies (c-ANCA)	Negative	N/A
Anti-GBM antibody	Negative	N/A
HIV serology	Negative	N/A
Hepatitis B surface antigen	Negative	N/A
Hepatitis B surface antibody	**Positive**	<10 IU/L
Hepatitis B core antibody	Negative	N/A
Hepatitis C antibody	**Positive**	N/A
Hepatitis C viral load	**High** (>800,000 IU/mL)	Undetectable
Serum protein electrophoresis	Normal	N/A

3 Discussion

Cryoglobulins are immune complexes that precipitate in cold temperatures and redissolve in higher temperatures [1]. There are three different subtypes of cryoglobulins. Type I is made up of monoclonal immunoglobulins and is usually caused by monoclonal gammopathies such as multiple myeloma. Type II and III are mixed and are most often secondary to chronic viral infection, particularly hepatitis C [2]. They can also be due to some lymphoproliferative disorders and autoimmune connective tissue diseases, such as systemic lupus erythematosus and Sjogren's syndrome [3]. They are antibodies directed against immunoglobulin G, which then form immune complexes and initiate an inflammatory immune response. This leads to endothelial injury and end-organ damage.

Some cryoglobulins are, by definition, rheumatoid factors, which are antibodies detected against the Fc portion of immunoglobulin G. A positive rheumatoid factor is often present in patients with mixed cryoglobulinaemia, and the presence of rheumatoid factor is not specific to rheumatoid arthritis and may be found in a variety of autoimmune and non-autoimmune conditions [4].

Cryoglobulins are more difficult to collect as a thermos must be collected from pathology to prewarm collection tubes to ensure the sample does not fall below 37° to avoid premature precipitation of cryoglobulin. Due to the complexity, it is usually only processed within usual working hours, and it has a long turnaround time as it takes a minimum of 72 hours to incubate.

It is important to consider the presence of cryoglobulins when faced with a positive rheumatoid factor in an acutely unwell patient with features similar to those discussed in the case, and in the context of known monoclonal gammopathy or risk factors for hepatitis or other chronic viral infection.

4 Other Gems

- Correct testing conditions for cryoglobulins are necessary to minimise false negatives.
- Type 1 cryoglobulinaemia is more often associated with hyperviscosity syndromes than vasculitis and may cause digital ischaemia and ulcers.
- 'Meltzer's triad' is a syndrome consisting of purpura, arthralgia and fatigue, and is commonly seen in mixed cryoglobulinaemia.

References

1. Ramos-Casals M, Stone JH, Cid MC, Bosch X. The cryoglobulinaemias. Lancet. 2012;379(9813):348–60. https://doi.org/10.1016/S0140-6736(11)60242-0.
2. Charles ED, Dustin LB. Hepatitis C virus-induced cryoglobulinemia. Kidney Int. 2009;76(8):818–24. https://doi.org/10.1038/ki.2009.247.
3. Boleto G, Ghillani-Dalbin P, Musset L, et al. Cryoglobulinaemia after the era of chronic hepatitis C infection. Semin Arthritis Rheum. 2020;50(4):695–700. https://doi.org/10.1016/j.semarthrit.2020.05.004.
4. Shmerling RH, Delbanco TL. The rheumatoid factor: an analysis of clinical utility. Am J Med. 1991;91(5):528–34. https://doi.org/10.1016/0002-9343(91)90190-9.

Part XVII
Drug Allergy and Immunology

Sulfonamide Cross-Reactivity

Jessica Plager and Elizabeth Phillips

1 Clinical Pearl

Sulfonamide antimicrobials and sulfonamide non-antimicrobials are not cross-reactive.

2 Clinical Case

A 52-year-old man presents to urgent care with a "red, swollen, painful bump" in his left axilla. He is clinically diagnosed with purulent cellulitis with no drainable abscess. Per guidelines, the antibiotic of choice would be sulfamethoxazole-trimethoprim (SMZ-TMP), but patient reports that he has a "sulfa allergy." He states that he had a flat itchy rash with furosemide about 10 years ago. While he did not require treatment and/or hospitalisation for this reaction, he was counselled to avoid all "sulfa drugs." Given this history, the practicing clinician prescribes doxycycline as an alternative. Unfortunately, his cellulitis continued to worsen on doxycycline therapy, and he presented to the Emergency Department 2 days later where he was admitted, placed on intravenous antibiotics; a wound culture ultimately grew a doxycycline-resistant methicillin-resistant *Staphylococcus aureus*.

J. Plager
Department of Medicine, Department of Pediatrics, Vanderbilt University Medical Center, Nashville, TN, USA

E. Phillips (✉)
Department of Medicine, Dermatology, Pathology, Microbiology and Immunology, Vanderbilt University Medical Center, Nashville, TN, USA

Department of Pharmacology, Vanderbilt University School of Medicine, Nashville, TN, USA

R. Junckerstorff et al. (eds.), *Beyond Evidence-Based Medicine*,
https://doi.org/10.1007/978-981-99-4440-8_118

3 Discussion

Sulfamethoxazole-trimethoprim (SMZ-TMP) is a common culprit of hypersensitivity reactions and other adverse drug reactions. While the most common reaction is a benign maculopapular eruption, SMZ-TMP can also cause immediate IgE-mediated reactions and severe cutaneous adverse reactions such as Stevens-Johnson syndrome, toxic epidermal necrolysis, drug reaction with eosinophilia and systemic symptoms and fixed drug eruption [1–3].

Despite the prevalence of SMZ-TMP allergy, much confusion exists surrounding sulfonamide allergy which is known colloquially as "sulfa allergy." [1] Sulfonamides, aka "sulfa" drugs can be divided into two groups: sulfonamide anti-microbials and non-antimicrobial sulfonamides. While both are derived from *p*-aminobenzesulfonamide and contain an-SO_2NH_2 moiety, they have key structural differences (namely, sulfonamide antimicrobials contain the immunogenic N1 heterocyclic ring and N4 aromatic amine whereas non-antimicrobials *do not* – see Fig. 1) such that sulfonamide anti-microbials and non-antimicrobial sulfonamides do *not* cross-react [1, 4].

Current expert guidance (as summarised in Table 1) recommends that patients with a history of reacting to a sulfonamide anti-microbial (e.g. SMZ-TMP) should avoid other sulfonamide anti-microbials (e.g. topical silver sulfadiazine) but *not* avoid sulfonamide non-antimicrobials (e.g. celecoxib) [1]. As for sulfonamide non-antimicrobials, there is *no* evidence for cross reactivity among sulfonamide non-antimicrobials (e.g., a patient with a reaction to furosemide may tolerate celecoxib), so no avoidance is necessary beyond avoiding the culprit drug [1].

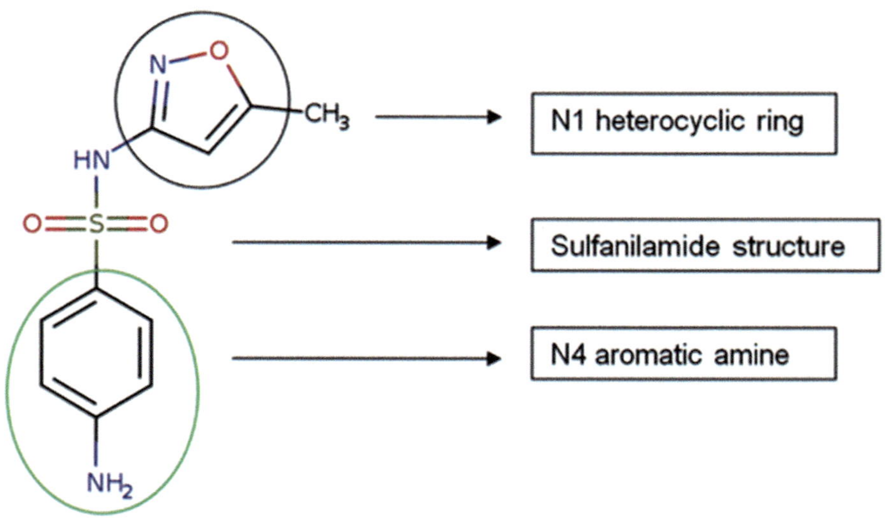

Fig. 1 Whereas sulfonamide antimicrobials and non-antimicrobials share a core sulfanilamide structure, sulfonamide non-antimicrobials lack the immunogenic N1 heterocyclic ring and N4 aromatic ring. (Adapted from Khan et al. [1])

Table 1 Cross reactivity of sulfonamides

Drug or compound	Drug class: drug	Comments
Sulfonamide non-antimicrobials	Alpha blocker: tamsulosin	There is no cross-reactivity among sulfonamide non-antimicrobials (e.g. celecoxib does not cross react with glimepiride)
	Antiarrhythmics: Ibutilide, sotalol	
	Anticonvulsants: Topiramate	
	Carbonic anhydrase inhibitors: Acetazolamide, metazolamide, dorzolamide, brinzolamide	
	COX-2 inhibitors: Celecoxib	
	Loop diuretics: Furosemide, bumetanide	There is no cross-reactivity between sulfonamide antimicrobials and non-antimicrobials
	Sulfonylureas: Glimepiride, glyburide, gliclazide	
	Thiazide diuretics: Hydrochlorothiazide, chlorthalidone, indapamide, metolazone, diazoxide	
	Triptans: Sumatriptan, naratriptan	
Sulfonamide antimicrobials	Sulfamethoxazole (oral/parental: cotrimoxazole, *Septra)*	There *is* cross-reactivity among sulfonamide antimicrobials
	Sulfasalazine (oral: *Salazopyrin*)	
	Sodium sulfacetamide (ophthalmic)	
	Silver sulfadiazine (topical: *Flamazine)*	
Other drugs	Dapsone (oral and topical)	Possible cross-reactivity with sulfonamide antimicrobials. Would exercise caution and recommend consultation of Allergy / Immunology specialist if available
	Darunavir (oral: *Prezista, Prezcobix)*	
	Fosamprenavir (oral: *Telzir)*	
	Sulfur	No sulfonamide moiety and therefore no cross-reactivity
	Sulfate (e.g. ferrous sulfate, magnesium sulfate)	
	Sulfites (e.g. sodium metabisulfite)	
	Trimethoprim	Should avoid in all patients who reacted to sulfamethoxazole-trimethoprim as it is unknown which component was the causative agent

4 Other Gems

- Sulfur, sulfate, and sulfites do *not* contain a sulfonamide moiety and thus do *not* need to be avoided in patients with a history of sulfonamide anti-microbial and/or non-antimicrobial allergy [1]
- While most SMZ-TMP allergy is mediated by the sulfonamide antimicrobial component, it is prudent to avoid trimethoprim as well [1]
- Patients with HIV have a high rate of sensitivity to SMZ-TMP ranging from 34–50%. Such patients often are negative on rechallenge when they have had immune reconstitution or response to antiretrovirals [3].

References

1. Khan DA, Knowles SR, Shear NH. Sulfonamide hypersensitivity: fact and fiction. J Allergy Clin Immunol Pract. 2019;7(7):2116–23.
2. Krantz MS, et al. Oral challenge with trimethoprim-sulfamethoxazole in patients with "sulfa" antibiotic allergy. J Allergy Clin Immunol Pract. 2020;8(2):757–760.e4.
3. Broyles AD, et al. Practical guidance for the evaluation and management of drug hypersensitivity: specific drugs. J Allergy Clin Immunol Pract. 2020;8(9):S16–S116.
4. Strom BL, et al. Absence of cross-reactivity between sulfonamide antibiotics and sulfonamide nonantibiotics. N Engl J Med. 2003;349(17):1628–35.

Non-IgE Mediated Immediate Reactions

Jessica Plager and Elizabeth Phillips

1 Clinical Pearl

Not all immediate reactions are IgE-mediated.

2 Clinical Case

A 67-year-old woman with multiple myeloma is admitted for chemotherapy. She is doing well initially however on hospital day 4 develops cough and shortness of breath, and a chest x-ray shows a left lower lobe infiltrate. The hospital team starts her on vancomycin and cefepime. When she gets vancomycin, she develops immediate onset flushing and itching with a few hives noted tracking along her intravenous line. When the team slows down the infusion and pre-medicates her with an antihistamine, she can tolerate the vancomycin without reaction. She turns to you and asks, "Am I allergic to vancomycin?"

J. Plager
Department of Medicine, Department of Pediatrics, Vanderbilt University Medical Center, Nashville, TN, USA

E. Phillips (✉)
Department of Medicine, Dermatology, Pathology, Microbiology and Immunology, Vanderbilt University Medical Center, Nashville, TN, USA

Department of Pharmacology, Vanderbilt University School of Medicine, Nashville, TN, USA

R. Junckerstorff et al. (eds.), *Beyond Evidence-Based Medicine*,
https://doi.org/10.1007/978-981-99-4440-8_119

3 Discussion

As a broad category, adverse drug reactions (ADRs) are defined as the unintended pharmacologic effects of a medication. This can be further subdivided into type A and type B reactions [2]. Type A reactions are also known as "on-target ADRs" and are dose-dependent and related known interaction of the drug with the known pharmacological target [2]. Type B reactions, also known as "off-target ADRs," can be dose-dependent or dose-independent, and arise due to an unknown interaction of the drug with a pharmacological target distant to where the drug exerts its mechanism of action. [2] These off-target reactions are further classified to help bridge the previous Gell-Coombs immunological classification with the more recent Rawlins pharmacological classification into those ADRs related to cellular toxicity, non-IgE mediated, antibody (including IgE-mediated) and T-cell mediated [2] (Fig. 1).

In a typical type I hypersensitivity reaction, a sensitised individual is re-exposed to an allergen which leads to cross-linking of receptors on mast cells and basophils, which in turn results in the subsequent release of mediators (e.g., histamine), leading to the clinical manifestations including anaphylaxis, angioedema, bronchospasm, urticaria, and hypotension [2].

In non-IgE mediated reactions (formerly known as pseudo-allergic or anaphylactoid), mast cells and basophils degranulate via non-IgE mechanisms. While the complete mechanisms underlying these reactions are still being elucidated, they can include activation of mast cells directly (through a non-IgE mediated mechanism) or activation of the complement cascade [3]. Common culprit medications of non-IgE mediated mast activation reactions include vancomycin, radiocontrast media, fluoroquinolones, opioids, local anaesthetics, chemotherapeutic agents, and neuromuscular blocking agents [4].

Although non-IgE mediated reactions appear symptomatically identical to IgE-mediated drug reactions, patients importantly do *not* require history of sensitisation and thus these reactions can occur in patients without a prior history of any prior drug exposure. Furthermore, non-IgE mediated mast cell activation also differs from IgE-mediated reactions by being variable, modifiable, and largely dose-dependent; in true IgE-mediated immediate reactions there is less dependency on dose as antigen is amplified through IgE-mediated mechanisms [2].

It is important for the general practitioner to be aware of non-IgE mediated reactions because their diagnosis, prognosis and prevention differs from immediate IgE-mediated hypersensitivity reactions. For intravenous drugs associated with non-IgE mediated mast cell activation such as vancomycin, radiocontrast dye, fluoroquinolones, neuromuscular blocking agents or opioids, these reactions importantly are importantly *infusion-rate dependent* and ameliorated by slowing the infusion and by pre-medication with antihistamines [5]. For example, as in the clinical case above, a patient with a vancomycin-induced flushing may be able to tolerate the infusion if the rate is slowed and/or preceded by antihistamine therapy.

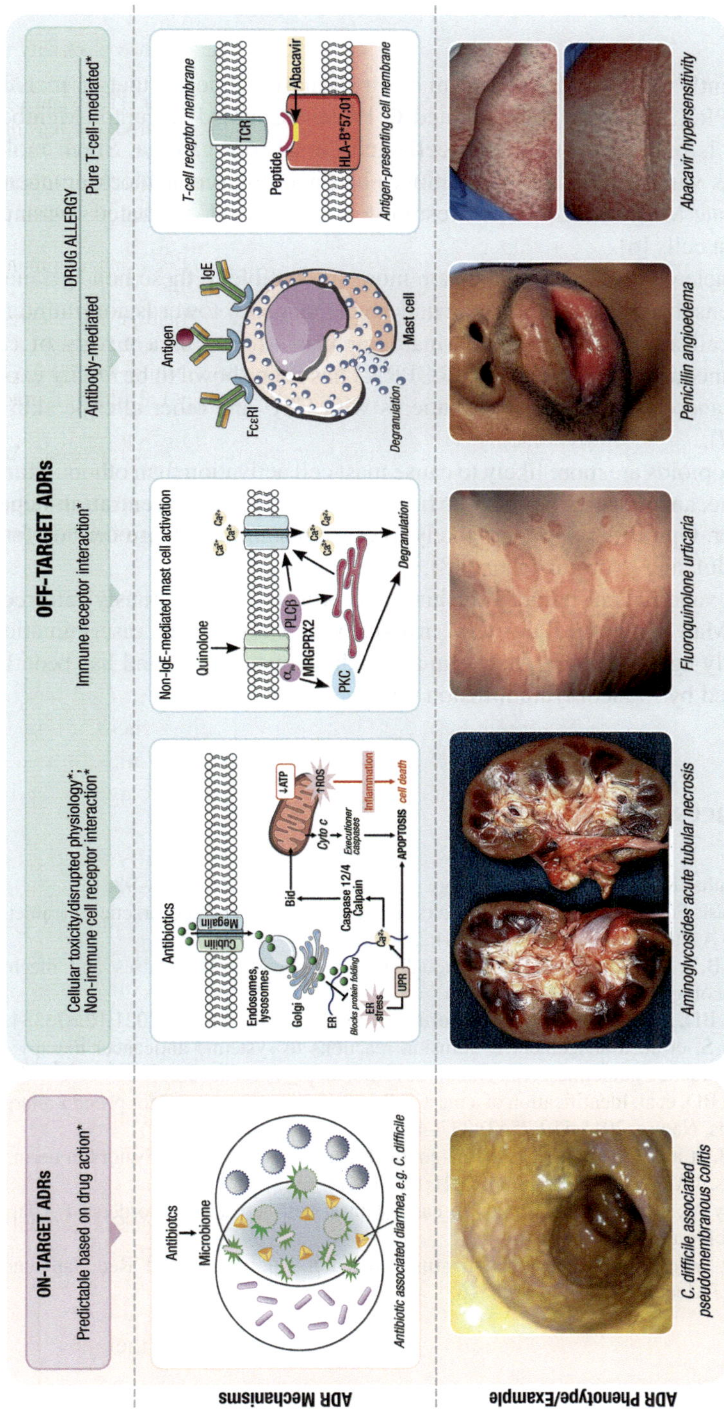

Fig. 1 Classification of on-target and off-target ADRs [1]

4 Other Gems

- A recently discovered mechanism of direct mast cell degranulation includes the MRGPRX2 receptor (Mas-Related G-Protein Coupled Receptor Member X2) which is only present on mast cells and dorsal root ganglia. Small molecules such as vancomycin, fluoroquinolones and neuromuscular blocking agents can stimulate MRGPRX2 directly, resulting in the non-IgE mediated degranulation of mast cells [6].
- It is unclear why some patients are more susceptible to these non-IgE mediated reactions than others. Clues to an underlying tendency towards non-immunologic mast cell activation include dermatographism as well as a history of chronic spontaneous urticaria (CSU). MRGPRX2 has been shown to be highly expressed on cutaneous mast cells from patients with CSU and other allergic skin disorders [7].
- Some opioids are more likely to cause mast cell activation than others. Morphine, codeine, and meperidine provoke histamine release in a concentration-dependent manner. Opioids that are less likely to cause histamine release include fentanyl, tramadol, and hydromorphone [8].
- While vancomycin-induced flushing and pruritis was previously referred to as "Red Man Syndrome," this term invokes both sex and racial discrimination particularly against Native American and Indigenous peoples and has been largely replaced by "vancomycin infusion reaction" [9].

References

1. Blumenthal KG, et al. Antibiotic allergy. Lancet. 2019;393(10167):183–98.
2. Joint Task Force on Practice Parameters. Drug allergy: an updated practice parameter. Ann Allergy Asthma Immunol. 2010;105(4):259–73.
3. Zhang B, et al. Drug-induced pseudoallergy: a review of the causes and mechanisms. Pharmacology. 2018;101(1-2):104–10.
4. McNeil BD. MRGPRX2 and adverse drug reactions. Front Immunol. 2021;12:676354.
5. Roselló S, et al. Management of infusion reactions to systemic anticancer therapy: ESMO clinical practice guidelines. Ann Oncol. 2017;28(suppl_4):iv100–18.
6. McNeil BD, et al. Identification of a mast-cell-specific receptor crucial for pseudo-allergic drug reactions. Nature. 2015;519(7542):237–41.
7. Kühn H, et al. Mas-related G protein–coupled receptor X2 and its activators in dermatologic allergies. J Allergy Clin Immunol. 2021;147(2):456–69.
8. Lepelley M, et al. Which opioids in case of mast cell activation disorders? J Allergy Clin Immunol Pract. 2019;7(4):1317–8.
9. Alvarez-Arango S, et al. Vancomycin infusion reaction—moving beyond "Red Man Syndrome". N Engl J Med. 2021;384(14):1283–6.

Medication Timeline is Important for Causality

Jessica Plager and Elizabeth Phillips

1 Clinical Pearl

Drawing a timeline of all implicated drugs within the last 8 weeks is critical for determining drug causality in severe cutaneous adverse drug reactions (SCARs).

2 Clinical Case

A 34-year-old woman with a history of hypertrophic cardiomyopathy requiring heart transplant is admitted to the hospital with fever, rash, and mouth pain. She had her heart transplant about 1 month ago and was started on prophylactic antibiotics including trimethoprim-sulfamethoxazole (TMP/SMX). Two days ago, she developed a painful rash on her face and upper chest. Since then, she has developed oral blisters which are making it hard to eat and stay hydrated. On exam, she is toxic appearing with erythematous, irregular shaped, dusky macules involving her face and chest as well as haemorrhagic erosions with crust involving her mouth.

J. Plager
Department of Medicine, Department of Pediatrics, Vanderbilt University Medical Center, Nashville, TN, USA

E. Phillips (✉)
Department of Medicine, Dermatology, Pathology, Microbiology and Immunology, Vanderbilt University Medical Center, Nashville, TN, USA

Department of Pharmacology, Vanderbilt University School of Medicine, Nashville, TN, USA

R. Junckerstorff et al. (eds.), *Beyond Evidence-Based Medicine*,
https://doi.org/10.1007/978-981-99-4440-8_120

3 Discussion

Delayed immune-mediated adverse drug reactions (ADRs) are defined as reactions occurring more than six hours after dosing [1]. While the most common delayed ADR are benign exanthems, severe cutaneous adverse drug reactions (SCARs) are potentially life-threatening reactions with varying clinical patterns and morbidity [2, 3]. Within the broad category of SCAR are Stevens-Johnson syndrome (SJS) and toxic epidermal necrolysis (TEN), drug reaction with eosinophilia and systemic symptoms (DRESS), as well as acute generalised exanthematous pustulosis (AGEP). Because SJS, TEN, and DRESS are life-threatening and can result in long-term severe sequelae, it is important for all physicians to feel comfortable with the diagnosis and basic management of SCARs.

Once a physician suspects and/or makes the diagnosis SCAR, a critical step in management is the prompt withdrawal of the culprit drug. Indeed, for SJS and TEN, early culprit drug discontinuation is associated with better prognosis [4]. In order to determine drug causality, one should consider the SCAR type, day of symptom onset, drug notoriety and time since drug intake [3]. The time since drug intake is of particular importance as the interval between exposure and SCAR onset differs according to SCAR type: typically within a few days for AGEP, 4–28 days for SJS/TEN, and 2–8 weeks for DRESS [2, 3]; see Fig. 2 for timeline of ADRs. For AGEP the timeline is typically very short (24–72 hours) for aminopenicillins and much longer (2–4 weeks) for some other drugs (e.g. calcium channel blockers and hydroxychloroquine). For DRESS although most cases will typically occur within 2–6 weeks, shorter latency DRESS (<2 weeks from starting drug) has been noted particularly with aminopenicillins and other beta lactams [5]. The clinical time course of the reaction is best visualised via the creation of a drug timeline with day 0 being the first day of symptoms (see Fig. 1) [2]. When reviewing the drug timeline, one can identify high culprit drug via utilising published tables of high risk medications [3], using various algorithms [6–8], or with the use of published validation scores such as EuroSCAR (for AGEP) and RegiSCAR (for DRESS). Of note, it is also important to consider drugs with long half-lives that were stopped prior to disease onset [2].

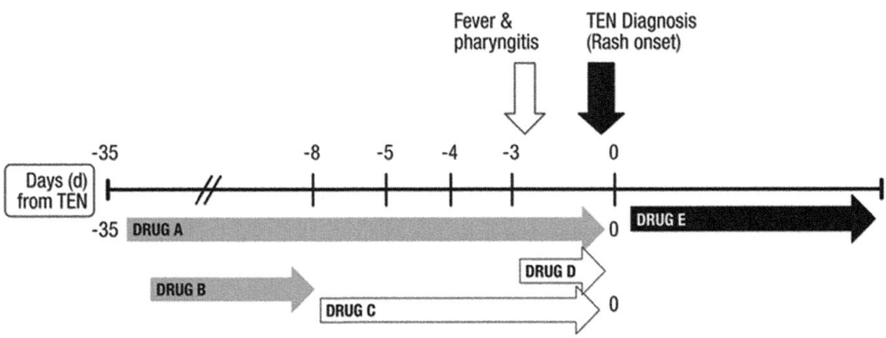

Fig. 1 Example drug timeline from Lehloenya et al. [2]

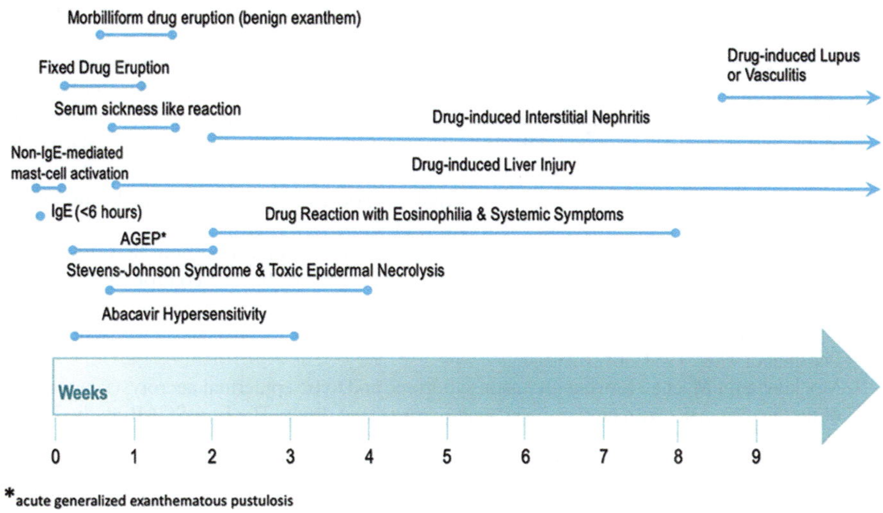

Fig. 2 Timeline of drug hypersensitivity reactions from Drug allergy: A 2022 practice parameter update [5]

4 Other Gems

- For SJS/TEN, high-risk small molecule medications include allopurinol, aromatic antiepileptic agents, anti-microbial sulfonamides, nevirapine, and oxicam NSAIDs (piroxicam, tenoxicam) [9].
- For DRESS, high-risk small molecule medications include allopurinol, aromatic anti-epileptic agents, anti-microbial sulfonamides, vancomycin, minocycline, nevirapine, anti-tuberculosis agents, and mexiletine [10, 11]
- For AGEP, high-risk medications include most commonly aminopenicillins but also other antibiotics, antimalarials (hydroxychloroquine), antifungals (terbinafine) and the calcium channel blocker diltiazem.
- *Mycoplasma pneumoniae* and other infections have been associated with SJS-like illnesses sometimes coined Mycoplasma induced rash and mucositis (MIRM) or reactive infectious mucocutaneous eruption (RIME), mainly in children and young adults [12]
- Although AGEP is less severe than SJS, TEN and DRESS, it is still classified as SCAR given its potential (albeit rare) for systemic involvement [2]

References

1. Phillips EJ, et al. Controversies in drug allergy: testing for delayed reactions. J Allergy Clin Immunol. 2019;143(1):66–73.
2. Lehloenya RJ, et al. Delabeling delayed drug hypersensitivity: how far can you safely go? J Allergy Clin Immunol Pract. 2020;8(9):2878–2895.e6.

3. Duong TA, et al. Severe cutaneous adverse reactions to drugs. Lancet. 2017;390(10106):1996–2011.
4. Garcia-Doval I, et al. Toxic epidermal necrolysis and Stevens-Johnson syndrome: does early withdrawal of causative drugs decrease the risk of death? Arch Dermatol. 2000;136(3):323–7.
5. Hama N, et al. Drug-induced hypersensitivity syndrome (DIHS)/drug reaction with eosinophilia and systemic symptoms (DRESS): clinical features and pathogenesis. J Allergy Clin Immunol Pract. 2022;10(5):1155–1167.e5.
6. Bégaud B, et al. Imputation of the unexpected or toxic effects of drugs. Actualization of the method used in France. Therapie. 1985;40(2):111–8.
7. Sassolas B, et al. ALDEN, an algorithm for assessment of drug causality in Stevens-Johnson syndrome and toxic epidermal necrolysis: comparison with case-control analysis. Clin Pharmacol Ther. 2010;88(1):60–8.
8. Naranjo CA, et al. A method for estimating the probability of adverse drug reactions. Clin Pharmacol Ther. 1981;30(2):239–45.
9. Mockenhaupt M, et al. Stevens–Johnson syndrome and toxic epidermal necrolysis: assessment of medication risks with emphasis on recently marketed drugs. The EuroSCAR-study. J Invest Dermatol. 2008;128(1):35–44.
10. Kardaun SH, et al. Drug reaction with eosinophilia and systemic symptoms (DRESS): an original multisystem adverse drug reaction. Results from the prospective RegiSCAR study. Br J Dermatol. 2013;169(5):1071–80.
11. Husain Z, Reddy BY, Schwartz RA. DRESS syndrome: Part I. Clinical perspectives. J Am Acad Dermatol. 2013;68(5):693.e1–14; quiz 706–8.
12. Tomaino J, et al. Stevens-Johnson syndrome after mycoplasma pneumonia infection in pediatric post-liver transplant recipient: case report and review of the literature. Pediatr Transplant. 2012;16(3):E74–7.

History-Based Drug Allergy Risk Stratification

Jessica Plager and Elizabeth Phillips

1 Clinical Pearl

History-based risk stratification is key to guide the drug allergy evaluation.

2 Clinical Case

A 36-year-old woman with a history of human immunodeficiency virus (HIV) infection and presumed secondary syphilis is admitted for rash, fever, and headache. She is recommended to start on intravenous penicillin therapy however she has a history of penicillin allergy. When asked about her history, she states that she thinks she had an itchy rash as a young child and was told by her parents never to take it again. In accordance with their inpatient drug allergy pathway, the team administers penicillin by direct challenge administering a single dose of 250 mg of amoxicillin which she tolerates without issue. She is now permanently delabelled of her penicillin allergy without the need for desensitisation and started on penicillin therapy per Infectious Disease recommendations.

J. Plager
Department of Medicine, Department of Pediatrics, Vanderbilt University Medical Center, Nashville, TN, USA

E. Phillips (✉)
Department of Medicine, Dermatology, Pathology, Microbiology and Immunology, Vanderbilt University Medical Center, Nashville, TN, USA

Department of Pharmacology, Vanderbilt University School of Medicine, Nashville, TN, USA

R. Junckerstorff et al. (eds.), *Beyond Evidence-Based Medicine*,
https://doi.org/10.1007/978-981-99-4440-8_121

3 Discussion

The first and most important step in a drug allergy evaluation is the clinical history. Historically, a formal drug allergy evaluation has consisted of skin testing followed by an ingestion or drug challenge reserved for skin-test negative cases [1, 2]. While this method is certainly safe and accurate and therefore advisable in patients with tenuous cardiopulmonary status and pregnancy, it has distinct disadvantages; skin testing is challenging to learn for the non-allergist, resource-intensive, and carries a risk of false positives particularly when the pre-test probability is low [2–6]. Additionally, skin testing is often unavailable – there are limited number of allergists to evaluate all the outpatient drug allergies, and even in hospitals with access to allergy consultation, skin testing is often unavailable to inpatients or available only for a limited number of drugs [2].

To surmount these disadvantages, risk stratification pathways have been developed to identify low-risk patients who may be able to skip skin testing and proceed directly to either direct challenges and/or test doses [4, 7–11]. Now extensively studied for beta-lactams and in particular penicillin, these pathways have proven safe and effective for both inpatients in need of antibiotic therapy (either by challenging the implicated penicillin or cephalosporin thereby "delabelling" the patient of any risk of an immediate allergy, or alternatively by performing a challenge to the indicated therapeutic beta-lactam which is most often a cephalosporin), as well as outpatients who are low-risk enough to skip the cumbersome step of skin testing [3, 11]. Building on this success, similar risk-stratification pathways have been developed for other antimicrobials such as TMP-SMX, where the higher risk reactions are severe cutaneous adverse reactions (SCAR) rather than anaphylaxis [12]. TMP-SMX is a good example where skin testing has not been validated and one or two-step where skin testing has been effectively used to remove the drug allergy label. Following a negative one or two dose challenge the risk of an immediate reaction has been ruled out and the risk of a delayed reaction is at the population baseline of 2–5% [12].

While a complete review of risk-stratification pathways is beyond the scope of this text, there are certain key aspects of the clinical history which are key in evaluating allergic risk. For allergists and general practitioners alike, it is important to determine whether the reaction was severe (e.g. anaphylaxis, angioedema, etc.) and/or recent (e.g., within the past 1–5 years), as both are associated with higher risk for true allergy [2]. On the other hand, certain aspects of the clinical history are highly suggestive of tolerance including mild non-IgE cutaneous reaction (e.g. morbilliform drug eruption (MDE), non-IgE symptoms (headache etc.), family history of drug allergy, and an unknown history [1, 3, 7, 11]. In this way, the clinical history can be used to risk stratify and guide subsequent drug allergy evaluation.

4 Other Gems

- Drug-allergy pathways have become an inpatient standard of care and essential part of antibiotic stewardship initiatives
- In the paediatric setting, evidence supports direct ingestion challenge for delabelling penicillin allergy in all children with a suspected amoxicillin-induced rash (exception: severe cutaneous adverse reactions, SCAR). Evidence additionally suggests that milder reactions in children such as serum-sickness like reaction can also be delabelled by direct oral challenge [13].
- For adults a well-validated easy-to-remember risk-stratification tool for penicillin allergy is PEN-FAST: penicillin allergy, five or fewer years ago (2 points), anaphylaxis or angioedema or SCAR (2 points) and treatment required for reaction (1 point). Patients with a cumulative score of 0, 1–2, 3, and 4–5 had a < 1%, 5%, 20% and 50% risk of penicillin allergy, respectively [14]. In a recent study, the PEN-FAST tool did not help identify low risk paediatric populations, however other evidence supports that milder reactions can be readily delabelled by direct oral challenge in children [15]. (Available on: https://www.mdcalc.com/calc/10422/penicillin-allergy-decision-rule-pen-fast)
- In the adult outpatient setting practice is moving towards one- or two-step ingestion challenge for low-risk penicillin allergy however engagement of primary health care providers will be necessary to provide the services to scale-up delabelling on a population level.
- At this point in time, although most cross-reactivity is thought to be driven by the R1 side chain, the cross-reactivity patterns relevant for severe delayed reactions such as SCAR or single organ involvement have not been clinically or mechanistically ascertained to a high evidence level therefore rechallenge is generally avoided across all penicillins and cephalosporins. Exceptions may occur if the benefit outweighs the risk and in this case, specialty services such as Allergy & Immunology and Dermatology should be involved when possible. Procedures such as slow reintroduction or desensitisation are not effective for SCAR reactions.

References

1. Broyles AD, et al. Practical guidance for the evaluation and management of drug hypersensitivity: specific drugs. J Allergy Clin Immunol Pract. 2020;8(9):S16–S116.
2. Plager J, Judd A, Blumenthal K. Role of clinical history in beta-lactam hypersensitivity. Curr Opin Allergy Clin Immunol. 2021;21(4):320–6.
3. Blumenthal KG, et al. Risk-based pathway for outpatient penicillin allergy evaluations. J Allergy Clin Immunol Pract. 2019;7(7):2411–2414 e1.
4. Chiriac AM, et al. Controversies in drug allergy: drug allergy pathways. J Allergy Clin Immunol Pract. 2019;7(1):46–60 e4.
5. Blumenthal KG, et al. Addressing Inpatient beta-lactam allergies: a multihospital implementation. J Allergy Clin Immunol Pract. 2017;5(3):616–625 e7.

6. Wolfson AR, Huebner EM, Blumenthal KG. Acute care beta-lactam allergy pathways: approaches and outcomes. Ann Allergy Asthma Immunol. 2019;123(1):16–34.
7. Stone CA, et al. Risk-stratified management to remove low-risk penicillin allergy labels in the ICU. Am J Respir Crit Care Med. 2020;201(12):1572–5.
8. Moreno EM, et al. Usefulness of an artificial neural network in the prediction of beta-lactam allergy. J Allergy Clin Immunol Pract. 2020;8(9):2974.
9. Mustafa SS, Conn K, Ramsey A. Comparing direct challenge to penicillin skin testing for the outpatient evaluation of penicillin allergy: a randomized controlled trial. J Allergy Clin Immunol Pract. 2019;7(7):2163–70.
10. Ramsey A, Caubet JC, Blumenthal K. Risk stratification and prediction in beta-lactam allergic patients. J Allergy Clin Immunol Pract. 2019;7(7):2182–4.
11. Blumenthal KG, et al. Outcomes from an inpatient beta-lactam allergy guideline across a large US health system. Infect Control Hosp Epidemiol. 2019;40(5):528–35.
12. Krantz MS, et al. Oral challenge with trimethoprim-sulfamethoxazole in patients with "sulfa" antibiotic allergy. J Allergy Clin Immunol Pract. 2020;8(2):757–760.e4.
13. Mill C, et al. Assessing the diagnostic properties of a graded oral provocation challenge for the diagnosis of immediate and nonimmediate reactions to amoxicillin in children. JAMA Pediatr. 2016;170(6):e160033.
14. Trubiano JA, et al. Development and validation of a penicillin allergy clinical decision rule. JAMA Intern Med. 2020;180(5):745.
15. Copaescu AM, et al. Validation of the PEN-FAST score in a pediatric population. JAMA Netw Open. 2022;5(9):e2233703.

History is the Key to Allergy Evaluation

Celia Zubrinich and Mark Hew

1 Clinical Pearl

The clinical history is the most valuable investigation in allergy assessment.

2 Clinical Case

A 23-year-old woman developed acute generalised urticaria, dyspnoea and a hoarse voice while lunching at a café. When the ambulance arrived, they found her systolic blood pressure to be 80 mmHg and treated her with intramuscular epinephrine (adrenaline) to good effect. She attributed the event to nuts in the pesto she consumed at lunch, despite having no prior history of nut allergy. After a period of observation in the Emergency Department, she was discharged with an adrenaline autoinjector (AAI) and advised to avoid all nuts.

At clinic review, careful history-taking elicited a self-initiated course of amoxicillin for a toothache, taking the first dose just before leaving home for the restaurant. She had not divulged this information earlier because—having intermittently used amoxicillin previously with no ill effects – she mistakenly assumed it could not possibly have caused her any harm. Testing revealed no evidence of food allergy, and she resumed an unrestricted diet. However, she had positive serum specific IgE against amoxicillin and was given appropriate avoidance advice. AAI carriage was discontinued.

C. Zubrinich (✉) · M. Hew
Allergy, Asthma and Respiratory Medicine, Alfred Health, Melbourne, VIC, Australia

R. Junckerstorff et al. (eds.), *Beyond Evidence-Based Medicine*,
https://doi.org/10.1007/978-981-99-4440-8_122

3 Discussion

Testing for IgE-mediated allergies involves blood testing for serum specific IgE, skin prick testing (SPT), or both. Tests are available for foods, insect venoms, latex and a very limited number of medications. Positive SPT or IgE indicate the ***probability*** of an allergy being present but do not predict the ***severity*** of each reaction [1]. The severity of an allergic reaction depends on a number of unpredictable clinical variables such as the 'dose' of allergen, the presence of a viral infection or uncontrolled asthma at baseline, or co-factors such as exercise or alcohol. Most individuals who experience more than one reaction do come to recognise that they vary in severity on each occasion. Allergy tests should be used carefully and informed by a meticulous clinical history of all circumstances and exposures preceding an allergic reaction, including—but not limited to—food. As occurred in the vignette above, follow-up testing allows accurate diagnosis that may be quite different to the initial provisional diagnosis. In our reported experience, ten of 48 patients presenting to ED (21%) had their diagnosis changed following clinic review, including testing [2].

Had the patient described in the vignette experienced symptom onset with postprandial exertion, then the unique clinical syndrome of Food-Dependent Exercise-Induced Anaphylaxis (FDEIA) would need to be considered, even if the same foods had been consumed on subsequent occasions without reaction [3]. FDEIA is rarely associated with nut allergy; instead, wheat and shellfish are the commonest causes. Alternatively, an unsuspected (or unreported) food allergen may have been the culprit, even though nuts and seafood are often suspected by patients as the trigger, sometimes even in the absence of any clear exposure. Possible exposures to occult food allergens need to be carefully considered, considering rarities such as lupin, goat cheese, buckwheat, linseed, cochineal, spices, or even crickets as a novel source of protein. Establishing these diagnoses requires careful attention to the clinical history before any testing is undertaken, to ensure relevant testing is not overlooked.

It is common for individuals to insist that a medication could not have triggered their reaction, assuming this because prior use had not provoked symptoms. On the contrary however, prior use provides the initial allergen exposure required for allergic sensitisation and subsequent development of clinical allergy. Intermittent medication use, as is typical for NSAIDs and antibiotics, then provides the opportunity for an allergic reaction to occur on the next exposure, seemingly "out of the blue". On the other hand, care mut be taken to avoid incorrectly blaming medications used continuously for long periods. The important exception to this rule is ACE inhibitor-induced angioedema, a non-allergic pharmacological adverse reaction which can occur at any stage—sometimes after years of use.

When requesting allergen tests, care should be exercised to undertake the relevant tests, and to avoid unnecessary tests with the potential to confuse the patient (and clinician) with false positive results. A prime example is skin prick testing to nuts. Many individuals have a false positive SPT to peanut [4], that is, they can eat nuts regularly without any allergic symptoms. Demonstrating a positive allergy test to peanut in this situation will only confuse the clinical assessment and is best avoided in the first place.

Access to an AAI is a valuable and lifesaving strategy for allergens that are difficult to avoid reliably and consistently i.e., foods and insect stings. However, for a confirmed medication allergy, the likelihood of inadvertent exposure is very low, and it is not usual to recommend AAI carriage, which can be restrictive and burdensome. An AAI is an appropriate safety net when there is diagnostic uncertainty. In our patient's case, establishing the correct diagnosis not only removed dietary restriction but also freed her from the need for AAI carriage.

4 Other Gems

- Individuals often try to understand, explain, or interpret their history in light of the 'usual suspects', but in doing so may omit crucial additional information.
- Investigations are only as good as the clinical history that informs them. Allergy tests must be interpreted appropriately in light of the clinical history. Inappropriate tests should not be performed in the first place.
- The initial suspected cause of an allergic reaction may not be the final diagnosis, so lifelong avoidances should be implemented based on clear evidence, not just assumptions.
- Unnecessarily avoiding an incorrectly suspected allergen is not just inconvenient, it is accompanied by ongoing risk because the true allergenic trigger has not been identified.
- Where immunotherapy is contemplated, such as with insect venom anaphylaxis, then accurate identification of the culprit insect is essential for effective therapy. This will also be the case for food allergen immunotherapy, which is on the near horizon.

References

1. Sampson HA. Utility of food-specific IgE concentrations in predicting symptomatic food allergy. J Allergy Clin Immunol. 2001;107(5):891–6.
2. Zubrinich C, Douglass J, Bartlett J, Patel M, Hew M. Anaphylaxis presentations to the emergency department: impending Victorian reporting legislation. Intern Med J. 2019;49(1):135–6.
3. Asaumi T, Ebisawa M. How to manage food dependent exercise induced anaphylaxis (FDEIA). Curr Opin Allergy Clin Immunol. 2018;18(3):243–7.
4. Martens M, Schnoor HJ, Malling HJ, Poulsen LK. Sensitization to cereals and peanut evidenced by skin prick test and specific IgE in food-tolerant, grass pollen allergic patients. Clin Transl Allergy. 2011;1(1):15.

Penicillin Allergy is Not Forever

Jessica Plager and Elizabeth Phillips

1 Clinical Pearl

Penicillin allergy is not forever.

2 Clinical Case

A 32-year-old G1P0 female at 37 weeks and 4 days estimated gestational age presents to the hospital in active labour. She tested positive for Group B *Streptococcus* (GBS) on rectovaginal culture at 35 weeks. While guidelines suggest intravenous penicillin G as the treatment of choice for intrapartum antibiotic prophylaxis against GBS, patient has a history of penicillin allergy. When asked to describe her allergy, she states that this reaction occurred in childhood, and she thinks she had an itchy rash but cannot remember the time course of the

J. Plager
Department of Medicine, Department of Pediatrics, Vanderbilt University Medical Center, Nashville, TN, USA

E. Phillips (✉)
Department of Medicine, Dermatology, Pathology, Microbiology and Immunology, Vanderbilt University Medical Center, Nashville, TN, USA

Department of Pharmacology, Vanderbilt University School of Medicine, Nashville, TN, USA

R. Junckerstorff et al. (eds.), *Beyond Evidence-Based Medicine*,
https://doi.org/10.1007/978-981-99-4440-8_123

reaction. She was not hospitalised or seen in urgent care for the reaction and did not require treatment. Following GBS antibiotic prophylaxis recommendations, the team starts clindamycin. While delivery was uncomplicated, patient subsequently developed profuse watery diarrhoea, abdominal pain, and fever after being discharged from the hospital, and was ultimately diagnosed with *Clostridioides difficile* colitis.

3 Discussion

β-lactam antibiotics, specifically penicillin and cephalosporins, are among the safest and most effective antibiotics, and are frequently the first-line antibiotics for many infections [1]. However, their use is often limited by a listed penicillin allergy label. Indeed, with prevalence rates ranging from 8–25% of the population (depending on region and treatment population), penicillin allergy is the most common reported drug allergy [2]. Contrary to popular belief, though, approximately 90–95% of patients with a reported penicillin allergy can in fact tolerate penicillin [2, 3]. This discrepancy stems from the misclassification of adverse drug reactions and/or infectious manifestations as an adverse drug reaction (i.e. the reaction never was a true penicillin allergy) as well as the waning of true penicillin allergy over time [4].

Although a penicillin allergy label is frequently overlooked in the setting of a busy clinical practice, the reality is that a penicillin allergy has important personal and public health consequences [3]. On an individual basis, a penicillin allergy label leads clinicians to prescribe inappropriately broad-spectrum antibiotics which are often less effective and associated with more toxic side effects [2, 5]. Furthermore, from a public health perspective, the avoidance of penicillin leads to increasing antibiotic resistance, higher rates of *C. difficile* infection, use of more expensive antibiotics, and increased hospital length of stay [2].

While Allergy and Immunology (A/I) specialists are often seen as the key stakeholder in solving the this this dilemma, there are simply not enough allergists to address the high burden of penicillin allergy. Thus, all clinicians must have basic knowledge of drug allergy, specifically as it relates to penicillin.

The first step is taking a clear, accurate drug allergy history. If the patient's reaction is consistent with a non-allergic side effect (headache, isolated gastrointestinal upset, etc.), the clinician should feel empowered to immediately remove the allergy from the patient's medical record and counsel the patient on the non-immunologic nature of their reaction [5]. That said, if the patient's index reaction is concerning for a hypersensitivity reaction (see Fig. 1 for classification of adverse drug reactions), the clinician can either refer to an allergist/immunologist, or alternatively, can utilise the numerous inpatient and outpatient risk stratification tools which have been developed to guide specialists and non-specialists alike in risk stratification and subsequent selection of safe antibiotics [7, 8].

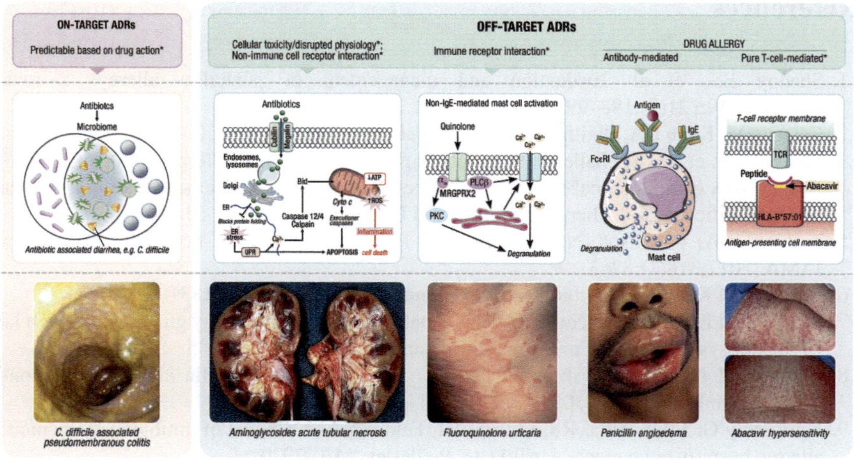

Fig. 1 Classification of on-target and off-target ADRs [6]

4 Other Gems

- In general, non-specialists may find it helpful to identify the reaction as a side-effect, an insignificant history (e.g., remote unknown reaction or family history of penicillin allergy) or a potential hypersensitivity reaction. If a potential hypersensitivity reaction, it is useful to classify these into 3 broad categories: IgE-mediated reactions (e.g. immediate lower-risk reaction such as urticaria or more severe reaction consistent with anaphylaxis), benign T-cell mediated reactions (e.g. delayed maculopapular rash), or severe cutaneous adverse reaction (e.g. Stevens-Johnson Syndrome) [1, 10]
- Reactions should undergo risk stratification that will help define appropriate management
- The medical record allergy section can often store lots of information! You can add comments regarding the index reaction and add any qualifying comments (e.g., “tolerates cephalexin”)
- When penicillin allergic patients were challenged with cephalosporins, less than 5% demonstrated cross-reactivity [11]. Most cross-reactivity with cephalosporins is thought to be based on the R1 side chain and related to the shared side-chain between aminopenicillins (amoxicillin/ampicillin) and aminocephalosporins (cephalexin, cefaclor, cefprozil and cefadroxil). For third and later generation cephalosporins, penicillin and cephalosporin cross-reactivity was less than 2% [12]. For cefazolin, a first-generation cephalosporin that shares no sidechains with penicillin, there is thought to be <1% cross-reactivity.

References

1. Shenoy ES, et al. Evaluation and management of penicillin allergy: a review. JAMA. 2019;321(2):188–99.
2. Castells M, Khan DA, Phillips EJ. Penicillin allergy. N Engl J Med. 2019;381(24):2338–51.
3. Stone CA Jr, et al. The challenge of de-labeling penicillin allergy. Allergy. 2020;75(2):273–88.
4. Broyles AD, et al. Practical guidance for the evaluation and management of drug hypersensitivity: specific drugs. J Allergy Clin Immunol Pract. 2020;8(9):S16–S116.
5. Trubiano JA, Adkinson NF, Phillips EJ. Penicillin allergy is not necessarily forever. JAMA. 2017;318(1):82–3.
6. Blumenthal KG, et al. Antibiotic allergy. Lancet. 2019;393(10167):183–98.
7. Blumenthal KG, et al. Outcomes from an inpatient beta-lactam allergy guideline across a large US health system. Infect Control Hosp Epidemiol. 2019;40(5):528–35.
8. Blumenthal KG, et al. Risk-based pathway for outpatient penicillin allergy evaluations. J Allergy Clin Immunol Pract. 2019;7(7):2411–2414 e1.
9. Kimberkly G, Blumenthal RS, Phillips EJ, Feldweg AM. Choice of antibiotics in penicillin-allergic hospitilized patients. UpToDate, Wellesley, MA; 2020.
10. Blumenthal KG, et al. Impact of a clinical guideline for prescribing antibiotics to inpatients reporting penicillin or cephalosporin allergy. Ann Allergy Asthma Immunol. 2015;115(4):294–300.e2.
11. Coker TR, et al. Diagnosis, microbial epidemiology, and antibiotic treatment of acute otitis media in children. JAMA. 2010;304(19):2161.
12. Campagna JD, et al. The use of cephalosporins in penicillin-allergic patients: a literature review. J Emerg Med. 2012;42(5):612–20.

GPSR Compliance

The European Union's (EU) General Product Safety Regulation (GPSR) is a set of rules that requires consumer products to be safe and our obligations to ensure this.

If you have any concerns about our products, you can contact us on ProductSafety@springernature.com

In case Publisher is established outside the EU, the EU authorized representative is:

Springer Nature Customer Service Center GmbH
Europaplatz 3
69115 Heidelberg, Germany

Batch number: 10732076

Printed by Printforce, the Netherlands